Drug-Resistant Infections

Rajesh Bhatia

Drug-Resistant Infections

Global Burden, Antimicrobial Stewardship, Prevention, and One Health Approaches

Springer

Rajesh Bhatia
Former Director Communicable Diseases,
WHO South-East Asia Region
New Delhi, India

Former Director National Institute of Biologicals,
Government of India
Noida, Uttar Pradesh, India

ISBN 978-981-92-4189-7 ISBN 978-981-92-4190-3 (eBook)
https://doi.org/10.1007/978-981-92-4190-3

This Springer imprint is published by the registered company Springer Nature Singapore Pte Ltd.
The registered company address is: 152 Beach Road, #21-01/04 Gateway East, Singapore 189721, Singapore

To Indu, Sangita, and Tushar—for being my life.

Foreword

Antimicrobial resistance (AMR) is widely recognized as one of the most significant threats to global public health, with far-reaching implications for clinical care, health systems, and sustainable development. The continued rise of resistant pathogens undermines the effectiveness of life-saving interventions and calls for coordinated, evidence-informed responses across sectors and regions.

This volume, *Drug-Resistant Infections: Global Burden, Antimicrobial Stewardship, Prevention, and One Health Approaches*, offers a timely and comprehensive examination of this complex challenge. It synthesizes diverse evidence to present a structured understanding of the global status of AMR, while highlighting critical gaps in. surveillance, stewardship, and access to appropriate diagnostics and therapeutics.

Dr. Rajesh Bhatia, the author of this book, has made long-standing contributions to the field, including leadership in advancing regional and global AMR strategies. His insight and experience are evident in the depth and coherence of this work. Drawing on extensive experience in policy development and programme implementation, the book offers valuable insights into operationalizing the One Health approach by integrating the human, animal, environmental, and community dimensions of antimicrobial resistance.

Particularly noteworthy is the balanced treatment of scientific, policy, and systems level considerations. The volume examines not only the epidemiological and clinical aspects of AMR but also the governance mechanisms, regulatory frameworks, and behavioural drivers that shape outcomes across contexts.

Over the last 10–15 years, several declarations and guidelines on AMR have been issued by national and international bodies. We need to move from rhetoric and general guidance to evidence-based practical solutions. I am sure that this book will serve as a valuable resource for a broad audience, including clinicians, researchers, public health practitioners, and policymakers. It makes an important contribution to the global effort to contain antimicrobial resistance and safeguard the effectiveness of antimicrobials for future generations.

I commend this volume as an authoritative and timely contribution to the global discourse on antimicrobial resistance.

Former Secretary to the Government of India, Department of Health Research and Director General, Indian Council of Medical Research
New Delhi, India
5 June 2026

V. M. Katoch

Foreword

The growing burden of antimicrobial resistance (AMR) poses a formidable challenge to health systems worldwide. Its implications extend beyond the management of infectious diseases, affecting economic stability, development trajectories, and global health security. Addressing AMR requires sustained commitment, strong governance, and coordinated action across sectors.

In this context, *Drug-Resistant Infections: Global Burden, Antimicrobial Stewardship, Prevention, and One Health Approaches*, offers a comprehensive, policy-relevant perspective on one of the defining public health issues of our time. The book situates AMR within a broader systems framework, examining patterns of antimicrobial use, health system capacities, regulatory environments, and socioeconomic determinants that influence resistance.

The author brings exceptional authority to this subject, having played a pioneering role in advancing the AMR agenda in India and significantly contributing to regional efforts during his tenure with the World Health Organisation South-East Asia Region. This experience is evident in the volume's analytical depth and practical orientation, which bridge global frameworks and country-level realities.

Adopting a One Health approach, the book highlights the interconnectedness of human, animal, and environmental health and underscores the importance of integrated surveillance, antimicrobial stewardship, infection prevention, and community engagement. It also reviews key global and national initiatives, identifying both progress achieved and areas requiring further attention.

This volume will be of considerable value to academics, policymakers, and practitioners working to address AMR. By combining evidence, experience, and policy insight, it contributes meaningfully to shaping informed and coordinated responses to antimicrobial resistance at national, regional, and global levels.

This work stands as a significant and practical contribution to advancing coherent and sustained action against antimicrobial resistance.

Former Vice Chancellor and Director,
Indian Veterinary Research Institute
Izzatnagar, Uttar Pradesh, India
5 June 2026

R. K. Singh

Preface

The discovery of antibiotics or antimicrobials—terms used interchangeably in this book—is often regarded as one of the most significant milestones in medical history. Their introduction in the mid-twentieth century revolutionized human health in ways that were previously unimaginable. Diseases that once caused countless deaths—like pneumonia, tuberculosis, meningitis, or even minor wounds that became septic—became manageable. Antibiotics offered new hope, making childbirth safer, enabling successful surgeries, cancer treatment, organ transplants, and intensive care. They have not only been life-saving drugs but also the foundation of modern healthcare.

This success has not been without several vulnerabilities. Almost as soon as antibiotics were widely used, bacteria began developing resistance. This was not surprising—microbes have existed for billions of years, constantly adapting to survive. What changed was the rapid growth of resistance, driven by human actions. The misuse and overuse of antibiotics—in hospitals, communities, livestock, aquaculture, and even crop production—have sped up this natural process. Antibiotics are often prescribed unnecessarily, sold without prescriptions, or used as growth promoters in animals. As a result, their effectiveness has been steadily declining, leading to a concerning reality: many infections are becoming increasingly difficult, and in some cases, impossible, to treat—a phenomenon known as antimicrobial resistance (AMR).

AMR is not merely a medical issue but a global challenge with significant social, economic, and developmental impacts. It threatens food security, undermines healthcare, and risks reversing decades of progress in reducing mortality and improving quality of life. Projections are stark: unless urgent coordinated action is taken, AMR could claim millions of lives annually by 2050, cripple health systems, and generate economic losses in the trillions of dollars.

This book, *Drug-Resistant Infections: Global Burden, Antimicrobial Stewardship, Prevention, and One Health Approaches*, aims to tell the story of antibiotics—their rise, promise, and the growing challenge of AMR. It combines historical insights, scientific explanations, real-world examples, and policy perspectives. The chapters aim to explain not only how antibiotics work and why resistance emerges but also the broader forces that lead to misuse, the consequences we already face, and the strategies being developed worldwide to confront this crisis.

The topic of AMR might seem technical, but its implications affect every individual. Whether one is a doctor treating patients, a policymaker creating regulations, a farmer raising livestock, or simply a parent caring for a child, antibiotics play a crucial role. Preserving their power is not the responsibility of scientists and health professionals alone; it is a shared duty of societies as a whole.

My hope in writing this book is twofold: first, to increase understanding of AMR by presenting it clearly, based on evidence and in an accessible manner; and second, to inspire collective responsibility and action. Combating AMR requires strong healthcare systems, rational antibiotic use, effective regulation, investment in innovation, and above all, a One Health approach linking human, animal, and environmental health.

Looking ahead, the challenge is formidable, but countering it is not impossible. By learning from history, applying science wisely, and acting urgently, we can still preserve the miracle of antibiotics for future generations.

Noida, Uttar Pradesh, India Rajesh Bhatia

Acknowledgements

This book compiles information from various presentations and interactions the author had over the past 20 years with policymakers, professionals, academics, students, and community representatives regarding antibiotics and antimicrobial resistance (AMR). It is not a textbook or a reference book but an informational resource that covers all aspects and provides an overview of the extensive scope and complexities of AMR. The author thanks everyone who shared their insights and input on this complex topic of AMR and possible actions to contain it.

The author used Grammarly software to improve the language and phrasing of some of the text in this book. The design, content selection, and distribution of information in 21 different chapters have been done by the author alone. No figure has been produced with AI assistance.

About the Book

The antibiotics have had an exciting journey from their discovery, success, misuse, decline, and the emergence of resistance in bacteria to these magic bullets. Antimicrobial resistance (AMR) has become one of the greatest public health challenges, threatening to derail the Sustainable Development Goals. The potential impact on human development has forced the UN General Assembly to have two special sessions to address it globally.

The book explores the dynamics of antimicrobial resistance (AMR) and its story, consequences, and solutions—presented in a way that bridges science, policy, and public awareness. Unlike many books that focus mainly on the medical aspects of AMR, this book integrates the interconnected drivers of resistance across humans, livestock, agriculture, and the environment. This makes it highly relevant to policymakers, veterinarians, public health specialists, and environmental scientists alike. It also explores policy frameworks, economic implications, and global initiatives. It combines science with practical governance.

AMR is an intricate subject. The book makes complex scientific ideas accessible to non-specialist readers, while still retaining depth and references for researchers and professionals. This dual readability broadens its audience beyond medical experts to students, civil society, and informed citizens.

Each chapter builds logically, covering scientific principles, irrational use, global initiatives, stewardship, challenges and solutions—a structured flow that few existing books capture in one volume.

This is a forward-looking book that provides practical solutions. Instead of stopping at the problem, the book emphasizes evidence-based strategies, WHO frameworks, and possible solutions. Readers are left with a sense of direction and optimism, rather than despair.

Authored by a global public health leader with extensive first-hand experience on AMR in the World Health Organisation (WHO), Food and Agriculture Organisation of the UN (FAO) and several developing countries. The book carries the authority of an insider perspective. This lends credibility and trustworthiness, distinguishing it from purely academic or journalistic accounts.

Contents

About the Author

Rajesh Bhatia, MBBS, MD, FRSPH is the former director of communicable diseases at the World Health Organization (WHO) South-East Asia Region, New Delhi, India. His areas of research interest and expertise include antimicrobial resistance surveillance, One Health approach, health policy development, capacity building, and community engagement for AMR containment. Dr. Bhatia has authored more than 180 scientific publications, including over 40 publications focused on antimicrobial resistance, and has contributed to several international technical reports, policy frameworks, and strategic documents on AMR. He has worked closely with global organizations, including WHO, FAO, UNEP, the Asian Development Bank, USAID, and multiple national governments, contributing to key initiatives such as the Global Action Plan on Antimicrobial Resistance, the Jaipur Declaration on AMR, and regional AMR strategies in South-East Asia. He played a key role in establishing India's first antimicrobial resistance surveillance networks in human health and animal sectors. Dr. Bhatia has received gold medals from the Indian Association of Medical Microbiologists, the Indian Association of Epidemiologists, and the Indian Vaccinologists Association for his contributions to public health. In 2025, he was elected a fellow of the Royal Society for Public Health (RSPH), United Kingdom.

Abbreviations

AMR	Antimicrobial Resistance
AMS	Antimicrobial Stewardship
AST	Antimicrobial Susceptibility Testing
ATC	Anatomical Therapeutic Chemical Classification
AWaRe	Access, Watch, Reserve
CDC	Centers for Disease Control and Prevention
CDDEP	Center for Disease Dynamics, Economics and Policy
CLSI	Clinical and Laboratory Standards Institute
COVID-19	Coronavirus Disease 2019
ECDC	European Centre for Disease Prevention and Control
EQA	External Quality Assessment
ESBL	Extended-Spectrum Beta-Lactamase
EUCAST	European Committee on Antimicrobial Susceptibility Testing
FAO	Food and Agriculture Organization of the UN
FDA	Food and Drug Administration (of USA)
GDP	Gross Domestic Product
GLASS	Global Antimicrobial Resistance and Use Surveillance System
GNB	Gram-Negative Bacteria
GNRAAC	Global Network for Rapid Antimicrobial Resistance Analysis and Control
HAI	Healthcare-Associated Infections
HICs	High-Income Countries
HIV	Human Immunodeficiency Virus
ICMR	Indian Council of Medical Research
IPC	Infection Prevention and Control
LMICs	Low- and Middle-Income Countries
MDR	Multidrug-Resistant
MDR-TB	Multidrug-Resistant Tuberculosis
MRSA	Methicillin-Resistant *Staphylococcus aureus*
NCDC	National Centre for Disease Control (India)
NGOs	Non-governmental Organizations

NHS	National Health Service
NPS	National Pharmaceutical System
OECD	Organisation for Economic Co-operation and Development
OTC	Over-the-Counter
PCR	Polymerase Chain Reaction
PHEIC	Public Health Emergency of International Concern
PPP	Public–Private Partnership
R&D	Research and Development
SDGs	Sustainable Development Goals
STGs	Standard Treatment Guidelines
TB	Tuberculosis
UK	United Kingdom
UN	United Nations
UNEP	United Nations Environment Programme
UNGA	United Nations General Assembly
US	United States
USAID	United States Agency for International Development
USD	United States Dollar
UTIs	Urinary Tract Infections
WB	World Bank
WHA	World Health Assembly
WHO	World Health Organization
WOAH	World Organization for Animal Health
WTO	World Trade Organization
XDR	Extensively Drug-Resistant

Part I
Foundations of Antibiotics and Antimicrobial Resistance

Chapter 1
Rise and Fall of Antibiotics: An Overview

Abstract The discovery and application of antibiotics in the twentieth century revolutionised medicine by significantly reducing death rates from bacterial infections and enabling modern medical procedures like surgery, cancer treatment, and organ transplants. Initially celebrated as "miracle drugs," antibiotics provided unmatched treatment of previously deadly diseases, significantly improving global health outcomes. However, their efficacy has been weakened by the rapid and relentless rise of antimicrobial resistance (AMR)—a natural yet accelerated evolutionary process caused by the misuse and overuse of antibiotics in humans, animals, agriculture, and the environment. Resistance mechanisms, often appearing soon after new drugs are introduced, have led to an increase in multidrug-resistant pathogens, known as "superbugs," which threaten medical progress. AMR has become a major global health concern, associated with rising illness, death rates, and healthcare costs, and if unaddressed, is projected to cause 10 million deaths annually by 2050. This will harm human health, food security, human development, and delay the achievement of several Sustainable Development Goals.

Keywords Anti-bacterial agents · Microbial drug resistance · One health · Global health · Public health · Zoonoses

Microorganisms including bacteria are the longest-living creatures on Earth. They appeared more than 3.5 billion years ago, faced numerous threats to their survival during that time, and developed the ability to undergo genetic changes in response to the deadly forces that threatened them. Unlike bacterial colonisation, the human population emerged on Earth around 200,000 years ago [1]. Survival benefits and evolutionary advantages have favoured bacteria. These continue to cause numerous infectious diseases in humans and animals causing significant mortality, morbidity, and economic loss.

Throughout human history, infectious diseases have played a critical role, even influencing major historical events. Bacterial pandemics like those due to cholera and plague led to widespread devastation, killing millions and prompting mass migrations away from outbreak areas. Until just under a century ago, there were few

R. Bhatia, *Drug-Resistant Infections*,
https://doi.org/10.1007/978-981-92-4190-3_1

artificial substances capable of destroying bacteria, preventing pandemics, or treating infections caused by these microorganisms.

The plagues of biblical times, the Black Death of the Middle Ages, and the 1918 "Spanish flu" pandemic are just a few examples of devastating pandemics. The 1918 flu pandemic claimed up to 50 million lives worldwide. In the pre-antibiotic era, infectious diseases caused up to 30–40% of all deaths globally. Bacterial infections were often untreatable and frequently fatal, resulting in a low life expectancy of typically 30–45 years [2].

History is witness to pneumonia being the top killer worldwide. Tuberculosis (TB) was once known as the "plague" and was responsible for millions of deaths annually. One in seven deaths in Europe was due to TB [3]. Diphtheria was a major cause of death in children before the vaccine and antitoxin became available. It was estimated that 15,000 children used to die annually in the USA due to diphtheria [4]. Frequent outbreaks of typhoid fever were once deadly. Scarlet fever was often fatal in children. Meningitis in young adults was rapidly lethal. Cholera caused large-scale epidemics, with extremely high mortality without rehydration.

Even today, numerous infectious diseases, primarily bacterial and viral, continue to be a leading cause of death and illness globally, especially in low-income countries and among young children. With bacteria becoming resistant to antibiotics—a subset of antimicrobial agents, even minor injuries that become infected could be fatal.

1.1 What Are Antibiotics, Antimicrobials, and Chemotherapeutic Agents?

Antibiotics are agents used to treat bacterial diseases in humans and animals. They are powerful medicines designed to combat or prevent bacterial infections. They work either by killing bacteria directly (*bactericidal*) or by stopping their growth and reproduction (*bacteriostatic*). It is important to know that antibiotics only work on target bacteria and are ineffective against viral infections like the common cold or flu.

Often, people use the terms antibiotics, antimicrobial agents, and chemotherapeutic agents interchangeably. However, they have subtle differences (Fig. 1.1). Chemotherapeutic agents are a broader class, encompassing any chemical substance used to treat disease, including anticancer drugs and antimicrobial agents. Antimicrobial agents are a broader category of substances that inhibit or kill microorganisms, including bacteria, fungi, viruses, and parasites. All antimicrobial agents are chemotherapeutic agents. All antibiotics are antimicrobial agents. Antibiotics are a subset of antimicrobial agents, specifically referring to substances produced by microorganisms that inhibit or kill other microorganisms [5].

Technically, an antibiotic is defined as a chemical substance produced by a living organism, generally a microorganism, that is detrimental to other microorganisms.

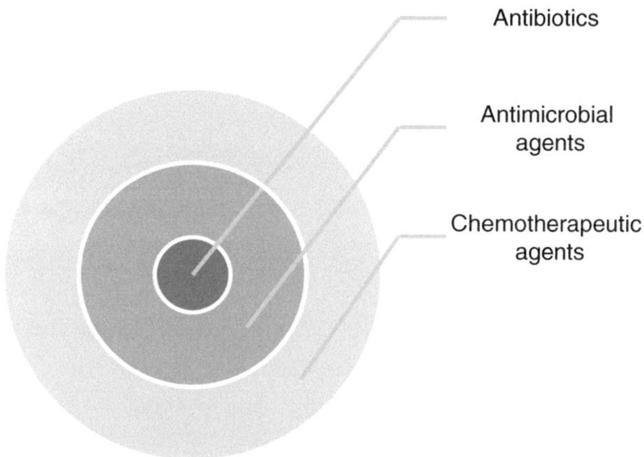

Fig. 1.1 Relationship between antibiotics, antimicrobial agents, and chemotherapeutic agents

Antibiotics are commonly produced by soil microorganisms and probably represent a means by which organisms in a complex environment, such as soil, control the growth of competing microorganisms. Microorganisms that produce antibiotics help prevent or treat diseases caused by bacteria and fungi [5].

Modern science has given rise to the synthetic production of antibiotics. They are antimicrobial agents entirely developed and manufactured in laboratories, rather than derived from natural microorganisms. Many of these function by inhibiting bacterial protein synthesis (bacteriostatic) or by disrupting bacterial membranes. Some examples of synthetic antibiotics include quinolones/fluoroquinolones (ciprofloxacin, norfloxacin), sulphonamides (sulphamethoxazole, trimethoprim), oxazolidinones (linezolid), and carbapenems. Their synthesis carries the advantage of often scalable, affordable, and, through structure-guided design, can overcome resistance mechanisms that render natural antibiotics ineffective.

1.2 Journey of Discovery of Chemotherapeutic Agents

In ancient times, herbal and mineral remedies were used to treat infectious diseases. These included arsenic compounds for curing various ailments despite their toxicity. Paul Ehrlich pioneered the concept of a "magic bullet"—a compound that targets disease-causing organisms without harming the host. He introduced the term chemotherapy, believing that chemicals could be used to treat infections. Salvarsan was the first effective chemotherapeutic agent against *Treponema pallidum*—the causative agent of syphilis.

The 1930s saw the discovery of Prontosil by Gerhard Domagk. This is claimed as the first commercially available antibacterial agent. It was followed by the discovery of sulphonamides, that was shown to inhibit bacterial folic acid synthesis.

The golden era of antibiotics commenced with the accidental discovery of penicillin by Alexander Fleming in 1928 [6]. It was purified for clinical use by Florey and Chain. Penicillin was widely used during the Second World War with remarkable success [7] in saving human lives.

Between 1940 and 1960, heralded by the discovery of streptomycin, several clinically useful antibiotics, including chloramphenicol, tetracyclines, erythromycin, rifampicin, etc., were discovered (Fig. 1.2). The introduction of antibiotics into clinical use was arguably the most significant medical breakthrough of the twentieth century. In addition to treating infectious diseases, antibiotics made many modern medical procedures possible, including cancer treatment, organ transplants, complex surgical procedures, e.g. open-heart surgery.

The pace of discovery of antibiotics gradually slowed down with the development and amplification of resistance against these agents in pathogens of public health importance, including *Mycobacteria*, *Salmonella*, *Staphylococcus*, and numerous Gram-negative and Gram-positive bacteria.

Numerous compounds have been, and continue to be, developed to expand the arsenal of antibacterial agents. Very few molecules successfully traverse the journey from discovery to clinical use. Many of the final products possess several characteristics, but the search for an ideal antibiotic [2, 5] with all desirable features (Table 1.1) remains ongoing.

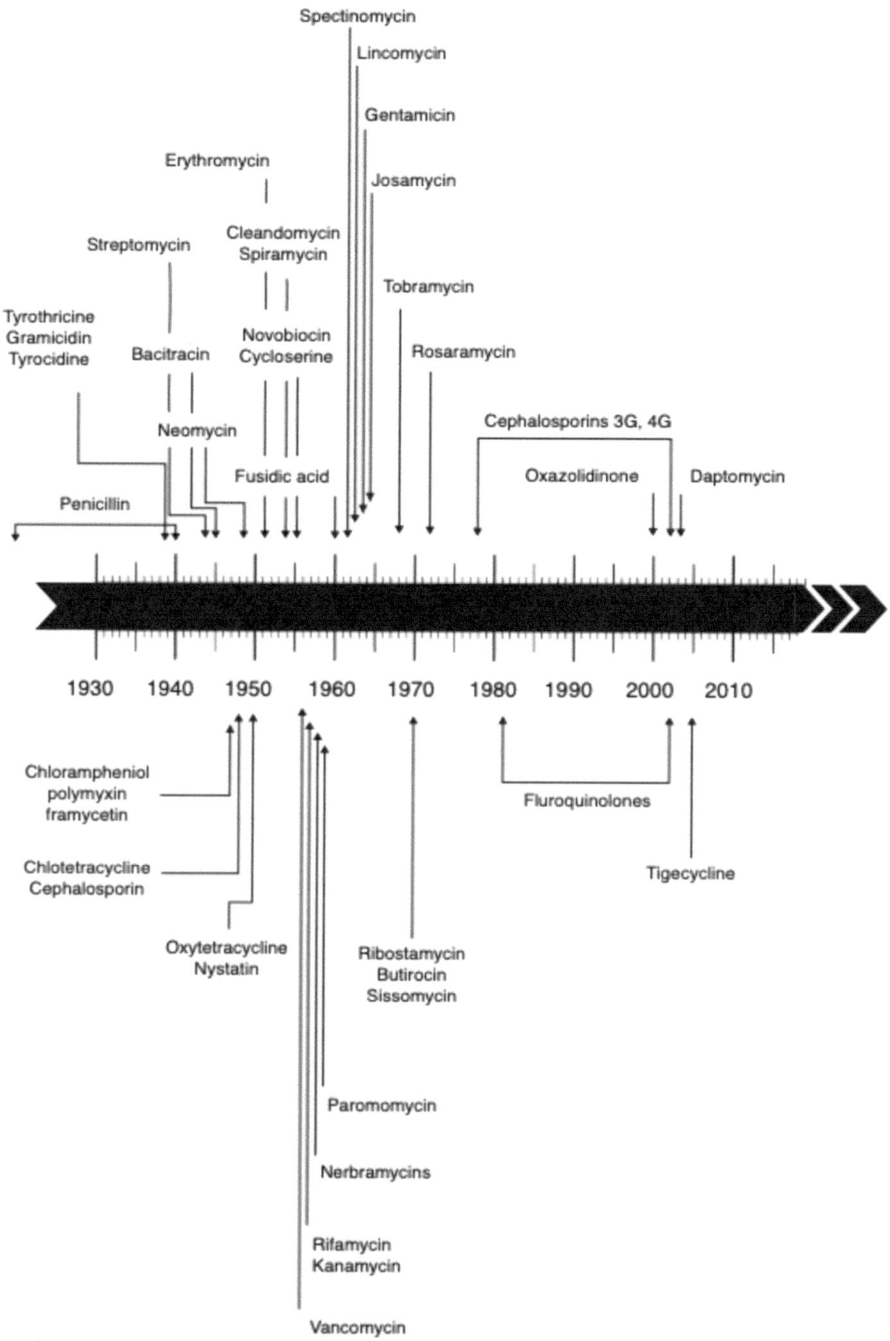

Fig. 1.2 Timeline of discovery of major antibiotics

Table 1.1 Desirable properties of an ideal antibiotic

Selective toxicity. Should act on pathogen without damaging the host tissue
Bactericidal in nature
Effective against a broad range of bacteria
Not allergenic
Active in plasma, other body fluids
Stable and preferably water soluble
Desired levels rapidly reached and maintained for adequate period of time
Avoid or delay giving rise to resistance in bacteria
Long shelf life
Affordable

Table 1.2 Sources of various antibiotics

Actinomycetes	Synthetic	Fungal	Other bacteria
Aminoglycosides Ansamycins Carbapenems Chloramphenicol Fosfomycin Glycopeptides Lincosamides Lipoglycopeptides Lipopeptides Macrolides Streptogramins Tetracyclines Tuberactinomycins	Azoles Nitrofurans Oxazolidinones Quinolones Sulphonamides	Cephalosporins Fusidic acid Penicillins Pleuromutilins	Monobactams Mupirocin Polymyxins Polypeptides

1.3 Sources of Antibiotics

The genus *Streptomyces*—a soil bacterium—was the source of almost all (55%) antibiotics discovered between 1945 and 1978 [8]. The chemicals produced by these soil organisms acted as weapons to kill competitors in the soil, either as a form of protection (defensive) or predation (offensive), or to facilitate interactions with eukaryotic hosts, such as insects and plants. Several other sources of antibiotics have been identified (Table 1.2).

1.4 Mechanism of Action of Antibiotics

Antibiotics target essential processes in bacteria that are different from those in human cells. Various mechanisms of action are illustrated in Figs. 1.3 and 1.4 for selected antibiotics [5]. Some antibiotics interfere with the building of the bacterial

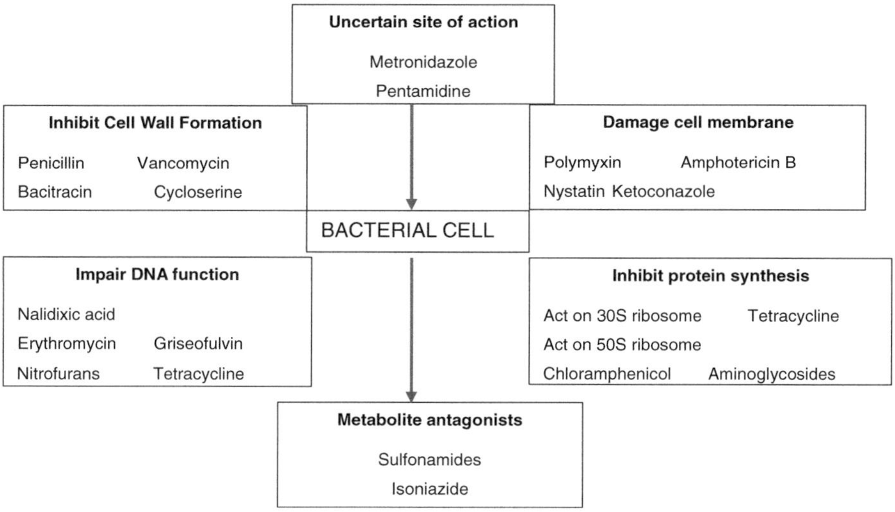

Fig. 1.3 Main actions of important antimicrobial agents on pathogens

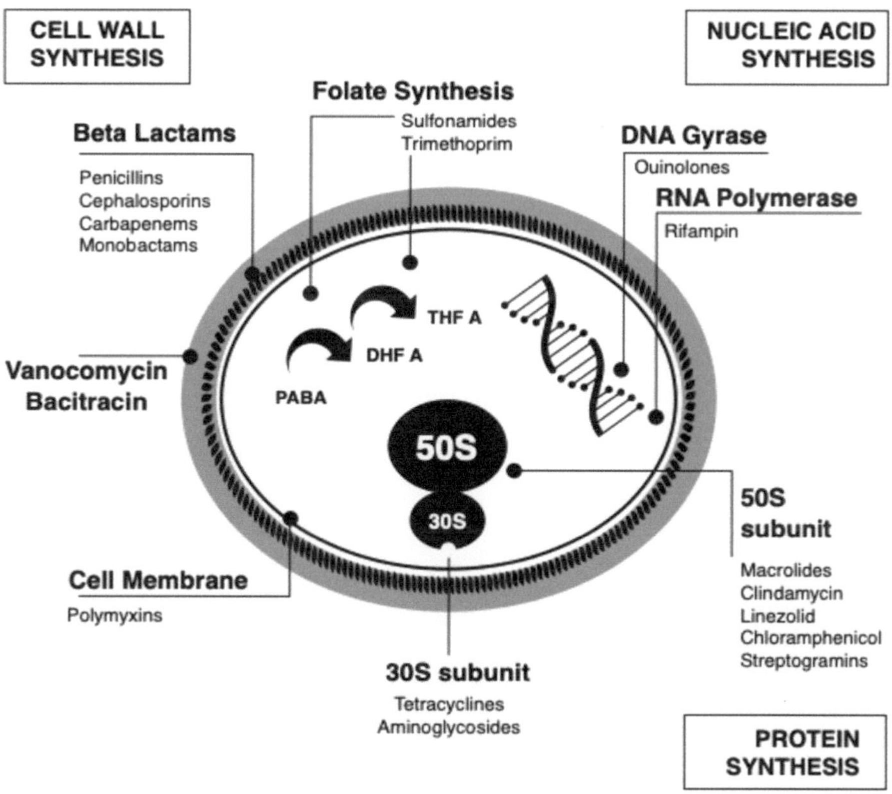

Fig. 1.4 Mechanism of action of antibiotics on various bacterial structures

cell wall, which is vital for its structural integrity, leading to cell death. Certain antibiotics can damage the bacterial cell membrane, leading to leakage and ultimately causing cell death. Many antibiotics block the production of proteins essential for bacterial survival and multiplication. Few antibiotics target the bacteria's DNA replication or RNA synthesis, preventing them from multiplying. A few antibiotics interfere with the bacterial ability to synthesis folic acid, a necessary nutrient for their growth.

1.5 Classification of Antibiotics

Antibiotics can be classified in several ways based upon their mechanism of action, spectrum of activity, and their chemical composition.

1.5.1 Mechanism of Action

This classification groups antibiotics based on how they target and inhibit or kill bacteria. It has been shown in Fig. 1.3.

1.5.2 Spectrum of Activity

This classification is based on the range of bacteria against which an antibiotic is effective.

- *Narrow-spectrum*: These antibiotics target a specific type or limited range of bacteria, such as penicillin G (primarily Gram-positive bacteria).
- *Broad-spectrum*: These are effective against a wide range of bacteria.
- *Extended-spectrum*: These are modified broad-spectrum antibiotics with enhanced activity against a wider range of organisms, potentially including some resistant strains.

1.5.3 Chemical Structure

Antibiotics with similar chemical structures often share identical mechanisms of action, effectiveness, toxicity, and potential for allergies (Table 1.3).

Table 1.3 Classification of antibiotics based upon their chemical structure

Chemical structure	Characteristics and examples
Beta-lactams	These include a beta-lactam ring in their structure and typically inhibit bacterial cell wall synthesis Examples: Penicillin, cephalosporins, and carbapenems
Macrolides	These have a macrocyclic lactone ring and primarily inhibit bacterial protein synthesis Examples: Erythromycin, clarithromycin, and azithromycin
Tetracyclines	Characterised by a four-membered ring structure, these antibiotics inhibit bacterial protein synthesis Examples: Tetracyclines, doxycycline
Fluoroquinolones	These are synthetic antibiotics with a fluoroquinolone ring structure that inhibit bacterial DNA synthesis Examples: ciprofloxacin, levofloxacin, moxifloxacin, gemifloxacin, norfloxacin, and ofloxacin
Sulphonamides	These synthetic antibiotics inhibit the bacterial production of folic acid Examples: Sulphadiazine, and sulphisoxazole
Glycopeptides	These have complex, multi-ring peptide core, often glycosylated, and with hydrophobic side chains in some cases Examples: Vancomycin and teicoplanin
Monobactam	This is characterised by monocyclic β-lactam ring structure, meaning the β-lactam ring is not fused to another ring system, unlike other β-lactams like penicillin and cephalosporins Example: Aztreonam
Carbapenems	These are characterised by a five-membered ring system fused to a beta-lactam ring, with a carbon atom replacing the sulphur found in penicillin Examples: Imipenem, meropenem
Lipopeptides	These are characterised by a fatty acid chain linked to a peptide (oligopeptide) structure. The peptide portion can be linear or cyclic, and the fatty acid chain is typically hydrophobic, interacting with cell membranes to disrupt them Example: Daptomycin

1.6 Impact of Antibiotics on Global Health

The global impact of antibiotics has been multifaceted. The antibiotics, along with vaccines and sanitation, have revolutionised healthcare by effectively treating bacterial infections, thereby dramatically reducing the mortality, morbidity, and economic losses caused by these infections (Fig. 1.5). Through their effective therapeutic role, antibiotics saved millions of lives [9].

Antibiotics have made routine medical procedures, such as surgeries and cancer treatments, safer by preventing infections and facilitating the successful and complication-free use of modern interventions.

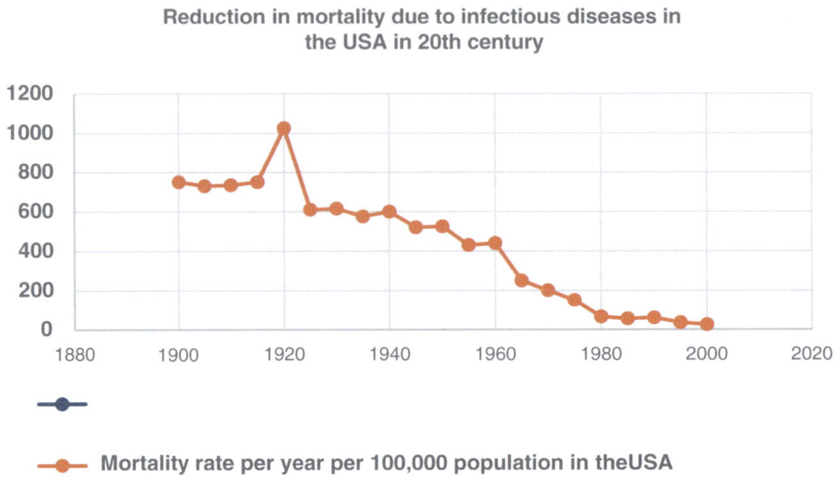

Fig. 1.5 Sharp decline in mortality due to infectious diseases in the USA in twentieth century

Efficient use of antibiotics in animals has simultaneously improved the health and productivity of these animals, thereby contributing to the nutrition security and economic well-being of rural populations.

The availability of antibiotics has significantly improved access to food in the world by facilitating the industrialisation of agriculture, increasing livestock productivity, and allowing for higher-density farming. Since the 1950s, antibiotics have been used to treat, prevent, and control diseases, as well as to enhance feed efficiency and promote growth in food animals. However, as in human health sector, indiscriminate extensive use of antibiotics in animals has facilitated emergence of antimicrobial resistance with severe public health implications.

1.7 Decline in Efficacy of Antibiotics Due to AMR

Microorganisms, including bacteria, appeared on Earth billions of years ago, before human beings. This gives them a survival advantage. The advent of antibiotics made bacteria face a formidable enemy and an existential crisis. A large number of mechanisms were evolved by bacteria to counteract the lethal or deleterious effects of antibiotics. The bacterial strains that resist the antibiotics usually appear immediately after the introduction of the antibiotics. Soon after penicillin was introduced into clinical use, reports began to appear on its resistance in certain bacterial species [10, 11]. This has primarily been due to the misuse of penicillin.

Sir Alexander Fleming had cautioned about the emergence of resistance in his Nobel Lecture. He warned that "It is not difficult to make microbes resistant to penicillin. The time may come when anyone in the shops can buy penicillin. Then there is the danger that the ignorant man may easily underdose himself and by exposing his microbes to nonlethal quantities of the drug make them resistant" [12]. His observation was based on publications in The Lancet [10] and Nature [11] regarding the detection of penicillin-resistant pathogens. This marked the beginning of recognition of antimicrobial resistance as a phenomenon of far-reaching importance for both human and animal health.

1.8 What Is Antimicrobial Resistance?

Antimicrobial resistance (AMR) is the ability of microorganisms to evade the effects of antimicrobial agents (antibiotics) in therapeutic doses, making it difficult to treat infectious diseases in humans and animals.

AMR is not an artificial process. It is a *natural biological unstoppable phenomenon* directly linked to antibiotic use and is very slow to reverse or may be irreversible. All antibiotics have the potential to select drug-resistant subpopulations of bacteria. Incontrovertible evidence now demonstrates that the inappropriate use of antibiotics in various sectors is the most significant driver of AMR (Fig. 1.6).

AMR has many serious consequences (Table 1.4). It leads to increased morbidity, longer stays in hospitals, and forced use of expensive diagnostic tests/toxic drugs. At clinical and public health platforms, patients with infections caused by drug-resistant bacteria are difficult to treat and may require long-term use of expensive and potentially toxic drugs.

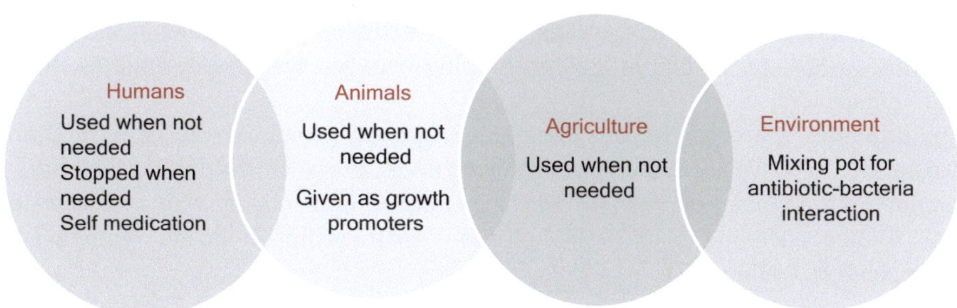

Fig. 1.6 Misuse of antibiotics in various sectors

Table 1.4 Impact of antimicrobial resistance on human health

Longer treatment
Longer duration of illness
Higher mortality
Treatment with expensive drugs
Greater use of diagnostics
Increased burden on the health system
Negates technological advances in the medical sector
Complex surgeries
Transplantations and other interventions
The patient acts as a reservoir of resistant organisms for a longer period with public health implications
Substantial impact on the economy and global human development

1.9 Use of Antibiotics in Animal Sector

All classes of antibiotics that are important for human medicine are used in significantly larger quantities in veterinary practices and animal husbandry worldwide. Antibiotics are extensively used in otherwise healthy livestock and poultry in lieu of biosecurity and sanitation issues on farms, and provide prophylaxis to animals against infectious diseases that may either kill them or stunt their growth [13]. Additionally, antimicrobials are added in low doses to promote growth and improve feed conversion efficiency, thereby facilitating faster growth in food animals [14]. It is estimated that by 2030, the global veterinary sector may consume 200,235 t of antibiotics [15]. Moreover, there is an impending threat of the inter-country spread of resistant pathogens from animals to humans. Extensive use of colistin in agriculture and pig rearing industry in China resulted in the manifestation of the resistant *mcr-1* gene in *Escherichia coli* in 2015. It subsequently spread rapidly to over 50 countries across six continents. This plasmid-mediated gene enables resistance to colistin—a last-resort antibiotic—by jumping between bacteria in animals, food, and humans [16].

Antibiotics are used for any therapeutic, growth promotion, food, agriculture use, and from pharmaceutical manufacturing units, along with antibiotic-containing residues, which find their way into the environment, into soil, air, water, wastewater and sediments, leading to antibiotic pollution, AMR seeding in the environment and subsequent recycling [17].

1.10 Drivers of Antimicrobial Resistance

The drivers of AMR are diverse and interconnected, spanning human, animal, and environmental sectors. Practices drive AMR at the intersection of human health, animal health and environment. This is why combating AMR requires a One Health approach, combining efforts across sectors with better policies, stewardship, and global collaboration.

Several drivers that facilitate the emergence, selection, and spread of resistant microorganisms have been summarised in Table 1.5.

Though AMR can be slowed down, the emergence of resistance is an unstoppable biological phenomenon. It is well-established that antimicrobial usage (AMU) is the most significant driver for AMR. It implies that a reduction in AMU shall have a corresponding mitigation in AMR. AMU is not limited to the human health sector. Antibiotics are also widely used in the animal health and agriculture sectors. Reduction in AMU is needed in all industries.

Antibiotic consumption for human health has been continuously increasing. Many times, antibiotics are administered to patients with viral infections, especially the common cold, where antibiotics have no role at all. In a study covering 67 countries, it was estimated that global antibiotic consumption increased by 16.3% between 2016 and 2023 and is likely to increase by 52.3% between 2023 and 2030 in terms of DDDs [18].

Self-medication with antibiotics is a major contributor to the global health crisis of AMR, deeply rooted in socio-economic disparities and, in turn, imposing significant economic and social burdens. This practice, driven by economic constraints, lack of education, and poor healthcare access, transforms from a personal attempt at saving money into a "tragedy of the commons" where individual actions lead to

Table 1.5 Drivers of antimicrobial resistance

Driver	Mechanism
Overuse and Misuse of Antibiotics	In humans: Unnecessary prescriptions, self-medication, use for viral infections, or incorrect dosage/duration In animals: Widespread use for growth promotion and disease prevention in livestock and aquaculture In crops and agriculture: Use of antibiotics as pesticides or to prevent bacterial plant diseases
Inappropriate prescription (>50% prescriptions by qualified physicians)	Lack of knowledge of disease & antibiotics Lack of investigation facilities Lack of standard guidelines Non-adherence to guidelines
Poor Infection Prevention and Control (IPC)	Inadequate hygiene and sanitation in healthcare facilities, animal farms, and communities Lack of effective hand hygiene, sterilisation of equipment, and isolation of infected patients
Inadequate Access to Clean Water, Sanitation, and Hygiene (WASH)	Facilitates the spread of resistant pathogens in hospitals, households, and communities Promotes the faecal-oral transmission of resistant organisms
Weak Health Systems and Diagnostic Gaps	Absence of diagnostic tools leads to overprescription and empirical use of broad-spectrum antibiotics Limited access to skilled healthcare providers and laboratory testing

(Continued)

Table 1.5 (Continued)

Driver	Mechanism
Unregulated Sale and Use of Antibiotics	Over-the-counter availability without prescription in many countries Online sales without proper controls Counterfeit or substandard drugs exacerbate resistance
Global Travel and Trade	Rapid movement of people, animals, and goods spreads resistant organisms across borders AMR can spread through food, animal feed, and water sources
Environmental Contamination	Pharmaceutical waste and antibiotic residues released into water bodies and soil from: Drug manufacturing plants Hospitals and households Agricultural runoff
Use of Antimicrobials in Animal Husbandry	Non-therapeutic use in poultry, cattle, and fish farming selects for resistant bacteria These bacteria can spread to humans via the food chain, environment, or direct contact
Lack of New Antibiotics and Incentives for R&D	Few new antimicrobials are in development due to poor return on investment Resistance is growing faster than the pipeline of new drugs
Lack of Public Awareness and Education	Misunderstanding among the public about when and how to use antibiotics Poor adherence to prescriptions and confusion between antibiotics and other medicines Self-medication
Inadequate Surveillance and Data Systems	Limited monitoring of AMR trends in humans, animals, and the environment Lack of integrated One Health AMR surveillance

collective harm. This practice is widely prevalent in developing and resource-starved countries and requires serious social analyses and sustainable communication leading to an affirmative behavioural change in the communities towards rational use of antibiotics.

According to the 2023 report of the World Organisation for Animal Health (WOAH), global antimicrobial use in animals has declined by 13% over the past 3 years. This represents a significant shift in the ongoing efforts to maintain the efficacy of these critical medicines [19]. The report further states that less than 20% of antimicrobials used in animals in 2019 were of critical importance for human health.

1.11 Magnitude of AMR

AMR is now globally recognised as the most significant public health challenge in humanity's fight against infectious diseases. If AMR persists or further increases and antibiotics fail, the world is likely to fall short of attaining several Sustainable Development Goals (SDGs), especially health-related SDG 3 and SDGs 1, 2, 3, 6, 8, 12 and 17 (Fig. 1.7), among others, which depend on ensuring the continuous efficacy of these life-saving drugs. AMR's role in hindering the achievement of the Sustainable Development Goals is a concern to policymakers and global leaders.

1.11.1 Global Impact of AMR

AMR is estimated to kill around 1.7 million people worldwide every year. In addition, around 4.5 million deaths are due to the indirect impact of AMR on human health; 20% of these deaths are in children [20], and without a stronger response, there will be an estimated average loss of 1.8 years of global life expectancy by 2035 [21]. The globally accepted projections on the impact of AMR estimate that, in the absence of urgent actions to contain AMR, it is likely to cause 10 million deaths globally every year by 2050 (Fig. 1.8).

The economic impact of AMR is staggering. By 2050, the cost of inaction in combating AMR is expected to approximate USD $100 trillion, resulting in a 3.5% decline in global gross domestic product (GDP) [22]. During this period, twenty-eight million people are likely to be pushed into poverty due to AMR. The World Bank estimates that AMR will cause an 11% reduction in food of animal origin. AMR could result in US$1 trillion of additional healthcare costs per year by 2050 [22]. The extra cost of treating patients with infections due to resistant bacteria is estimated to be around USD 412 billion annually. Recent data show a higher impact of AMR in developing countries, including those in Asia. Some of the data have been reflected in Table 1.6.

A Lancet study [23] reveals that from 1990 to 2021, while the deaths from AMR decreased by more than 50% among children younger than 5 years, these increased by over 80% in adults 70 years and older. Better IPC and vaccination for children have begun yielding positive results.

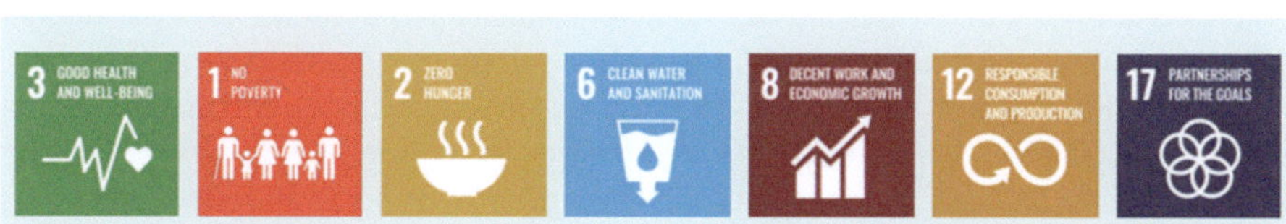
3 GOOD HEALTH AND WELL-BEING
1 NO POVERTY
2 ZERO HUNGER
6 CLEAN WATER AND SANITATION
8 DECENT WORK AND ECONOMIC GROWTH
12 RESPONSIBLE CONSUMPTION AND PRODUCTION
17 PARTNERSHIPS FOR THE GOALS

Fig. 1.7 AMR and SDGs

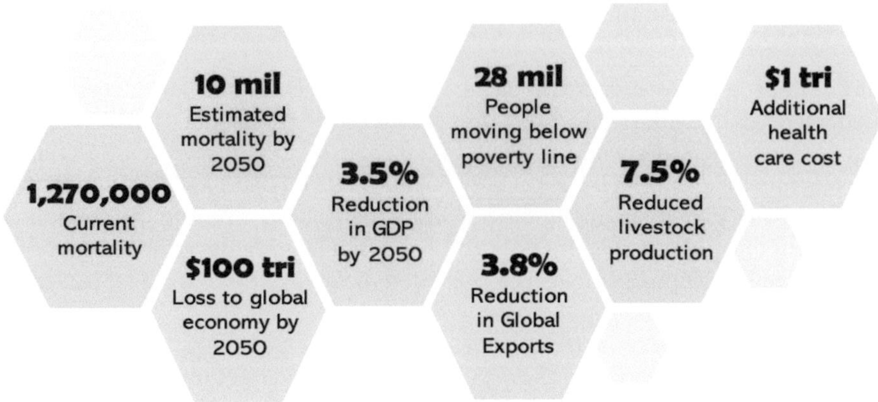

Fig. 1.8 Projected public health and economic impact of AMR if no action by 2050

Table 1.6 Deaths attributable and associated with bacterial AMR in South-East Asia in 2019 (obtained from Ref. [23])

Country	Attributable cause of death	Attributable cause of death/million population	Associated cause of death	Associated cause of death/million population
Bangladesh	26,200	158.8	98,800	598.78
India	297,000	211.74	1,042,500	743.58
Indonesia	34,500	126.3	133,800	490.10
Nepal	6400	225.35	23,200	816.90
Sri Lanka	2300	102.67	8800	392.85
Thailand	10,800	152.11	43,900	618.30

Table 1.7 AMR pathogens in descending order of impact on human health

AMR pathogens in descending order of impact on human health
Staphylococcus aureus
Acinetobacter baumannii
Escherichia coli
Klebsiella pneumoniae
Streptococcus pneumoniae
Pseudomonas aeruginosa

It also supports the WHO list of critical pathogens and demonstrates the impact of the six most important pathogens for AMR in descending order (Table 1.7).

The common hospital-infection-causing multi-resistant bacterium, methicillin-resistant *Staphylococcus aureus (MRSA)*, has increased the most globally. Among Gram-negative bacteria, resistance to the carbapenem group of antibacterial agents increased more than any other antibiotic class. The pathogen with the most substantial decline was *S. pneumoniae*.

The study [23] has also estimated that by 2050, there will be a substantial increase in the worldwide number of deaths attributable to resistant pathogens (~70%), in addition to a 67% rise in fatalities associated with AMR. Most of these deaths would be in South Asia, Latin America, and the Caribbean, hitting hard the developing countries.

Most of these deaths are preventable. Through evidence-based better care, an estimated 92.0 million deaths could be cumulatively averted between 2025 and 2050 [23]. The global community should strive to implement evidence-based strategies to prevent these deaths.

The Global Leaders Group, in its latest report, has estimated that the global community needs to invest USD46 billion every year to contain AMR. This investment is projected to yield a return of USD13 for every USD invested [21]. This thus makes a strong case for pooling and utilisation of appropriate resources worldwide to respond to this global public health challenge.

1.12 Mechanism of Resistance in Bacteria

The basis of drug resistance emergence in bacteria can be genetic or non-genetic (Fig. 1.9).

Resistance in bacteria is also classified as constitutional (intrinsic) resistance and acquired resistance. The intrinsic resistance is primarily due to basic structural/functional properties of the bacterium. These include a lack of target, lack of penetrability, and the constitutional production of antibiotic-degrading enzymes.

In acquired resistance, a sensitive bacterium becomes resistant through genetic alteration, mutation (vertical transmission), or the acquisition of extraneous genes (horizontal acquisition).

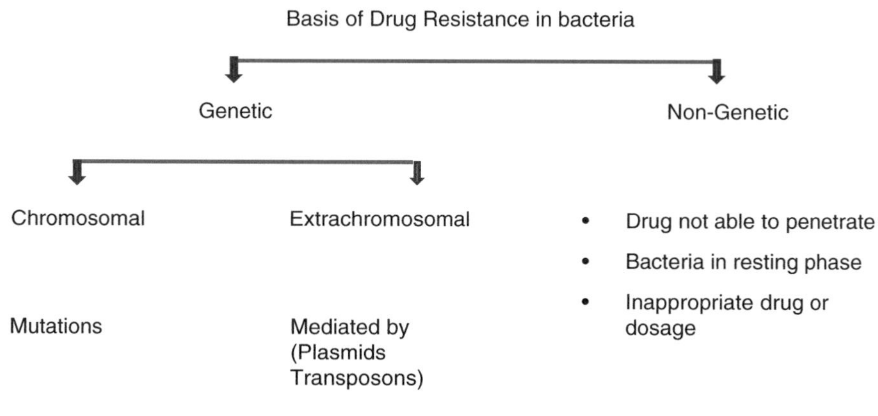

Fig. 1.9 Basis of drug resistance in bacteria

1.12.1 Origin of Drug-Resistant Strains

Drug-resistant strains originate through natural evolutionary processes (mutation and gene transfer) accelerated by human activities, including misuse and overuse of antimicrobials in humans, animals, and agriculture. Selective pressure kills sensitive pathogens, allowing resistant, mutated strains to survive, multiply, and spread.

Irrespective of the process, it culminates in a sensitive organism receiving the genetic material (part of DNA) from a resistant organism. This part of DNA carries information on the mode of inducing resistance against one or multiple antibiotics. Drug resistance can arise by random mutation. When an organism becomes resistant to an antibiotic, the continuous use of that drug selects for the resistant organisms and allows them to multiply, thus making them the dominant population.

1.12.2 Transmissible (Infectious) Drug Resistance

Apart from chromosomal resistance, extrachromosomal material—called as plasmids is capable of conferring resistance (*r determinant*) through the process of conjugation[1] or transduction.[2] This transmission of resistance is also known as infectious drug resistance. Through this mechanism, resistance to single or multiple antibiotics can be transferred. This is the common mode of drug transfer in bacteria that belong to the Gram-negative category, including *Acinetobacter baumannii*, *Escherichia coli*, *Klebsiella pneumoniae*, and *Pseudomonas aeruginosa*. Resistance in *Staphylococcus aureus* is usually due to a plasmid that produces penicillinase. This plasmid is transferred through bacteriophage by a process known as transduction.

1.12.3 Biochemical Mechanism of Drug Resistance

The biochemical changes that are seen in bacteria that have become resistant due to mutation are:

- Increased synthesis of the drug antagonist

---

[1] Bacterial conjugation is a mechanism of horizontal gene transfer where genetic material (usually a plasmid) is transferred from a donor bacterium to a recipient cell through direct physical contact, often via a structure called a pilus. It is a key method for sharing antibiotic resistance and is often considered a form of bacterial "sexual reproduction" or mating.

[2] Transduction in bacteria is a horizontal gene transfer process where a bacteriophage (a virus that infects bacteria) carries bacterial DNA from one bacterium (donor) to another (recipient), incorporating it into the recipient's genome, essentially acting as a genetic delivery system.

Table 1.8 Plasmid-mediated drug resistance

Antimicrobial agent	Mechanism of resistance
Sulphonamides	Reduced permeability
Erythromycin	Modification of ribosomes
Lincomycin	Ribosomal modification
Tetracycline	Reduced permeability
Neomycin	Phosphorylation of antibiotic
Chloramphenicol	Acetylation of antibiotic
Kanamycin	Phosphorylation of antibiotic
Streptomycin	Adenylation of antibiotic
Penicillin	Hydrolysis of beta-lactam ring

Table 1.9 Distinguishing features between resistance conferred by mutation and plasmid-mediated drug resistance

Feature	Mutation	Plasmid-mediated resistance
Number of antibiotics to which resistance is conferred	Usually one	Multiple. Can be up to 100
Degree of resistance	Low	High
Can be overcome by increasing dose	Yes	No
Preventable by combination of antibiotics	Yes	No
Transferable	No	Yes
Metabolically defective	Yes	Normal
Virulence of bacteria	Low	Not decreased

- Decreased permeability to the drug
- Increased destruction of the inhibitor
- Induction of different relative affinities of substrate and antagonist.

The mechanism of drug resistance induced by plasmids differs from that seen in mutated resistant organisms (Table 1.8) [5 , p. 63].

There are a few important differences (Table 1.9) between drug resistance induced by mutation and transferable drug resistance [5 , p. 64].

The complexity of antimicrobial resistance in its emergence and spread, along with its tremendous impact on human health and development, has made AMR a global challenge requiring concerted action by all countries to avert and delay the world slipping into the dreadful post-antibiotic era.

1.13 Spread of AMR

The emergence of resistance in bacteria, due to mutation or the acquisition of plasmids, can occur in the human body, animals, their environment, and in nature. Antibiotics exert selective pressure, allowing resistant strains to become the

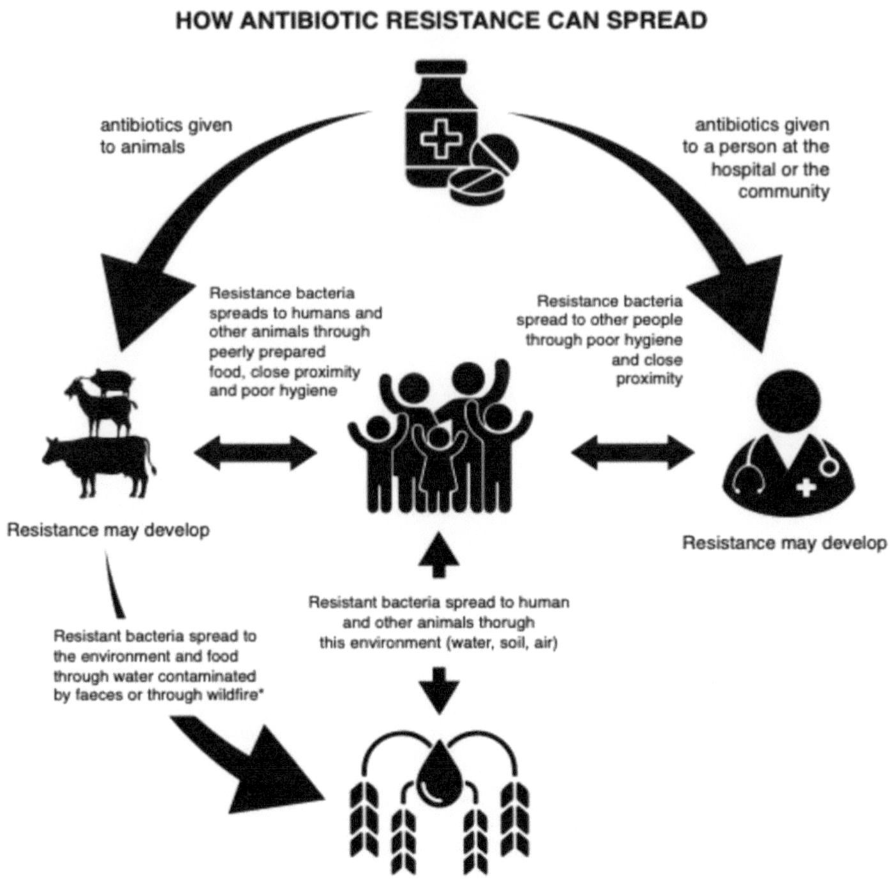

Fig. 1.10 Spread of resistant bacteria between humans, animals, and the environment

dominant population. However, the resistant strains do not persist in humans, animals, or the environment. They can easily move from one sector to another (Fig. 1.10) either through direct contact or as food-borne infections due to resistant pathogens.

1.14 Multidrug-Resistant Organisms

Multidrug-Resistant Organisms (MDROs) are bacteria that have developed resistance to at least one agent in three or more antimicrobial classes, rendering conventional antibiotics ineffective. These bacteria often cause infections in healthcare settings, spreading via contact with contaminated surfaces or bodily fluids. While sometimes defined simply as resistance to one or more antimicrobial classes, MDROs are specifically recognised for their ability to withstand multiple, often unrelated, antibiotic types.

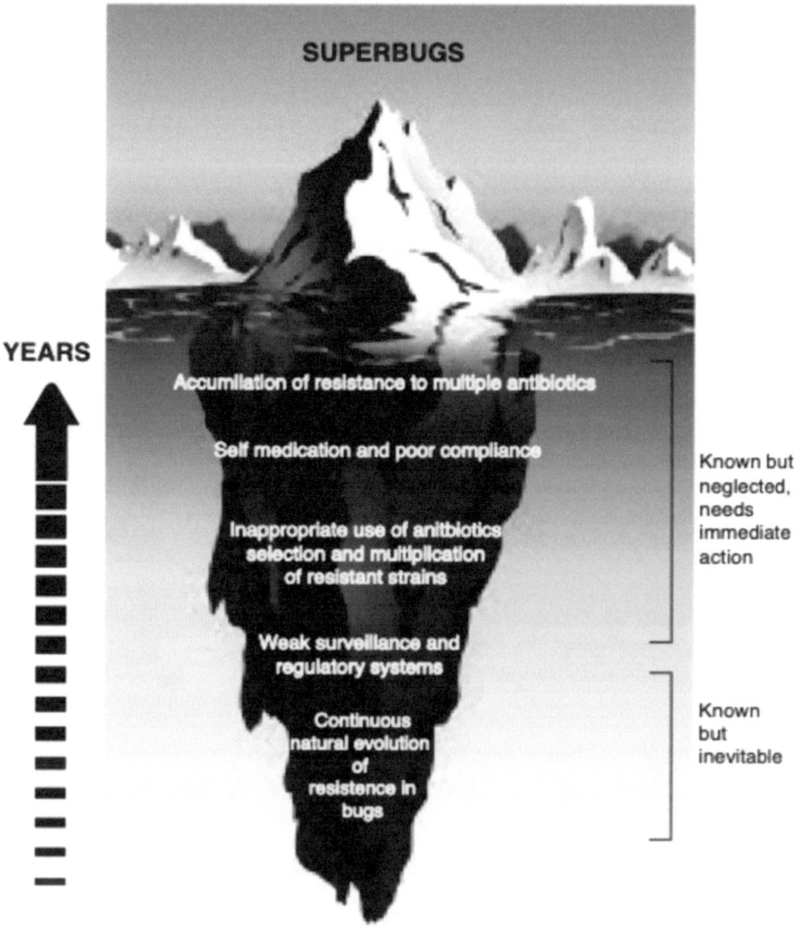

Fig. 1.11 Appearance of superbugs is a culmination of long-time misuse of antibiotics

Antimicrobial-resistant bacteria emerge, are selected, amplified, shared and spread across humans, animals, plants, and the environment. At the same time, the resistance becomes incremental: monoresistance to resistance against multiple antibiotics, i.e. multidrug-resistant organisms (MDRO), which in common language have been referred to as superbugs.

MDRO infections are hard to treat, leading to increased morbidity, mortality, and extended hospital stays. Examples include methicillin-resistant *Staphylococcus aureus* (MRSA), vancomycin-resistant Enterococci (VRE), extended-spectrum *β*-lactamases (ESBLs), carbapenem-resistant *Enterobacteriaceae* (CRE), and multidrug-resistant *Acinetobacter baumannii*.

Superbugs are visible manifestations of our prolonged failure to preserve antibiotics. These are the tip of the iceberg, which carries with it prolonged misuse of antibiotics (Fig. 1.11).

References

1. Chan EKF, Timmermann A, Baldi BF, et al. Human origins in a southern African palaeo-wetland and first migrations. Nature. 2019;575:185–9. https://doi.org/10.1038/s41586-019-1714-1.
2. Adedeji WA. The treasure called antibiotics. Ann Ib Postgrad Med. 2016;14(2):56–7.
3. Prinzi A. Ending-tuberculosis-in-the-face-of-antimicrobial. https://asm.org/articles/2023/march/ending-tuberculosis-in-the-face-of-antimicrobial-r#:~:text. Accessed 2 Sep 2025.
4. Najera RF. Three US Presidents lost their children to diphtheria. https://historyofvaccines.org/blog/three-us-presidents-lost-their-children-to-diphtheria. Accessed 4 Aug 2025.
5. Bhatia R, Ichhpujani RL. Essentials of medical microbiology. 4th ed. New Delhi: Jaypee Medical Publishers.
6. Fleming A. On the antibacterial action of cultures of a penicillium, with special reference to their use in the isolation of *B. influenzæ*. Br J Exp Pathol. 1929;10(3):226–36.
7. Lobanovska M, Pilla G. Penicillin's discovery and antibiotic resistance: lessons for the future? Yale J Biol Med. 2017;90(1):135–45.
8. Hutchings MI, Truman AW, Wilkinson B. Antibiotics: past, present and future. Curr Opin Microbiol. 2019;51:72–80. https://doi.org/10.1016/j.mib.2019.10.008.
9. Ventola CL. The antibiotic resistance crisis: part 1: causes and threats. P T. 2015 Apr;40(4):277–83.
10. Chain E, Florey H, Gardner AD, Heatley NG, Jennings MA, Orr-Ewing J, Sanders AG. Penicillin as a chemotherapeutic agent. Lancet. 1940;236(6104):226–8.
11. Abraham E, Chain E. An enzyme from bacteria able to destroy penicillin. Nature. 1940;146:837.
12. Rosenblatt-Farrell N. The landscape of antibiotic resistance. Environ Health Perspect. 2009;117(6):A244–50. https://doi.org/10.1289/ehp.117-a244.
13. Klein EY, Van Boeckel TP, Martinez EM, Pant S, Gandra S, Levin S, Goossens H, Laxminarayan R. Global increase and geographic convergence in antibiotic consumption between 2000 and 2015. Proc Natl Acad Sci. 2018;115(15):E3463–70. https://doi.org/10.1073/pnas.1717295115.
14. Food and Agriculture Organization of the United Nations. Thirty-ninth session: Status report on antimicrobial resistance. 2015. http://www.fao.org/3/a-mm736rev1e. Accessed 15 Jul 2025.
15. Van Boeckel TP, Glennon EE, Chen D, Gilbert M, Robinson TP, Grenfell BT, et al. Reducing antimicrobial use in food animals. Science. 2017;357:1350–2. https://doi.org/10.1126/science.aao1495.
16. Wang R, van Dorp L, Shaw L, et al. The global distribution and spread of the mobilized colistin resistance gene mcr-1. Nat Commun. 2018;9(1):1179. https://doi.org/10.1038/s41467-018-03205-z.
17. Pareek S, Mathur N, Singh A, Nepalia A. Antibiotics in the environment: a review. Int J Curr Microbiol App Sci. 2015;4(11):278–85.
18. Klein EY, et al. Global trends in antibiotic consumption during 2016–2023 and future projections through 2030. Proc Natl Acad Sci USA. 2024;121(49):e2411919121. https://doi.org/10.1073/pnas.2411919121.
19. WOAH: New report reveals global decrease in antimicrobial use. https://www.woah.org/en/new-report-reveals-global-decrease-in-antimicrobial-use-in-animals/. Accessed 1 Feb 2025.
20. World Bank. Drug-resistant infections: a threat to our economic future. Washington, DC: World Bank; 2017. License: Creative Commons Attribution CC BY 3.0 IGO. Accessed 4 Feb 2025.
21. Global Leaders Group Report on AMR. 2024. https://www.amrleaders.org/resources/m/item/glg-report. Accessed 7 Jan 2025.
22. O Neill (Chair). The review on antimicrobial resistance. Tackling drug-resistant infections globally. Final report and recommendations. https://amr-review.org/sites/default/files/160525_Final%20paper_with%20cover.pdf. Accessed 9 Jan 2025.
23. GBD 2021 Antimicrobial Resistance Collaborators†. Global burden of bacterial antimicrobial resistance 1990–2021: a systematic analysis with forecasts to 2050. Lancet. 2024;404:1199–226. https://doi.org/10.1016/S0140-6736(24)01867-1.

Chapter 2
Rational Use of Antibiotics

Abstract Antibiotics have revolutionised medicine by enabling effective treatment of infections and supporting advanced medical interventions, yet their benefits are increasingly threatened by irrational use. Irrational antibiotic use—comprising inappropriate prescribing, self-medication, incorrect dosing, unsupervised access, and agricultural misuse—has become a primary global driver of antimicrobial resistance (AMR). There are multifaceted determinants of irrational use across patients, prescribers, health systems, pharmaceutical markets, and the veterinary and environmental sectors. There are severe consequences of misuse, including treatment failures, increased morbidity and mortality, economic burden, and erosion of public trust in health systems. The World Health Organisation (WHO) has outlined comprehensive frameworks to promote rational use, including the Global Action Plan on AMR, the AWaRe classification of antibiotics, and facility-level antimicrobial stewardship programmes. Key strategies include enhanced surveillance, strengthened diagnostics, improved regulatory enforcement, education of prescribers and patients, and multisectoral collaboration through a One Health approach. Despite progress, significant challenges persist in raising awareness, enforcing regulations, ensuring access to diagnostics, and striking a balance between stewardship and equitable access to essential antibiotics. Several context-specific, programmatic solutions integrate governance, behavioural interventions, agricultural regulation, and research to safeguard antibiotic efficacy for future generations.

Keywords Antimicrobial resistance · Antimicrobial stewardship · AWaRe classification · Diagnostic capacity · Regulatory enforcement · One Health · Public engagement

Since the discovery of penicillin, antibiotics have transformed medicine, preventing bacterial infections that have killed millions of people and facilitating sophisticated procedures, chemotherapy, and neonatal care. However, widespread irrational use—overuse, misuse, underuse, incorrect prescribing, and unsupervised access—threatens to undermine their benefits by accelerating the development and spread of antimicrobial resistance (AMR). AMR is recognised as a significant

R. Bhatia, *Drug-Resistant Infections*,
https://doi.org/10.1007/978-981-92-4190-3_2

global public health concern that hinders the effective prevention and treatment of an increasing number of infections. To combat irrational antibiotic usage, coordinated measures must be implemented, along with an understanding of its drivers at the human, clinical, societal, economic, and system levels. There are several World Health Organisation (WHO), World Organisation for Animal Health (WOAH) and Food and Agriculture Organisation of the United Nations (FAO) guidelines and recommendations to promote rational use of antibiotics, which look at the leading causes of irrational antibiotic use, describe the health, social, and economic repercussions and recommend rational use of various antibiotics in humans and animals [1, 2].

2.1 Defining “Irrational” Antibiotic Use

“Irrational” antibiotic use is an umbrella term encompassing patterns of antibiotic administration that are inappropriate, unnecessary, sub-optimal, or not evidence-based. This includes prescribing antibiotics for viral infections, using broad-spectrum agents when narrow-spectrum drugs are indicated, improper dosing or duration, self-medication, obtaining antibiotics without a prescription, and incomplete courses or incorrect adherence. Irrational use exists across the community, in outpatient clinics, hospitals, and in the veterinary and agricultural sectors—the latter also contributing to resistance through selection pressure in animals and the environment [2].

Rational antibiotics use is defined as patients taking or administered appropriate drugs as per their needs, at the correct dose, adequate duration, and at an affordable cost. According to the WHO, more than 50% of all medicines are prescribed, dispensed, or sold inappropriately and half of the patients fail to take it appropriately [3].

Antibiotics have an indispensable role in maintaining the health of patients. Therefore, increasing access to antibiotics and their rational use can improve health status and secure development gains. The WHO had developed the core components of drug use indicators. According to these, there is an extensive irrational antibiotics use through polypharmacy, inappropriate indication, dose and route, especially in the developing countries [4].

2.2 Impact of Irrational Use of Antibiotics

The increasing irrational use of antibiotics worldwide is leading to a surge in antibiotic resistance, creating a significant risk and reducing the effectiveness of many affordable antibiotics against prevalent bacterial infections. The 2022 Global Antimicrobial Resistance and Use Surveillance System (GLASS) report [5] highlights concerning levels of resistance in common bacterial pathogens. Median reported rates of 42% for third-generation cephalosporin-resistant *Escherichia coli* and 35% for methicillin-resistant *Staphylococcus aureus* in 76 countries are alarming. In 2020, one in five cases of urinary tract infections caused by *E. coli* exhibited diminished sensitivity to conventional antibiotics, including ampicillin, co-trimoxazole, and fluoroquinolones. This is complicating the effective treatment of typical infections.

The Global Antibiotic Resistance Surveillance Report (2025) shows further deterioration in resistance patterns across several organisms. It presents a global analysis of antibiotic resistance prevalence and trends, drawing on more than 23 million bacteriologically confirmed cases of bloodstream infections, urinary tract infections, gastrointestinal infections, and urogenital gonorrhoea. Data were reported by 104 countries in 2023 and by 110 countries between 2016 and 2023. The report revealed that antimicrobial resistance (AMR) is now widespread and rising globally, based on standardised data from 104 countries and over 23 million infection cases. In 2023, roughly one in six bacterial infections were resistant to commonly used antibiotics, with resistance highest in urinary tract infections and bloodstream infections. Between 2018 and 2023, resistance increased in over 40% of monitored pathogen–antibiotic combinations, with key pathogens such as *E. coli* and Klebsiella pneumoniae showing high resistance to essential drugs such as third-generation cephalosporins. Resistance is especially severe where health systems are weak, notably in parts of South-East Asia and the Eastern Mediterranean, where there is an urgent need for strengthened surveillance, improved diagnostics, responsible antibiotic use, and coordinated global action to contain AMR [6].

In an extensive study of the primary healthcare system in China [7], of all eligible 209,662 antibiotic prescriptions, 147,758 (70.5%) were deemed inappropriate. Upper respiratory tract infections, acute bronchitis, and non-infectious gastroenteritis accounted for 68.9% of inappropriately prescribed antibiotics. Highly inappropriate antibiotic prescribing rates were observed among children aged 0–5 years and patients living in economically underdeveloped areas (77.5%). 82.2% of all prescribed antibiotics were broad-spectrum, with second-generation cephalosporins (15.1%) and third-generation cephalosporins (14.6%) being the most commonly prescribed subgroups.

2.3 Drivers for Irrational Use of Antibiotics

The causes of irrational antibiotic use are multifactorial and interact across multiple levels, including patient/community, prescriber/clinical, health system, commercial, and regulatory, as well as broader socio-cultural or structural drivers (Fig. 2.1).

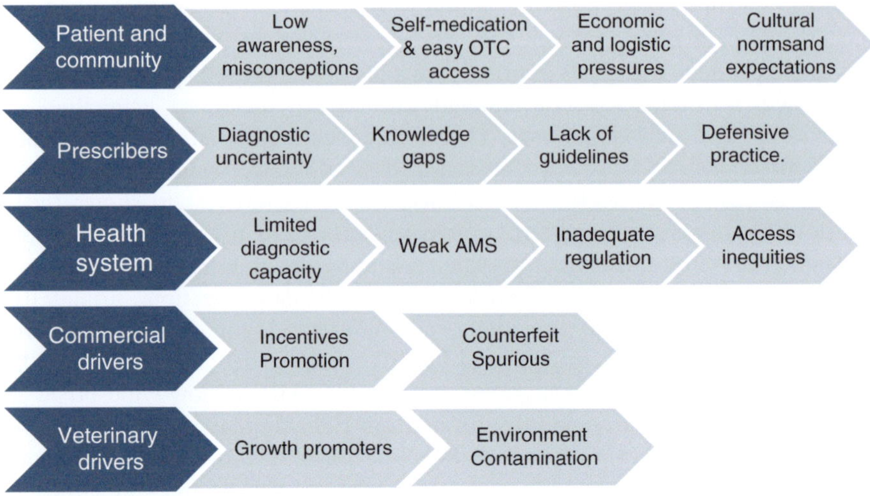

Fig. 2.1 Drivers of irrational use of antibiotics

2.3.1 Patient and Community Drivers

Many individuals mistakenly think that antibiotics are a cure-all for a variety of illnesses and that they also work well against viral infections (flu, colds). Even though antibiotics are ineffective against viral infections, this misperception fuels demand for them [8]. Antibiotics are available without a prescription in pharmacies, unlicenced drug dealers, or markets in many low and middle-income countries (LMICs). Based on previous experiences, recommendations from friends and family, or with a sense of urgency, consumers self-treat. This results in improper duration, dosage and selection of resistant strains [9].

Rapid relief from symptoms, mainly fever, is essential to wage-earning households, and using antibiotics is erroneously considered a quick remedy in LMICs. One-time purchases or early terminations are frequent due to limited access to diagnostic services and the associated expenses and hassles of follow-up.

In certain cultures and environments, it is customary to get medication during a clinical visit, particularly injections or antibiotics. Prescriptions for needless antibiotics may result from providers feeling under pressure to meet expectations. Another factor is social norms that encourage sharing medications [10].

Across the world, irrational antibiotic use is strongly influenced by patient and community factors. Limited awareness leads to the belief that antibiotics cure all fevers and respiratory infections. Patients often demand quick relief, stop treatment early, self-medicate, or share leftover medicines. Community norms encourage use of "strong" drugs, injections, and advice from peers or informal providers. Easy over-the-counter access, weak regulatory enforcement, and poor trust in health systems worsen misuse. Social factors such as poverty, time constraints, low health literacy, and barriers to quality care drive reliance on antibiotics, underscoring the need for community-centred behaviour change, regulation, and health system strengthening. It reinforces the core concept that AMR control needs *behaviour change communication, community engagement, strong pharmacy regulation, and trust-building—not just clinical guidelines.*

2.3.2 Prescriber and Clinical Factors

In several developing countries, physicians lack access to reliable information for rational antibiotic prescription. Hence, their decisions are imperfect. Lack of access to timely microbiology, limited point-of-care diagnostics, and the non-specific presentation of many infections incline prescribers to give "just in case" antibiotics, especially when a bacterial infection cannot be confidently excluded [11]. Some prescribers lack up-to-date training in stewardship, local resistance patterns, or guideline-based choices (such as drug, dose, and duration). Where guidelines exist, awareness and implementation may be poor [2]. Clinicians may prescribe antibiotics to avoid the unfounded risk of bacterial complications, address malpractice concerns, or shorten the perceived recovery time. This is particularly prominent in high-risk patients or in settings with limited follow-up capabilities [11]. High patient volumes and short consultations reduce the time available for history-taking, patient education, and arranging diagnostics, thereby increasing the likelihood of empirical or broad-spectrum prescribing [6].

In addition to the above constraints, even qualified prescribers face multiple constraints that limit rational antibiotic use. Diagnostic uncertainty due to poor access to microbiology and rapid tests leads to empirical, broad-spectrum prescribing. Heavy workloads and time pressure reduce opportunities for patient counselling and watchful waiting. Prescribers often respond to patient expectations and fear of dissatisfaction, complaints, or loss to follow-up. Limited antibiotic stewardship support, weak access to local resistance data, and variable training further affect prescribing quality. Systemic factors such as pharmaceutical promotion, fragmented care, and incentive structures prioritising volume over quality underline the need for strengthened diagnostics, stewardship programmes, and supportive health system reforms.

2.3.3 Health System and Policy Drivers

Most LMICs have inadequate laboratory and surveillance capacity. Without local antimicrobial susceptibility data, empirical prescribing is less targeted. Weak surveillance also undermines stewardship programmes and national benchmarking. Many facilities lack a functional antimicrobial stewardship programme (AMSP), which leads to prescribing oversight or inadequate feedback mechanisms. Where stewardship exists, enforcement and resources vary widely [11]. Inadequate regulation and weak enforcement fail to restrict over-the-counter (OTC) antibiotic sales and poor pharmaceutical distribution controls. Weak enforcement of prescription laws fuels inappropriate community access, leading to greater AMR [9]. In most settings, both over-access (unregulated availability) and inadequate access to appropriate antibiotics coexist. Stock-outs of first-line, narrow-spectrum agents may prompt prescribers to use broader-spectrum agents; the lack of affordable diagnostics perpetuates the use of empirical therapy [1].

All components of the health system, especially in the developing world, influence AMR. Health system deficiencies in developing countries significantly facilitate antimicrobial resistance. Weak regulation allows over-the-counter sales and inappropriate distribution of antibiotics. Limited laboratory capacity and poor surveillance restrict evidence-based prescribing and monitoring of resistance patterns. Inadequate infection prevention and control in health facilities increases antibiotic demand. Shortages of trained health workers, high patient loads, and fragmented care promote empirical and prolonged antibiotic use. Supply chain gaps lead to substandard or falsified medicines. Insufficient stewardship programmes, poor enforcement of treatment guidelines, and underinvestment in primary care and public health create systemic conditions that accelerate the emergence and spread of AMR.

2.3.4 Commercial and Pharmaceutical Influences

Pharmaceutical marketing, incentives for prescribers, and profit motives for pharmacies can bias antibiotic selection and lead to increased inappropriate use. In settings with direct provider-industry relationships, promotional activities may favour newer or broader agents [2]. Poor-quality and substandard antibiotics can lead to therapeutic failure and encourage repeated or escalated antibiotic use, thereby indirectly promoting resistance [12].

The pharmaceutical industry influences antimicrobial resistance (AMR) through several interconnected mechanisms. Promotional practices that emphasise broad-spectrum or newer antibiotics encourage their use even when narrow-spectrum or non-antibiotic options are appropriate. Incentives, sponsorships, and biased educational materials can subtly shape prescribing behaviour and weaken adherence to standard treatment guidelines. In many developing countries, industry links with distributors and pharmacies contribute to easy availability of antibiotics without prescriptions. Market-driven production and sales targets prioritise volume over stewardship, increasing community-level exposure to antibiotics. At the same time, limited commercial incentives for developing new antibiotics, rapid diagnostics, and stewardship-support tools result in overreliance on existing drugs. Weak regulation of pharmaceutical promotion, distribution, and conflict-of-interest disclosure allows these influences to persist. Collectively, these factors promote inappropriate antibiotic use and accelerate the emergence and spread of antimicrobial resistance.

2.3.5 *Veterinary, Agricultural, and Environmental Drivers*

The routine use of antibiotics for growth promotion or prophylaxis in livestock and poultry creates selection pressure for resistant bacteria that can be transferred to humans through food, animals, or the environment (Chap. 1; Fig.1.10). Weak regulation and monitoring in the animal sectors exacerbate this problem [13].

Discharge of antibiotics and resistant organisms from pharmaceutical manufacturing, hospitals, farms, and communities contaminates water systems and soils, creating reservoirs of resistance [13].

2.4 Consequences of Irrational Antibiotic Use

The irrational use of antibiotics has wide-ranging, severe clinical, public health, economic, and social consequences (Table 2.1) (also see Table 1.3).

2.4.1 *Clinical Consequences*

The primary direct consequence is the accelerated selection and spread of resistant pathogens, including multidrug-resistant organisms (MDROs). Common examples include ESBL-producing *Enterobacterales*, carbapenem-resistant *Enterobacterales* (CRE), methicillin-resistant *Staphylococcus aureus* (MRSA), and multidrug-resistant tuberculosis. Resistance increases treatment failures, morbidity, and mortality [1].

Resistant infections require second-line or combination therapies that may be less effective, toxic, and more costly. Patients experience prolonged illness, complications (e.g. sepsis), longer recovery times, and a higher risk of death.

Rising resistance undermines the safety of routine surgeries, cancer chemotherapy, organ transplantation, and neonatal care—procedures that rely on effective

Table 2.1 Consequences of irrational use of antibiotics

	Types of consequences	Major impact
1	Clinical consequences	Increased antimicrobial resistance Treatment failures and complications Negation of modern high-tech and complex medical interventions
2	Public health and societal consequences	Transmission of resistant strains Increased healthcare utilisation Equity implications
3	Economic consequences	Direct medical cost Macroeconomics impact
4	Wider implications	Threat to public trust and health security

perioperative and prophylactic antibiotics. This could reverse decades of medical progress.

2.4.2 Public Health and Societal Consequences

Resistant organisms can spread within hospitals, communities, and across borders. Outbreaks of MDROs increase pressure on health systems and require costly infection-control measures [14]. Resistant infections lead to extended hospital stays, increased admissions, the need for isolation, and repeat clinic visits, thus straining health services and diverting resources [12].

Vulnerable populations (low-income groups, people in LMICs, and those with limited access to advanced care) bear a disproportionate burden of AMR due to limited treatment options and health system constraints.

2.4.3 Economic Consequences

Treatment of resistant infections is costlier due to the use of expensive drugs, prolonged inpatient care, additional diagnostics, and increased use of intensive care. Estimates indicate substantial additional per-patient costs associated with MDRO infections. AMR also carries a macroeconomic impact. It can reduce workforce productivity through illness and premature death, affecting GDP. Modelling studies project significant economic losses worldwide if AMR is not controlled [12].

2.4.4 Wider Implications

Failure to control AMR undermines trust in the health system and threatens overall health security, raising the risk of uncontrollable spread of untreatable infections.

2.5 WHO Recommendations and Frameworks for Rational Antibiotic Use

WHO has articulated a comprehensive, multi-layered approach to promote rational use of antibiotics, combining global guidance, classification tools, stewardship frameworks, surveillance, and policy recommendations [15]. Below are the main elements and recommendations in these guidelines.

2.5.1 Global Action Plan on Antimicrobial Resistance (2015)

The WHO Global Action Plan (GAP), adopted in 2015 [16], set five strategic objectives:

(a) improve awareness and understanding of AMR;
(b) strengthen knowledge through surveillance and research;
(c) reduce incidence of infection through adequate sanitation, hygiene, and infection prevention;
(d) optimise use of antimicrobial agents; and
(e) ensure sustainable investment in countering AMR.

The GAP emphasises a One Health approach (human, animal, environment) and asks countries to develop respective national action plans aligned with GAP objectives, with a focus on optimal use of antibiotics.

2.5.2 AWaRe Classification and WHO Antibiotic Book

To guide selection of antibiotics and stewardship, WHO developed the AWaRe classification (Access, Watch, Reserve) [17]. AWaRe categorises antibiotics into three groups:

Access Group: These antibiotics are considered the first- or second-line choices for common infections, possessing activity against a wide range of susceptible pathogens and lower resistance potential. They should be readily available, affordable, and quality-assured. Examples include amoxicillin and penicillin.

Watch Group: These antibiotics have a higher resistance potential and include agents of high priority among critically important antimicrobials for human medicine. They are generally broader-spectrum and should be used cautiously, prioritising stewardship programmes and monitoring to preserve their effectiveness. Examples include azithromycin, ciprofloxacin, and ceftriaxone.

Reserve Group: These antibiotics are "last resort" options reserved for confirmed or suspected infections due to multidrug-resistant organisms. Their use should be strictly limited to specific situations when all other options have failed or are unsuitable. They are key targets for high-intensity national and international stewardship programmes. Examples include colistin and linezolid.

The AWaRe framework helps countries monitor antibiotic consumption, set targets (e.g. percentage of use from the Access group), and design stewardship policies. WHO updates the AWaRe classification every 2 years to support antibiotic stewardship efforts. The 2023 update recommends 41 essential antibiotics for over 30 clinical infections, as well as assigning AWaRe groups to an additional 257 antibiotics not included on the WHO Essential Medicines List [18]. WHO also published the AWaRe-aligned Antibiotic Book [19], which provides concise, evidence-based choices, doses, and durations for common infections to support clinicians [20].

The WHO recommends that at least 60% of total antibiotic consumption should be from the Access group to promote rational use. Rational use of antibiotics, guided by the WHO AWaRe classification, is essential to preserve the effectiveness of these life-saving medicines and mitigate the threat of antimicrobial resistance.

2.5.3 Antimicrobial Stewardship Programmes

Antimicrobial stewardship programmes (AMSP) are organised efforts to promote the optimal use of antimicrobial drugs, including antibiotics, thereby improving patient outcomes, minimising the development of AMR, and reducing adverse events [21]. These programmes involve a range of strategies and interventions implemented at various levels (individual, hospital, community) to ensure that antimicrobials are used appropriately.

2.5.3.1 Goals of AMSP

The following are the goals of any AMSP

- To improve patient outcomes by ensuring that patients receive the most effective treatment for their infections.
- To reduce AMR, AMSP aims to optimise antibiotic use, thereby slowing the development and spread of resistance.
- To minimise adverse events by using antibiotics appropriately, AMSP can reduce the risk of side effects and other complications associated with antibiotic use.
- To reduce healthcare costs by optimising antibiotic use, AMSP can help mitigate unnecessary expenses associated with inappropriate prescribing.

Key components of AMSP have been shown in Box 2.1.

Box 2.1 Key Components of AMSP

Optimal Antimicrobial Selection

Choosing the right antibiotic for the specific infection, considering factors like the pathogen, patient's condition, and local resistance patterns

Appropriate Dosage and Duration

Administering the correct dose and for the appropriate duration of therapy to ensure effectiveness and minimise the risk of resistance development

Monitoring and Evaluation

Tracking antibiotic use, resistance patterns, and patient outcomes to assess the effectiveness of the programme and identify areas for improvement

(continued)

Box 2.1 (continued)

Education and Training

Providing education and training to healthcare professionals on appropriate antimicrobial use and the principles of stewardship

Infection Prevention and Control

Implementing measures to prevent infections in the first place, reducing the need for antibiotics

Collaboration and Communication

Fostering collaboration between different healthcare professionals (physicians, pharmacists, nurses, etc.) and ensuring effective communication about antimicrobial use

Optimal Antimicrobial Selection

Choosing the right antibiotic for a specific infection involves considering factors such as the pathogen, the patient's condition, and local patterns of antibiotic resistance.

Appropriate Dosage and Duration

Administering the correct dose and for the appropriate duration of therapy to ensure effectiveness and minimise the risk of resistance development.

Monitoring and Evaluation

Tracking antibiotic use, resistance patterns, and patient outcomes to assess the effectiveness of the programme and identify areas for improvement.

Education and Training

Providing education and training to healthcare professionals on appropriate antimicrobial use and the principles of stewardship.

Infection Prevention and Control

Implementing measures to prevent infections in the first place reduces the need for antibiotics.

Collaboration and Communication

Fostering collaboration between different healthcare professionals (physicians, pharmacists, nurses, etc.) and ensuring effective communication about antimicrobial use.

WHO and partner guidance recommend facility-level AMSP to optimise antibiotic use. Core elements should include:

- Leadership commitment and dedicated resources.
- Multidisciplinary stewardship teams (physicians, pharmacists, microbiologists, infection preventionists).
- Evidence-based guidelines, local antibiograms and formulary management.

- Prospective audit with feedback, pre-authorisation for selected agents, and decision support.
- Education and training for prescribers and clinical staff.
- Surveillance of antibiotic use and resistance, with regular reporting and benchmarking.
- Integration with infection prevention and control (IPC) efforts.

2.5.4 Surveillance, Diagnostics, and Laboratories

WHO emphasises strengthening laboratory capacity and surveillance systems. Routine, quality-assured antimicrobial susceptibility testing should be performed to generate local antibiograms, guiding empirical therapy. Surveillance networks should be expanded to monitor trends and inform national and provincial antibiotics policy. There is a need to encourage development, production and use of reliable point-of-care diagnostics and rapid tests to reduce diagnostic uncertainty and unnecessary antibiotic use.

2.5.5 Regulatory and Policy Measures

WHO recommends national actions to curb inappropriate access and commercial drivers of AMR through strengthening of regulatory frameworks to restrict OTC antibiotic sales and to ensure that prescriptions are required where appropriate. National authorities should ensure the availability and affordability of first-line, narrow-spectrum antibiotics to avoid default use of broad-spectrum agents. The regulatory authorities should monitor and regulate antibiotic use in agriculture, phase out their non-therapeutic uses (e.g. growth promotion), and harmonise veterinary and human antibiotics use policies (One Health) [13].

2.5.6 Public Awareness, Behaviour Change, and Education

Public communication campaigns aimed at correcting misconceptions about antibiotics are central to the WHO's strategy [22]. Behavioural interventions for patients and prescribers—including delayed prescriptions where appropriate, shared decision-making, and adherence counselling—can reduce inappropriate demand and use. Education of healthcare workers, pharmacists and animal-health practitioners is emphasised (see Chap. 20).

2.5.7 Access and Equity Considerations

WHO emphasises balancing stewardship with access: policies must avoid restricting necessary access to antibiotics for those who need them. Measures should ensure a reliable supply of appropriate agents, especially in resource-constrained settings, while curbing inappropriate availability.

2.6 Challenges in Assuring Rational Use of Antibiotics

Significant challenges in assuring rational antibiotic use are summarised below:

- Inadequate awareness among prescribers and users.
- Weak regulatory enforcement, which allows the availability of antibiotics of questionable quality, along with easy access from licenced and unlicenced sources.
- Resource constraints in LMICs limit laboratory capacity, staffing for AMSP, and enforcement.
- Cultural norms and commercial incentives.
- Global inequities in access to diagnostics, vaccines, and newer antimicrobials complicate the development of balanced policy.
- Environmental contamination and agricultural uses continue to pose challenges for regulation across jurisdictions.

2.7 Possible Solutions and Way Forward

The WHO's frameworks for promoting the rational use of antibiotics are comprehensive. Their successful implementation requires a systematic, programmatic approach that is adapted to suit local contexts, with judicious use of available resources. Some of these have been summarised in Box 2.2 and illustrated with major action points that follow.

2.7.1 Strengthen National Governance and Financing

- Develop or update national action plans aligned with the WHO GAP and One Health principles.
- Allocate sustainable funding for surveillance, laboratories, stewardship, and public engagement.
- Establish intersectoral coordinating mechanisms that encompass the human health, veterinary, agricultural, and environmental sectors.

2.7.2 *Scale up Antimicrobial Stewardship Programmes at All Healthcare Levels*

- Implement AMSP in tertiary hospitals, and then adapt core elements for smaller facilities and primary care settings.
- Use AWaRe targets (e.g. percentage Access use) as measurable metrics.
- Incorporate digital tools (electronic prescribing, decision support) where feasible to prompt guideline-aligned choices. Digital health, telemedicine, and decision support tools can extend the reach of stewardship.

Box 2.2 Implementation of Frameworks to Ensure Rational Use of Antibiotics

- Strengthen the national governance mechanism and allocate adequate resources
- Establish or scale up AMSP in all health facilities
- Improve diagnostic capacity and facilitate the use of point-of-care rapid diagnostics
- Enforce effective, relevant national regulations
- Engage with communities for behavioural change
- Advocate antimicrobial stewardship in the veterinary and environmental sectors

2.7.3 *Improve Diagnostic Capacity and Use of Rapid Tests*

- Invest in laboratory networks with quality management systems and data linkage between laboratories and clinicians.
- Promote validated point-of-care tests (where evidence supports) to reduce empirical prescribing for viral illnesses.

2.7.4 *Regulatory Enforcement and Supply Chain Management*

- Reinforce prescription-only regulations and pharmacy practice standards; combine enforcement with education for pharmacists.
- Secure supply chains for essential *Access* category of antibiotics to reduce substitution with broader agents.

2.7.5 Behavioural and Community Interventions

- Deploy targeted public campaigns to correct beliefs about antibiotics; focus on caregivers, parents, and frequent antibiotic users.
- Engage communities and pharmacists as partners; train pharmacy staff to provide appropriate advice and referrals rather than antibiotics.

2.7.6 Stewardship in Agriculture and Environment

- Phase out the routine use of medically necessary antibiotics for growth promotion of animals and regulate and monitor veterinary prescriptions.
- Promote good animal husbandry practices, biosecurity, and vaccination to minimise the need for antibiotics in livestock.
- Monitor pharmaceutical effluents to ensure compliance with environmental regulations and limit contamination.

2.7.7 Monitoring, Targets, and Research

- Establish measurable targets (e.g. AWaRe Access target, reductions in specific inappropriate prescriptions).
- Support operational research into effective behavioural interventions, diagnostic algorithms, and implementation science to scale interventions equitably.

The irrational use of antibiotics is driven by a complex mix of knowledge gaps, diagnostic uncertainty, patient expectations, commercial incentives, weak regulation, and systemic weaknesses across human, animal, and environmental sectors. The consequences—rising AMR, treatment failures, increased healthcare costs and threats to modern medical practice—are profound. Countries must follow WHO's guidance, which combines strategic global goals (Global Action Plan), practical tools (AWaRe and the Antibiotic Book), and recommended interventions (antimicrobial stewardship, surveillance, regulatory action, public education, and One Health coordination). Implementing these recommendations requires political will, sustainable investment, multisectoral collaboration, and context-adapted strategies. With coordinated action, rational antibiotic use can be promoted without compromising access to those in need, thus preserving antibiotic efficacy for current and future generations.

References

1. WHO. Antimicrobial resistance. https://www.who.int/news-room/fact-sheets/detail/antimicrobial-resistance. Accessed 7 Feb 2025.
2. Hossain MJ, Jabin N, Ahmmed F, Sultana A, Abdur Rahman SM, Islam MR. Irrational use of antibiotics and factors associated with antibiotic resistance: findings from a cross-sectional study in Bangladesh. Health Sci Rep. 2023;6(8):e1465. https://doi.org/10.1002/hsr2.1465.
3. World Health Organization. Rational use—WHO policy perspectives on medicines. https://www.who.int/teams/health-product-policy-and-standards/medicines-selection-ip-and-affordability/medicines-policy/rational-use. Accessed 2 Feb 2026.
4. Amsalu W, Tilahun Z, Bekele F. Evaluation of drug use pattern using WHO drug use indicators at Tikur Anbessa Specialized Hospital, Addis Ababa, Ethiopia. HSOA J Commun Med Public Health. 2022.; https://doi.org/10.24966/CMPH-1978/100118.
5. WHO. Global Antimicrobial Resistance and Use Surveillance System: GLASS. https://www.who.int/publications/i/item/9789240062702. Accessed 9 Feb 2025.
6. WHO. The Global Antibiotic Resistance Surveillance Report.2025. https://www.who.int/publications/i/item/9789240116337?utm_source=chatgpt.com. Accessed 1 Feb 2026.
7. Fu M, Zhiwen G, Yuezhen Z, Li C, Zhou Y, Hu L, et al. Inappropriate antibiotic prescribing in primary healthcare facilities in China: a nationwide survey, 2017–2019. Clin Microbiol Infect. 2023;29:602–9. https://doi.org/10.1016/j.cmi.2022.11.015.
8. Wang X, Liu C, Zheng S, Zhang X, Lin R, Duan L, Wang D, Wang Q, Zhong W, Ding X. The public's irrational use of antibiotics for upper respiratory tract infections: a cross-sectional study based on the health belief model. Sci Rep. 2025;15(1):17220. https://doi.org/10.1038/s41598-025-01767-9.
9. Nahar P, Unicomb L, Lucas PJ, et al. What contributes to inappropriate antibiotic dispensing among qualified and unqualified healthcare providers in Bangladesh? A qualitative study. BMC Health Serv Res. 2020;20:656. https://doi.org/10.1186/s12913-020-05512-y.
10. Melaku T, Assegid L. Prescription in peril: the sociology of antibiotics and antimicrobial resistance in low resource settings. Discov Soc Sci Health. 2025;5:71. https://doi.org/10.1007/s44155-025-00225-1.
11. Khadse SN, Ugemuge S, Singh C. Impact of antimicrobial stewardship on reducing antimicrobial resistance. Cureus. 2023;15(12):e49935. https://doi.org/10.7759/cureus.49935.
12. Keenan K, Silva Corrêa J, Sringernyuang L, Nayiga S, Chandler CIR. The social burden of antimicrobial resistance: what is it, how can we measure it, and why does it matter? JAC Antimicrob Resist. 2025;7(2):dlae208. https://doi.org/10.1093/jacamr/dlae208.
13. Wernli D, Harbarth S, Levrat N, Pittet D. A 'whole of United Nations approach' to tackle antimicrobial resistance? A mapping of the mandate and activities of international organisations. BMJ Glob Health. 2022;7(5):e008181. https://doi.org/10.1136/bmjgh-2021-008181.
14. Zujbe Z, Tabassum N, Kibria G, et al. The burden of hospital-acquired infections and antibiotic resistance in Bangladesh: current trends and policy implications. Discov Public Health. 2025;22:290. https://doi.org/10.1186/s12982-025-00665-9.
15. Mudenda S, Daka V, Matafwali SK. World Health Organization AWaRe framework for antibiotic stewardship: where are we now and where do we need to go? An expert viewpoint. Antimicrob Steward Healthc Epidemiol. 2023;3(1):e84. https://doi.org/10.1017/ash.2023.164.
16. WHO. Global action plan on antimicrobial resistance. https://www.who.int/publications/i/item/9789241509763. Accessed 11 Feb 2025.
17. WHO. Web Annex C. WHO AWaRe (access, watch, reserve) classification of antibiotics for evaluation and monitoring of use, 2023. In: The selection and use of essential medicines 2023: Executive summary of the report of the 24th WHO Expert Committee on the Selection and Use of Essential Medicines, 24–28 April 2023. Geneva: World Health Organization; 2023. (WHO/MHP/HPS/EML/2023.04). Licence: CC BY-NC-SA 3.0 IGO.
18. WHO. AWaRe classification of antibiotics for evaluation and monitoring of use, 2023. https://www.who.int/publications/i/item/WHO-MHP-HPS-EML-2023.04#:~. Accessed 11 Feb 2025.

19. WHO. Web Annex. Infographics. In: The WHO AWaRe (Access, Watch, Reserve) antibiotic book. Geneva: World Health Organization; 2022. (WHO/MHP/HPS/EML/2022.02). Licence: CC BY-NC-SA 3.0 IGO.
20. Zanichelli V, Sharland M, Cappello B, Moja L, Getahun H, Pessoa-Silva C, Sati H, van Weezenbeek C, Balkhy H, Simão M, Gandra S, Huttner B. The WHO AWaRe (access, watch, reserve) antibiotic book and prevention of antimicrobial resistance. Bull World Health Organ. 2023;101(4):290–6. https://doi.org/10.2471/BLT.22.288614.
21. WHO. Antimicrobial stewardship programmes in health-care facilities in low- and middle-income countries. A practical toolkit. Geneva: World Health Organization; 2019. Licence: CC BY-NC-SA 3.0 IGO.
22. WHO. WHO multi-country survey reveals widespread public misunderstanding about antibiotic resistance. https://www.who.int/news/item/16-11-2015-who-multi-country-survey-reveals-widespread-public-misunderstanding-about-antibiotic-resistance. Accessed 10 Feb 2025.

Chapter 3
Challenges and Possible Solutions to Contain AMR

Abstract Antimicrobial resistance (AMR) is one of the most significant global public health challenges, threatening the effective treatment of infectious diseases and endangering health, development, and economic stability. Despite increasing awareness, nations continue to encounter difficulties in establishing sustainable and coordinated strategies to manage AMR. The multifaceted nature of AMR obstructs its control. Political commitment is insufficient, with AMR frequently prioritised lower than other prominent health concerns. Limited and unsustainable financial resources undermine the execution of national action plans. Technical deficiencies, such as inadequate surveillance systems, poor diagnostic capabilities, and insufficient infection prevention and control measures, exacerbate the challenges. Programmatic issues, including inadequate integration across sectors, weak governance, and insufficient connections with preventive health initiatives, impede advancement. Regulatory deficiencies permit the overuse, misuse, and distribution of substandard antimicrobials, while a lack of educational programmes and professional training contributes to irrational prescribing practices. Weak multisectoral collaboration, underutilisation of community involvement, and insufficient engagement from the private sector further intensify the crisis. Innovation in research and development, combined with international collaboration, is essential for sustaining progress. To contain AMR, strong political will, adequate resources, effective governance, One Health collaboration, and community engagement are necessary to prevent a post-antibiotic era.

Keywords Antimicrobial resistance · AMR surveillance · Diagnostic capabilities · Insufficient IPC · AMR regulations · National AMR response

Antimicrobial resistance (AMR) is the biggest threat the world faces in controlling infectious diseases. It already affects the entire world. Inaction to combat AMR may culminate in a horrific post-antibiotic era. Containing AMR requires sustained national efforts and worldwide collaboration to generate the resources needed to

R. Bhatia, *Drug-Resistant Infections*,
https://doi.org/10.1007/978-981-92-4190-3_3

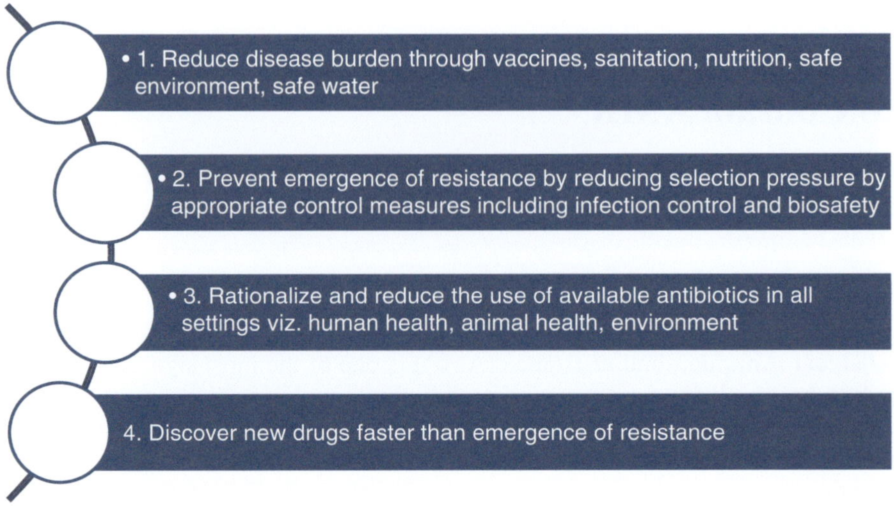

Fig. 3.1 Four broad approaches to combat AMR

preserve the efficacy of antimicrobials and to create new diagnostic and therapeutic tools to protect the health of all people, as enshrined in the UN Sustainable Development Goals and articulated in paragraph 26 of the political declaration on these goals17 [1]. It is a battle that must be vigorously fought and won.

The global, societal, and individual impacts of AMR, as well as the numerous drivers of its emergence and spread, have been summarised in Chap. 1 (Tables 1.3 and 1.4). These exemplify the complexity and consequences of AMR. The emergence and spread of AMR are the outcome of several naturally occurring and human-induced actions.

Logically, and based upon scientific knowledge currently available, the following are four major action areas to reduce the impact of AMR (Fig. 3.1).

To achieve these objectives, several challenges must be addressed simultaneously on a sustainable basis over a long period to reduce the prevalence of AMR in both healthcare facilities and the community. The challenges have a broad spectrum. Box 3.1 articulates major issues that are being experienced, especially in developing countries, in the fight against AMR. Box 3.1 also reinforces the multidimensional and complex nature of AMR, necessitating corresponding whole-of-society actions.

Box 3.1: Multidimensional Challenges in Containing AMR
Global unrestricted movement of resistant pathogens.

Complexity in understanding the genesis and spread of AMR.
Political challenge in allocating resources vis-à-vis competing priorities.
Economic challenge in revenues generated or saved by the use of antibiotics.
Technical challenge in the development of diagnostic and therapeutic tools.
One Health coordinating challenge with other sectors using antibiotics.
Regulatory challenge on the use, development and disposal of antimicrobials.
Legal challenge in gathering data and enforcing regulations.
Environmental challenge in protecting it from contamination.
Educational challenge in giving sound knowledge to professionals.
Behavioural change in antimicrobial users, i.e. communities.
Challenges in aligning national policies with international standards.

Despite various national, regional, and global initiatives, these challenges and major issues continue to persist and require vigorous and sustained addressing by the respective country, with technical assistance from international development partners.

3.1 Major Issues in AMR Containment

The significant challenges in combating AMR can be broadly categorised into several key areas. However, all categories are linked with each other and are interdependent (Fig. 3.2). These include: political commitment and prioritisation, appropriate financial allocation on a sustainable basis, technical challenges, programmatic issues, regulatory inadequacies, educational shortcomings, multisectoral response with One Health approach, Research & development and innovations, community engagement and intercountry and global coordination.

These issues need to be prioritised at the country level, and solutions that are most appropriate in the local context should be implemented vigorously. A brief description of challenges and directive suggestions to address these are given below.

3.1.1 Political Commitment and Prioritisation

The political and decision-making leadership of several countries has yet to recognise the global and national critical importance of AMR and its dire consequences for the country's development. In competing with other health priorities for resource

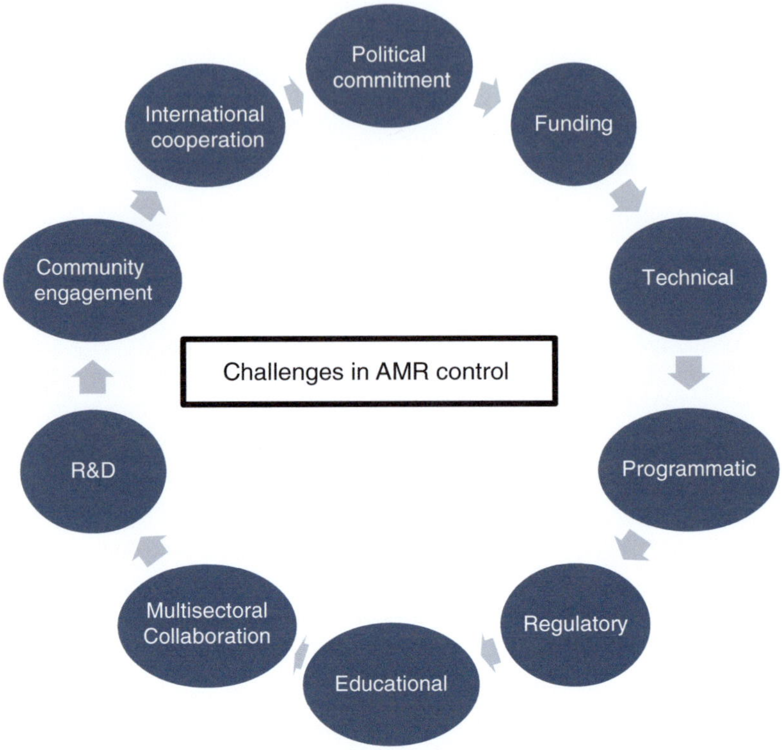
Political commitment
Funding
Technical
Programmatic
Regulatory
Educational
Multisectoral Collaboration
R&D
Community engagement
International cooperation
Challenges in AMR control

Fig. 3.2 Major inter-dependent issues and challenges in AMR control

allocations, AMR remains secondary to established priorities, such as tuberculosis, malaria, acute respiratory infections, HIV/AIDS, diarrhoeal diseases, zoonoses, and post-COVID-19 pandemic preparedness and response. One of the reasons is the invisibility of AMR in contrast with patients with tuberculosis, malaria, typhoid fever, etc., who are visible and can be quantified. Political priority thus moves towards the latter set of ailments.

Insufficient awareness and visibility of the public health importance of AMR have resulted in low prioritisation of AMR within the national health agenda. Several resolutions and recommendations from global high-level organisations, including the United Nations General Assembly (UNGA), World Health Organisation (WHO), Food and Agriculture Organisation of the UN (FAO), G20, G7, and various regional political and economic platforms, should be leveraged to advocate for elevating AMR control on the national agenda. The targets established by the UNGA in 2024 [2] (Chap. 4, Table 4.2) should motivate national authorities to speed up the development and implementation of national action plans to combat AMR and to meet the UNGA targets within the specified timeframe.

Because AMR is a complex, multisectoral problem, there are no easy solutions. Stopping its spread requires a strong political commitment that enables local, evidence-based solutions, as the factors contributing to it are context-specific. National and international cross-sectoral coordination mechanisms that engage all government agencies, the private sector, civil society and professional groups need to be harmonised to address AMR.

National authorities need to address the rising threat of AMR through a holistic and multisectoral implementation in the true spirit of the One Health approach (Chap. 5), integrating primarily human and animal health and encompassing a wide array of environmental concerns [3].

Containing AMR requires a whole-of-society approach, with significant roles for various sectors that warrant continuous coordination through a high-level governing mechanism under the purview of the highest national authority.

A step-by-step approach to a national strategy, carried out through a well-designed and adequately funded programme focusing on generating evidence to inform action, guided by a contextualised and prioritised roadmap, endorsed by top political and administrative authorities, will be the suitable approach.

A strong political commitment, an effective governance mechanism and sustained appropriate funding shall facilitate the impactful implementation of national action plans to contain AMR (NAP). Multisectorality of complex implementation of AMR requires a high-level multistakeholder steering committee or monitoring mechanism that can keep a close eye on the progress of NAP and suggest corrective measures.

Political commitment at the highest level in any country is the quiet superpower and fountainhead of all initiatives required for effective AMR control. National authorities must take AMR seriously because of its socio-economic and developmental dimensions and put into motion policy and programmatic level actions in the right evidence-based direction. AMR must be recognised as a developmental issue for the country and not merely a technical challenge.

Placing AMR on the national priority list indicates political commitment. This translates into clear policies, funded national action plans, and accountability across ministries—health, agriculture, environment, and finance. High-level endorsement helps break silos and enables a true One Health approach that encompasses a whole-of-society approach with active participation of private sector and communities—the ultimate beneficiaries.

Bringing AMR higher on the national agenda sends out positive signals to the provinces/states in a federated country like India, where implementation of all activities about human and animal health has been constitutionally delegated to them. This ripple effect of heightened awareness strengthens AMR control activities at the state level, thus encompassing the entire country.

Political backing is essential for development and effective enforcement of regulations on production, sale, use and disposal of antibiotics in the most rational way. This includes controlling over-the-counter antibiotic sales, regulating pharmaceutical promotion, improving prescription practices, and enforcing standards in animal husbandry and food production—areas that often face resistance without political will.

It is well established that any political commitment at the top drives system-wide coordination and monitoring. It empowers institutions to set targets, track antibiotic use and resistance trends, and publicly report progress, creating pressure for performance and reform.

A visible political leadership shapes public and professional norms. When leaders communicate AMR as a national threat (as was recently done in 2026 by the Prime Minister of India in one of his national telecasts) and link it to health security, economic productivity, and pandemic preparedness, it legitimises behaviour change among prescribers, farmers, industry, and communities. It sends out strong signals to all stakeholders to pursue AMR containment on priority.

3.1.2 Financial Allocation on a Sustainable Basis

Political commitment unlocks sustainable financing. Governments that prioritise AMR are more likely to allocate domestic budgets for surveillance, laboratories, infection prevention and control, and stewardship programmes, instead of relying only on short-term donor support. Predictable funding allows systems to mature and scale and facilitate effective implementation of respective national action programmes.

National Action Plans to control AMR (NAP) have been developed by a large number of countries. These align with the WHO Global Action Plan on Antimicrobial Resistance (Chap. 4). Their implementation has not been as expected, primarily due to inadequate funds being made available for the implementation of NAPs. As of 2024, only 11% of the NAPs have been funded by the national authorities [2].

Limited financial resources pose challenges to implementing all AMR control measures, such as surveillance systems, stewardship programmes, and infection prevention and control (IPC) initiatives. National authorities, having made firm commitments at regional and global levels, must ensure the provision of appropriate resources for the efficient implementation of their respective NAPs.

There has been a drastic reduction in financial support from international agencies (e.g. WHO, FAO) and several established donors (e.g. Fleming Fund) due to internal constraints. This necessitates the allocation of greater domestically generated resources to execute multisectoral activities essential to contain AMR.

3.1.3 Technical Challenges

Implementing NAPs faces several technical challenges, including data collection and analysis, surveillance, and the need for robust monitoring and evaluation frameworks. Furthermore, the complexity of AMR containment, requiring multisectoral coordination and integration across various sectors, adds to the challenge [4].

Lack of standardised data collection and analysis methods makes many countries struggle to collect comprehensive and reliable data on AMR, including surveillance data, antimicrobial consumption, and resistance patterns. Existing surveillance systems are not adequately capturing the full extent of AMR, potentially leading to underestimation of the problem and hindering effective interventions.

AMR data often resides in different sectors (human health, animal health, environment) and is not easily integrated for a comprehensive overview.

Many countries lack the trained personnel, laboratory infrastructure, and resources to conduct effective AMR surveillance. National surveillance systems for tracking AMU and AMR are often underdeveloped or non-existent in many countries. AMR surveillance is entirely laboratory-based. The laboratories in most of the developing countries have remained neglected over the years. Enhancing laboratory-based surveillance infrastructure is essential for monitoring trends, detecting emerging resistance patterns, and informing policy decisions. The capacity to undertake AMU in various sectors is minimal, and the data generated is frequently questionable, making them unsuitable for policy formulation. Integrated surveillance is yet to commence in most countries. Contribution to the WHO Global Antimicrobial Resistance and Use Surveillance System (WHO GLASS) has been limited.

The capacity of the health system in peripheral geographical areas in most countries is limited due to resource constraints in procuring and utilising laboratory tools, including point-of-care (PoC) tests, as well as a lack of standard treatment guidelines for infectious diseases. IPC and antimicrobial stewardship programmes (AMSP) are grossly inadequate in these health facilities. Both access to antibiotics in remote areas and excessive unnecessary use of antibiotics in health facilities have been recognised as significant challenges to the health system.

Several developing countries have weak or minimal national monitoring and evaluation frameworks. Without robust monitoring and evaluation mechanisms, it is challenging to track progress, identify bottlenecks, and adjust strategies accordingly. Many NAPs lack specific, measurable indicators to track progress on key activities, making it difficult to assess the effectiveness of interventions.

Integrating AMR-related activities into existing public health programmes (e.g. infectious disease control, immunisation) can be complex and require significant coordination.

Technical challenges also include a shortage of trained healthcare professionals, which is essential for implementing AMR interventions such as infection prevention and control, antimicrobial stewardship, and surveillance. Optimising antimicrobial use in human and animal health is crucial for reducing the emergence and spread of AMR. Strengthening IPC practices, which are critical for preventing the spread of AMR in healthcare settings and communities, and ensuring the availability of appropriate technical tools to enhance public awareness and understanding of AMR for their effective engagement [4].

Inadequate IPC measures in healthcare settings contribute to the spread of resistant pathogens. Implementing and enforcing robust IPC practices is essential to reducing healthcare-associated infections and the need for antimicrobial treatment. Limited surveillance data from various national networks in developing countries indicate a high and increasing prevalence of hospital-associated infections, as well as the emergence and persistence of multidrug-resistant organisms within the health facility environment. The absence of a designated national focal point on AMR to implement a programmatic approach is a critical gap in AMR containment. The implementation of IPC interventions requires an enabling environment and continuous training of healthcare workers. These areas are severely lacking in primary and secondary healthcare facilities.

Limited access to affordable and accurate diagnostic tests hampers efforts to promote appropriate antimicrobial use. Improving access to diagnostics, including rapid PoC tests, can help clinicians prescribe antimicrobials more judiciously, especially in managing viral infections, e.g. common cold and flu. These services are not widely available in developing countries.

AMSPs, which promote the prudent use of antimicrobials in healthcare settings, are lacking or ineffective in most healthcare facilities in many countries. Training of healthcare workers and coordination between various departments under the overall supervision of the Hospital Infection Control Committees is inadequate. While some tertiary care health facilities in both the public and private sectors are implementing evidence-based AMSP, numerous secondary and primary care units remain unaware of this initiative.

Human health, veterinary, agriculture, and environment systems often operate in silos with different governance, data standards, and priorities. Technical mechanisms for data sharing, joint risk assessment, and coordinated response are either absent or weak. The private sector in several countries plays an important technical role in prevention and spread of AMR. Unfortunately, this sector is not fully engaged in synergising national efforts against AMR.

Most developing countries lack systems to measure antibiotic consumption in hospitals, pharmacies, community settings, and livestock. Informal markets and unregulated sales further complicate data capture, limiting the ability to target high-risk use.

Even when policies exist, technical capacity to enforce prescription-only antibiotic use, regulate pharmaceutical promotion, and monitor veterinary practices is weak, particularly at subnational levels.

NAP activities are often donor-driven, fragmented, and time-bound, with limited domestic financing. This leads to pilot-heavy implementation without long-term institutionalisation.

Almost all technical challenges in combating AMR stem from weak health systems, limited capacity, and contextual constraints. These technical challenges in NAP implementation reflect broader health-system weaknesses—limited diagnostics, data, workforce, and coordination—making AMR control complex and slow unless these foundational capacities are strengthened alongside policy commitments.

Addressing these technical challenges requires a comprehensive approach that includes strengthening surveillance systems, building capacity comprehensively, promoting multisectoral coordination, and implementing evidence-based interventions.

3.1.4 Programmatic Issues

Globally, there has been a suboptimal implementation of NAPs. Till 2024, 178 countries had developed multisectoral national action plans on AMR, only 52% of countries had a functioning multisectoral coordinating mechanism, and only 68% were implementing their action plans [2]. Only 11% of countries have dedicated funding in their national budgets and were engaged in implementing multisectoral national action plans on AMR (Fig. 3.3).

These plans encompass strategies for governance, prevention, surveillance, stewardship, education, and regulation across the human health, animal health, environmental, and agricultural sectors. However, over the past eight years, there has been little progress in implementing these NAPs. Notwithstanding the COVID-19 pandemic, which posed a significant hurdle to the implementation of non-pandemic public health activities, the implementation of NAPs has been hindered by a weak programmatic approach and a grossly inadequate allocation of funds, especially in the developing world.

Fig. 3.3 Global status of NAPs, 2024. (Political Declaration, UNGA Special Session, Sept 2024 [2])

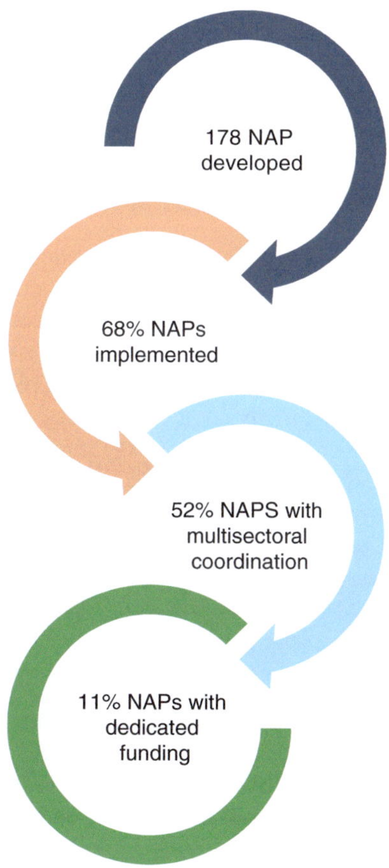

Data generated by surveillance networks on AMR and AMU are rarely utilised for understanding the dynamics of AMR and for the development of antibiotic policy/standard treatment guidelines at local and regional levels. Mechanisms to correlate AMR and AMU are not in practice. There is hardly any attempt to integrate surveillance data from different sectors and analyse the same for better epidemiological understanding and burden of resistance in defined geographical areas in the developing world.

Reducing the burden of communicable diseases is essential to prevent the use of antibiotics and the development of AMR. Promoting safe food, safe water, safe sex, safe blood, and a clean environment creates conditions that lower the incidence of these diseases. Vaccination rates for children and adults are suboptimal, leaving a large susceptible population. National programmes on immunisation, WASH, control of other infectious diseases, and nutrition need further strengthening.

Prevention of AMR has strong linkages with several other health programmes. The insufficient contribution of programmes strengthening the "prevention" of AMR promotes the occurrence and spread of AMR. These linkages should be operationalised and sustained. The WHO document on the people-centred approach [5] provides valuable guidance on integrating these preventive services in the overall process of AMR containment.

The comprehensive AMR control programme should include several actions directed towards improved healthcare infrastructure, ethical drug promotion, surveillance of AMR and antibiotic use in all sectors, prudent antibiotic use in humans and animals, effective IPC practices, AMSP in all healthcare facilities, and appropriate management of patients with resistant organisms through an efficient health system.

The health system must ensure equitable access to antibiotics, their optimal use at all levels, surveillance and effective regulatory mechanisms. Insufficient access to antibiotics remains a significant concern in many resource-poor settings. The number of children dying because of inadequate access to simple, affordable antibiotics is around half a million per year [6]. The programme must ensure an uninterrupted supply of life-saving antibiotics and complement the efforts being made through Universal Health Coverage initiatives nationwide.

Surveillance of AMR and antibiotic consumption is an ideal indicator for monitoring the dynamics of AMR and providing information on trends and magnitude. These activities require appropriate infrastructure, skilled human resources and accepted methodologies for the continuous generation of reliable data on the burden of AMR and the impact of interventions.

To assist countries in establishing a comprehensive programmatic approach in the health sector, WHO, in 2023, published a people-centred approach [5].

WHO's People-Centred Strategy for Addressing Antimicrobial Resistance

WHO views AMR control not only as a microbiological issue but also as a social and behavioural challenge—one that can only be solved by placing people at its centre. Accordingly, it developed, in 2023, a people-centred approach against AMR.

This WHO's people-centred strategy for addressing AMR prioritises individuals, families, and communities in prevention and response efforts. Recognising that daily behaviours significantly influence antibiotic consumption and resistance, it moves beyond solely technical or regulatory solutions to focus on informed choice, shared responsibility, and building trust between health systems and the public.

Central to this approach is *empowering and educating patients*. WHO emphasises health literacy, ensuring that people understand when antibiotics are necessary, such as avoiding their use for viral infections, and recognise the risks of misuse, including treatment failure and drug-resistant bacteria. Well-informed patients are more likely to follow prescriptions, avoid self-medication, and resist social pressure to use unnecessary antibiotics.

The strategy also highlights the importance of *people-centred healthcare services—ensuring* timely diagnosis, affordable, quality medicines, and accessible primary care reduces reliance on informal providers and over-the-counter antibiotics. When services are respectful, responsive, and accessible, inappropriate demand decreases.

Community engagement plays a key role, with WHO encouraging collaboration with community leaders, civil society, farmers' groups, and patient organisations to develop culturally relevant and context-specific AMR interventions. This is especially vital in low- and middle-income countries, where community norms greatly influence antibiotic use in humans and animals.

Furthermore, the approach connects AMR efforts to *equity and trust*, acknowledging that poverty, weak regulations, and limited healthcare access contribute to irrational antibiotic use. By addressing these structural issues and involving communities as active partners, WHO's strategy aims to make AMR containment more sustainable, ethical, and effective.

This approach has 13 interventions (Table 3.1) that encompass major interventions for containment of AMR.

3.1.5 Regulatory Issues

Most developing countries suffer from weak regulatory frameworks and inefficient enforcement. Regulatory frameworks are inadequate or inconsistently enforced, leading to overuse and misuse of antibiotics in human health, animal husbandry, and agriculture. Strengthening and effectively enforcing regulations around AMU and sales has not been accorded priority by the national authorities. Antibiotics of questionable quality are widely available in most countries. The regulatory authorities are understaffed and lack adequate infrastructure, particularly for assessing the quality of antibiotics. Spurious antibiotics are widely and readily available, thus facilitating the selection of resistant strains [7].

Poor-quality antibiotic preparations facilitate the emergence of resistance in pathogens. The functional regulatory mechanisms are prerequisites to ensure the availability of drugs that are potent, safe, sold in ethical ways and prescribed in

Table 3.1 Interventions suggested in WHO people-centred approach to contain AMR [5]

	Intervention no.	Core intervention as per people-centred approach
Foundation step Effective governance, awareness and education	1	AMR advocacy, governance, accountability, one health
	2	Awareness raising, education and behaviour change of prescribers and users
Foundation step Strategic information through surveillance and research	3	National AMR surveillance network to generate good quality data for patient care and action on AMR
	4	Surveillance of antimicrobial consumption to guide patient care
	5	Research and innovation including behavioural and implementation science
Pillar 1 Prevention	6	Universal access to WASH and waste management
	7	Implementation of IPC to mitigate AMR
	8	Access to vaccine and expanded immunisation to manage AMR
Pillar 2 Access to essential health services	9	Access to affordable diagnostic and management services
	10	Uninterrupted supply of essential quality assured antimicrobials and health products
Pillar 3 Timely accurate diagnosis	11	Good quality lab services and diagnostic stewardship
Pillar 4 Appropriate quality assured treatment	12	Evidence based treatment guidelines and programmes for antimicrobial stewardship
	13	Regulation to restrict sales of non-prescription antimicrobials

accordance with evidence-based guidelines. Given the dismal status of regulatory mechanisms in several developing countries, many of these may require international support to establish efficient regulatory systems in the health and veterinary sectors.

The availability of antibiotics without prescription, along with prevailing myths on how to take antibiotics, has fuelled rampant misuse of these medicines by communities that are not aware of AMR and its ramifications.

Substantial investments are needed in almost all countries for a comprehensive strengthening/revamping of the entire regulatory system in accordance with global best practices as advocated by the WHO. Adequate emphasis needs to be placed on regulating antibiotic use in the animal health sector, as well as various products that are widely used in this sector, such as animal feed.

3.1.6 Educational Needs for AMR Control

The lack of emphasis on AMR in the curricula of health professionals and allied workers is a malaise that affects nearly all developing countries [8]. Most of these countries have been using the age-old curriculum for teaching and training doctors, dentists, nurses, pharmacists, and allied healthcare professionals. These curricula do not adequately emphasise AMR and the rational use of antibiotics, thus providing a weak foundation for this critical component of their professional work. There are limited in-service trainings with very few dedicated to AMR prevention and control. Continuous Medical Education (CME) activities are mostly disease-centred and rarely focus on AMR and rational use of medicines.

A similar situation exists in the teaching and training of veterinary professionals and workers. Quality education in this sector can substantially reduce the irrational use of antibiotics, especially by reducing the growth-promoting use of antibiotics in animals.

The education of professionals (health, animal health and dentistry) is also essential. Continuing education and inclusion of this subject in the curriculum of graduate education will inculcate behaviour change that will enable optimal use of antimicrobials. Professional associations can provide a valuable platform for imparting information and ensuring best practices in the prudent use of these medicines by providing guidelines and updating them periodically, especially in settings where antimicrobial susceptibility services are not available. Still, antibiotics should be accessible to people and practitioners to save lives [8].

School-going children need to be empowered with information on the rational use of antibiotics for compliance not only by them but also through them to convey the message on completing the antibiotic course as prescribed and avoiding self-medication by the family.

3.1.7 Multisectoral Collaboration

AMR is recognised as a huge public health problem. Contributors to this global challenge are several stakeholders other than the health sector, including the animal health sector and the environmental domain. Bringing together all sectors with a common objective of reducing AMR is the essence of One Health. However, this approach has been under-recognised.

In alignment with the global action plan on AMR, all NAPs have been based on the One Health principle of a multisectoral, coordinated and collaborative approach. However, in practice, very few jointly planned and executed activities have been conducted by the health, veterinary and environment sectors. The silo approach continues [9].

Collaboration and coordination among different sectors (e.g. health, agriculture, environment) are essential for addressing AMR. However, fragmented governance structures and a lack of intersectoral coordination have been major hindrances impacting AMR control. Encouraging One Health approach is essential.

There is hardly any active and sustained engagement of the private sector in surveillance and for the rational use of antibiotics, as well as in building its capacity for containment of AMR. Productive collaboration between the private sector and the surveillance of AMR and AMU is virtually non-existent. Apart from collecting data from the private sector, it is vital to strengthen their capacity in prescribing antibiotics and implementing IPC.

The private sector plays a significant role in delivering healthcare to people in many countries. In some settings, such as India, more than two-thirds of all healthcare, including that for the poorest people, is provided by private and other non-state actors [10]. All these extensively use antibiotics and thus have a potential role in containing the spread of AMR. Any national effort directed towards AMR should necessarily engage the private sector in both the thought process and action to achieve tangible results.

In most countries, the role of the environment is least understood in the context of AMR. It has broad ramifications. Environmental contamination with antimicrobial agents and microorganisms is widespread. However, the countries lack adequate, affordable technologies, regulations, awareness, and the intent to reduce/prevent the discharge of effluents, sewage, and solid waste rich in antimicrobial agents, antimicrobial-resistant genes, and microorganisms into the environment. The contaminated environment serves as a mixing vessel, providing a conducive environment for the transfer and amplification of resistance. Subsequently, the environment acts as a reservoir for resistant pathogens for humans and animals through the food chain [11].

3.1.8 Research & Development and Innovations

Research and development (R&D) and innovation are crucial in the fight against AMR. This includes developing new drugs, diagnostics, and vaccines, optimising the use of existing antimicrobials, and improving IPC interventions. R&D is essential for understanding how AMR emerges and spreads (basic research), and for developing strategies to mitigate its impact (operational research) [8].

A primary focus of R&D should be on developing novel antibiotics, antivirals, antifungals, and antiparasitics that can overcome existing resistance mechanisms. This includes exploring new drug classes and developing new formulations of existing drugs with improved properties.

Rapid and accurate diagnostic tests are needed to identify the specific pathogen causing an infection and its antibiotic susceptibility profile. This helps physicians prescribe the right antibiotic, optimising treatment and reducing the risk of resistance development.

Vaccines can reduce the overall burden of infectious diseases, thereby decreasing the need for antimicrobial use and the selection pressure for resistant strains (Chap. 16).

Innovations are needed to introduce and strengthen AMSP, which involves optimising the use of existing antibiotics to ensure they are used effectively and appropriately, minimising the development of resistance. This includes strategies to reduce overuse and misuse of antimicrobials in human and animal health.

Research is underway on alternative therapies, such as phage therapy and antibiofilm drugs, which could offer new options for treating infections caused by bacteria that are resistant to antibiotics. This needs further encouragement. A big field of traditional medicine remains unexplored.

Artificial intelligence and machine learning can accelerate drug discovery, improve diagnostics, and enhance antimicrobial stewardship.

The global community has already initiated several steps to promote and encourage R&D. It is essential to engage the private sector, especially in the development of new molecules. WHO has suggested a bacterial priority pathogens list to prioritise research and development efforts for the most concerning drug-resistant bacteria (Table 3.2) in 2024. The list includes Gram-negative bacteria resistant to last-resort antibiotics, drug-resistant *Mycobacterium tuberculosis*, and other high-burden resistant pathogens such as *Salmonella*, *Shigella*, *Neisseria gonorrhoeae*, *Pseudomonas aeruginosa*, and *Staphylococcus aureus*. The inclusion of these pathogens in the list highlights their significant global impact in terms of burden, as well as issues related to transmissibility, treatability, and available prevention options. It also reflects the R&D pipeline of new treatments and emerging resistance trends [12].

Table 3.2 WHO recommended list of bacterial pathogens for R&D

Critical group	High group	Medium group
Enterobacterales Carbapenem-resistant	*Salmonella typhi* Fluoquinolone-resistant	Group A streptococci Macrolide-resistant
Enterobacterales Third-generation cephalosporin–resistant	*Shigella species* Fluoquinolone-resistant	*Streptococcus pneumoniae* Macrolide-resistant
Acinetobacter pneumoniae Carbapenem-resistant	*Enterococcus faecium* Vancomycin-resistant	*Haemophilus influenzae* Ampicillin-resistant
Mycobacterium tuberculosis *Rifampicin-resistant*	Non-typhoidal *Salmonella* Fluoquinolone-resistant	Group B streptococci Penicillin-resistant
	Neisseria gonorrhoeae Third generation cephalosporin and/or fluoroquinolone-resistant	
	Staphylococcus aureus Methicillin-resistant	
	Pseudomonas aeruginosa Carbapenem-resistant	

Global Antibiotic Research & Development Partnership (GARDP) [13] focuses on developing new antibiotics for drug-resistant infections. This is in accordance with the WHO bacterial priority list. Combating Antibiotic-Resistant Bacteria Biopharmaceutical Accelerator (CARB-X) also supports the development of new antibacterial products [14]. CARB-X has the objective of accelerating the development of novel antibiotics and other innovative approaches to address drug-resistant bacterial infections.

Several challenges continue to plague AMR R&D. These include a lack of financial incentives accompanied by the high cost of developing new drugs and diagnostics, and the relatively low return on investment for antibiotics, leading to a decline in R&D for these products.

Researchers and the pharmaceutical industry have frequently experienced regulatory hurdles. Navigating the regulatory landscape for new antimicrobial products can be a challenging and time-consuming process.

Despite global deliberations, there have not been any significant advances in the discovery of new antimicrobial agents. There are only 97 antimicrobials in the pipeline, and just 12 of those are considered novel. Only 4 of these 12 are active against at least 1 pathogen identified as "critical" by WHO. There are also significant gaps regarding products for children, oral agents for outpatient treatment, and agents capable of addressing the rising resistance [15].

AMR cannot be solved solely by the development of new classes of antimicrobial medicines. However, new drugs against multi-resistant pathogens are urgently needed to reduce the burden of diseases and to provide access to effective therapeutic options against infections. The discovery, development, and distribution of novel antimicrobials, along with their associated business models, face unique technical, financial, and ethical challenges. Because drug development is a resource-intensive process, the developed world must lead in this area. It is also crucial that new drugs are made accessible and affordable for the developing world.

The collaboration between the pharmaceutical industry and academia, encouraged by national authorities, can reignite the development of new classes of antimicrobials or alternatives to keep pace with the emergence of resistance. Public—private partnerships should be explored and encouraged, particularly in the context of regulatory activities, to enhance the interface between industry and academia and accelerate the development of affordable antibiotics [8].

3.1.9 Community Engagement

Public awareness about the risks of AMR and the importance of responsible antimicrobial use is low across the world, especially in developing countries. This is a behavioural challenge that needs a systematic scientific approach to alter it towards the rational use of antibiotics. National campaigns and educational initiatives are often limited in their ability to raise awareness among the general public, healthcare providers, and policymakers [16].

Community engagement is crucial for addressing AMR effectively and sustainably. By raising awareness, promoting behaviour change, developing context-specific solutions, strengthening health systems, and fostering collaboration, community engagement can empower communities to play an active role in tackling AMR and building a healthier future (Chap. 20).

Self-medication by consumers and failure to adhere to recommended regimens are widespread, especially in developing countries. Consumers often have a poor understanding of antimicrobial medicines and the diseases they are used to treat. However, changing human behaviour to ensure optimal use of medicines is highly challenging. It requires concerted efforts, utilising the skills of behavioural scientists, to change norms and practices. Civil society that is firmly engaged with communities can play a vital role in facilitating behavioural change in the use of antimicrobial medicines. The role of civil society in national planning and implementation activities is also essential. Mass media have a powerful voice that most people hear. The need for sustained partnerships with mass media cannot be overemphasised [8].

3.1.10 International Cooperation

AMR is a global problem that requires coordinated action across borders. However, there has been suboptimal worldwide coordination and cooperation. Inadequate international collaboration and information sharing can impede efforts to address AMR effectively. Limited efforts are being made to share best practices and lessons learnt in the implementation of NAPs by different countries. While WHO and FAO are providing technical assistance to countries in the development and implementation of NAPs through capacity building and information sharing, much more needs to be done. Other development partners, such as the World Bank, Asian Development Bank, USAID, and the Fleming Fund, which have been active in a few countries in the past, have been providing limited support to AMR containment activities.

The challenges mentioned above continue to persist and require addressing by the respective country, with technical assistance from international development partners. AMR has a multidimensional and complex nature, necessitating corresponding whole-of-society actions.

AMR is clearly a One Health issue—human health, animal health and environment sectors have equally important and critical roles to play in finding solutions. The rational use of antibiotics by all prescribers and users alike is essential to prevent the world from sliding into a dreadful post-antibiotic era. AMR is a global problem—but solutions must be found at both national and local levels to preserve efficacy and prolong the life of antibiotics [2].

References

1. UNGA: A/RES/74/4. Available at https://docs.un.org/en/A/RES/74/4#. Accessed 3 Mar 2025.
2. UNGA: Political declaration on AMR. Available at https://www.un.org/pga/wp-content/uploads/sites/108/2024/09/FINAL-Text-AMR-to-PGA.pdf. Accessed 5 Mar 2025.
3. Bhatia R, Katoch VM, Inoue H. Creating political commitment for antimicrobial resistance in developing countries. Indian J Med Res. 2019;149(2):83–6. https://doi.org/10.4103/ijmr.IJMR_1980_17.
4. Bhatia R, Walia K. Combating antimicrobial resistance in India: technical challenges & opportunities. Indian J Med Res. 2017 Dec;146(6):683–7. https://doi.org/10.4103/ijmr.IJMR_19_17.
5. WHO: WHO People-Centred Approach to Addressing AMR in the Human Health, 2023. Available at: https://www.who.int/publications/i/item/9789240082496. Accessed 10 Mar 2025.
6. ReAct. Available at https://www.reactgroup.org/news-and-views/news-and-opinions/year-2019/address-antibiotic-resistance-and-poverty-to-empower-children-their-families/. Accessed 23 Aug 2025.
7. Hedayatullah E. Antibiotic resistance in developing countries: emerging threats and policy responses. Public Health Chall. 2025;4:e70034. https://doi.org/10.1002/puh2.70034.
8. Ahmed SK, Hussein S, Qurbani K, Ibrahim RH, Fareeq A, Mahmood KA, Mohamed MG. Antimicrobial resistance: impacts, challenges, and future prospects. J Med Surg Publ Health. 2024;2:100081. https://doi.org/10.1016/j.glmedi.2024.100081.
9. Velazquez-Meza ME, Galarde-López M, Carrillo-Quiróz B, Alpuche-Aranda CM. Antimicrobial resistance: one health approach. Vet World. 2022;15(3):743–9. https://doi.org/10.14202/vetworld.2022.743-749.
10. Hunter BM, Murray SF, Marathe S, Chakravarthi I. Decentred regulation: the case of private healthcare in India. World Dev. 2022;155:105889. https://doi.org/10.1016/j.worlddev.2022.105889.
11. United Nations Environment Programme. Environmental dimensions of antimicrobial resistance: summary for policymakers. 2022. Available at https://wedocs.unep.org/bitstream/handle/20.500.11822/38373/antimicrobial_R.pdf. Accessed 13 Mar 2025.
12. WHO. Bacterial Priority Pathogens List, 2024. Available at (WHO: https://www.who.int/publications/i/item/9789240093461). Accessed 12 Mar 2025.
13. Global Antibiotic Research & Development Partnership GARDP.: Available at https://gardp.org. Accessed 9 Mar 2025.
14. CARB X.Combating antibiotic-resistant bacteria. Available at https://carb-x.org/.0. Accessed 8 Mar 2025.
15. World Health Organization. 2023 Antibacterial agents in clinical and preclinical development: an overview and analysis. Geneva: World Health Organization; 2024. Available at https://www.who.int/publications/i/item/9789240094000. Accessed 7 Mar 2025.
16. World Health Organization. Raising community awareness of antimicrobial resistance and enabling behavioural change. Available at https://www.who.int/europe/activities/raising-community-awareness-of-antimicrobial-resistance#. Accessed 5 Mar 2025.

Part II
Global Policy and One Health Approaches to AMR Control

Chapter 4
Global Initiatives to Combat AMR

Abstract Antimicrobial resistance (AMR) has become one of the most critical global health and development issues, endangering humans, animals, and the environment. Over the last 30 years, numerous initiatives at international, regional, and national levels have aimed to control its spread. Awareness was initially raised during World Health Day 1997, followed by the WHO's first Global Strategy for Containment of AMR in 2001. Later efforts enhanced collaboration through initiatives like the Transatlantic Taskforce on AMR, the FAO–WOAH–WHO–UNEP Quadripartite Agreement, and the Jaipur Declaration in South-East Asia. Campaigns such as World Health Day (2011) and the establishment of annual World Antimicrobial Awareness Week boosted advocacy. Political action was exemplified by the U.S. Presidential Executive Order (2014), the UK's AMR Review, and the Antibiotic Resistance Coalition. Frameworks like the 2015 Global Action Plan, the 2016 UN General Assembly declaration, the SDGs, and the IACG offer structured responses. More recent efforts include the Global Leaders Group, G20 commitments, UNGA High-Level Meeting with defined targets (2024), pooled funding mechanisms, and the WHO's people-centred approach. These initiatives highlight AMR as a One Health issue requiring coordinated governance, sustainable funding, strong surveillance, and community involvement. Despite notable progress, gaps remain in implementation, demanding increased accountability and political will worldwide.

Keywords Antimicrobial resistance · Global AMR Action Plan · One Health · Global Leaders Group · Sustainable Development Goals, UNGA

Antimicrobial resistance (AMR) has long been viewed as a silent pandemic, which, until about 30 years ago, did not receive the attention it deserved. Recently, it has become clear that AMR poses significant challenges not only to human health but also to nutrition security. Its implications are now recognised as multidimensional, affecting health, the economy, development, nutrition security, as well as financial and political issues that impact various aspects of human progress. Global leaders acknowledge that AMR has far-reaching consequences, including adverse effects

R. Bhatia, *Drug-Resistant Infections*,
https://doi.org/10.1007/978-981-92-4190-3_4

on human health, economic stability, food security, and overall human development (Chap. 1). The World Health Organisation (WHO) also identified AMR as one of the top ten global public health threats, alongside communicable diseases, air pollution, and flu pandemics [1]. Over the past 30 years, numerous initiatives have been launched globally, regionally, and nationally. Some of these efforts are summarised here in chronological order.

4.1 World Health Day on Emerging Infectious Diseases (1997)

Global awareness of AMR was initiated on World Health Day 1997, which had the theme of "Emerging Infectious Diseases." This theme highlighted the growing threat of new and re-emerging infectious diseases, including those resistant to antimicrobial drugs. The day aimed to raise awareness about the factors contributing to the emergence of these diseases and to promote strategies for prevention and control, particularly in the context of increasing global interconnectedness. This event catalysed a thinking process on the growing problem of drug-resistant bacteria, viruses, fungi, and parasites, which was also a significant concern, threatening the effectiveness of antibiotics and other antimicrobial treatments. The event called for "Global Alert and Global Response" to emerging infectious diseases and AMR.

4.2 WHO Global Strategy for Containment of AMR (2001)

WHO published the first comprehensive strategy for containment of AMR in 2001 [2]. This strategy addressed several issues related to AMR and made numerous recommendations for various sectors to initiate activities aimed at understanding and containing AMR. The approach, however, could not be efficiently advocated to the national health authorities and thus failed to gather much traction, and consequently could not be implemented at any level.

The WHO Global Strategy for Containment of Antimicrobial Resistance (AMR), released in 2001, was the first comprehensive global framework to address AMR as a public health threat. It emphasised strengthening AMR surveillance and laboratory capacity, promoting rational use of antimicrobials through treatment guidelines and stewardship, improving infection prevention and control, and ensuring regulation and quality assurance of medicines. Importantly, it recognised the role of antimicrobial use in animals and agriculture, called for public and professional education, and highlighted the need for research and development of new drugs, diagnostics, and vaccines. The strategy implicitly adopted a multisectoral perspective, predating the formal articulation of the One Health approach.

Despite its technical strength, the strategy achieved limited implementation. It was only an advisory document and was non-binding because of a lack of political ownership, with no enforcement, financing mechanism, or reporting requirements. At the time, AMR was viewed largely as a technical health issue, not a political, economic, or security concern, resulting in low political prioritisation. The strategy lacked operational guidance, costing, and implementation roadmaps, making it difficult for resource-constrained countries to act. Weak inter-sectoral coordination, limited engagement beyond the health sector, and low public visibility further undermined uptake.

It was perhaps ahead of its time in terms of vision and long-term global needs. Lessons from the 2001 strategy directly informed later initiatives, notably the WHO Global Action Plan on AMR (2015), which placed stronger emphasis on political commitment, national action plans, and accountability.

4.3 The Transatlantic Taskforce on AMR (2009)

The Transatlantic Task Force on Antimicrobial Resistance (TATFAR), a collaborative effort among the United States, Canada, the European Union, Norway, and the United Kingdom, was established to combat the growing threat of AMR. TATFAR focuses on strengthening cooperation and sharing best practices in areas like appropriate antimicrobial use, surveillance, and the development of new drugs and diagnostics [3].

TATFAR was created in 2009 after the U.S.-EU Summit to strengthen collaboration against AMR. It began with the U.S. and the EU, and later expanded to include the UK, Canada and Norway.

TATFAR emphasises the responsible use of antimicrobials by promoting proper antibiotic use in human and veterinary medicine. It supports surveillance and prevention of drug-resistant infections, implements strategies to stop them, and encourages innovations to develop new antimicrobial drugs, diagnostics, and alternative therapies.

TATFAR has finalised standardised evaluation measures for hospital stewardship programmes, created a roadmap for developing comparable stewardship programmes and data, and increased public awareness of proper antibiotic use through Antibiotic Awareness Day. TATFAR continues to assess progress, identify challenges, and explore new areas for collaboration to combat the global AMR threat.

4.4 The FAO-WHO-WOAH-UNEP Quadripartite Agreement (2010–)

The Food and Agriculture Organization of the UN (FAO), World Health Organization (WHO), World Organization for Animal Health (WOAH, formerly OIE), and the United Nations Environment Programme (UNEP) [4] have collaborated under a quadripartite agreement for years to manage risks at the human-animal ecosystem interface, formalising their partnership in 2010 through the FAO/OIE/WHO Tripartite Agreement [5]. This tripartite collaboration among FAO, WOAH, and WHO focused on AMR as a key area of action across the globe, at the regional and local levels [6].

The Tripartite Agreement promoted effective collaboration across multiple sectors, disciplines, and regions at local, national, regional, and global levels. It followed a multidisciplinary and multisectoral approach, aligned with the One Health concept, for effectively preparing for, detecting, assessing, and responding to emerging and endemic zoonotic diseases, including AMR. This approach provided valuable insights and technical expertise in AMR, resulting in more robust, efficient, and cost-effective solutions to this complex issue. The Tripartite Agreement established guidelines to support the implementation of national-level actions [6].

The UNEP became part of the Tripartite agreement with FAO, WHO, and WOAH, formalising the Quadripartite collaboration for One Health [7]. This partnership, confirmed through a Memorandum of Understanding, demonstrates a commitment to a more unified approach to addressing health issues across humans, animals, and ecosystems.

The MoU among the four organisations has created a framework to improve coordination, strengthen health systems at both national and regional levels, and address emerging issues like AMR and zoonotic diseases. The Quadripartite partners also promote the One Health approach at global platforms, including G20 summits, the United Nations Climate Change Conference, and the World One Health Congress.

The FAO–WHO–WOAH–UNEP Quadripartite Agreement has become the main global platform for promoting the One Health approach, especially since 2021. Recent efforts have emphasised coordinated actions across human, animal, plant, and environmental health sectors. A key milestone was the launch of the Quadripartite One Health Joint Plan of Action (2022–2026), which provides a shared operational framework with six action areas, including zoonotic diseases, antimicrobial resistance (AMR), food safety, and environmental health.

The Quadripartite has enhanced global AMR governance by harmonising surveillance systems like WHO-GLASS, FAO-InFARM, and WOAH-WAHIS, and supporting countries in implementing their National Action Plans on AMR. It has increased capacity-building efforts within One Health, developed guidance on integrated surveillance, and supported pandemic prevention through initiatives like the Pandemic Fund[1] and PREZODE.[2] UNEP's involvement has renewed focus on

[1] The Pandemic Fund is the first multilateral financing mechanism dedicated exclusively to strengthening critical pandemic prevention, preparedness, and response (PPR) capacities at the local, regional, and global levels, with a focus on low- and middle-income countries. The World Bank is the trustee for the Pandemic Fund, while the WHO is the technical lead.

[2] PREZODE (Preventing ZOonotic Disease Emergence) is an international initiative, bringing together a community of members to provide a scientific framework for pandemic prevention. It aims to enhance prevention, early detection, and resilience to prevent or respond rapidly to emerging infectious diseases of animal origin that can become pandemics.

environmental factors driving AMR, pollution, and biodiversity loss. Overall, the Quadripartite has transitioned from a conceptual framework to a coordinated mechanism for implementation at both global and national levels.

4.5 The Jaipur Declaration on AMR (2011)

As a regional initiative within the WHO South-East Asia Region, the Jaipur Declaration on AMR was adopted in 2011 by Health Ministers from 11 countries across this region[3] [8]. It committed the leaders of these countries to prioritise the prevention and containment of AMR. The declaration highlighted the risks associated with the emergence and spread of resistance to antimicrobials, which threaten human health, and identified irrational antimicrobial use as a key driver. It called for a comprehensive, multidisciplinary approach to address AMR, including: developing and implementing national policies to regulate antimicrobial use, fostering multisectoral collaboration involving private healthcare, industry, and communities, enacting laws to prevent the production and sale of counterfeit antibiotics, promoting preventive measures and healthy lifestyles to decrease infectious disease incidence and thus reduce antimicrobial demand, establishing systems to monitor resistance patterns, and supporting research for new drugs, diagnostics, and innovative solutions.

The Jaipur Declaration marked an important step in increasing awareness and securing regional political commitment to tackle the global threat of AMR. It also laid the foundation for future actions at both national and international levels, such as the development of a Global Action Plan on AMR (see Sect. 4.11).

4.6 World Health Day on AMR (2011)

In 2011, the theme for World Health Day was "Antimicrobial Resistance: No Action Today, No Cure Tomorrow" [9]. Celebrated annually on April 7th, this day aims to raise awareness about the increasing global threat of AMR and the urgent need for action. The WHO highlighted that, without intervention, the world could enter a post-antibiotic era where infections become more complicated or impossible to treat.

The WHO emphasised the global nature of the problem, noting that AMR was a worldwide issue, not confined to any specific region. It called on governments, healthcare providers, industries, civil society, and individuals to act swiftly to preserve antimicrobial medicines for the future. This includes slowing the spread of resistance and minimising its impact.

---

[3] In 2011, WHO South-East Asia Region comprised of Bangladesh, Bhutan, DPR Korea, India, Indonesia, Maldives, Myanmar, Nepal, Sri Lanka, Thailand and Timor Leste.

The WHO pointed out that the misuse and overuse of antimicrobials in humans, animals, and agriculture significantly contribute to the problem, leading to prolonged illnesses, an increased risk of death, and making it more difficult to treat common infections.

On this day, the WHO launched a six-point policy package aimed at combating the spread of AMR [9]. The package comprised of followings:

1. Establishing a national plan with funding and accountability.
2. Improving surveillance and laboratory capabilities.
3. Guaranteeing reliable access to essential, quality medicines.
4. Promoting the responsible use of medicines in both human and animal health and ensuring appropriate patient care.
5. Strengthening measures for preventing and controlling infections.
6. Encouraging research and development for new tools to fight AMR.

The package served as a guide for governments and partners to take immediate and coordinated steps to maintain the effectiveness of antimicrobial agents.

4.7 USA Presidential Executive Order on AMR (2014)

In 2014, then-President Barack Obama issued an Executive Order highlighting the global significance of AMR [10]. This order urged governments, academia, industry, healthcare providers, agriculture, and international partners to collaborate in detecting, preventing, and controlling AMR. It directed the USA Federal Government to take domestic and global actions to reduce the emergence and spread of antibiotic-resistant bacteria, aiming to prevent illness and death caused by such infections and to maintain the availability of effective treatments for bacterial infections.

4.8 UK Review on AMR (2014–2016)

In 2014, UK Prime Minister David Cameron initiated an independent Review on Antimicrobial Resistance, led by macroeconomist Jim O'Neill. The review aimed to assess the growing threat of AMR from an economic viewpoint and to propose solutions [11]. Co-sponsored by the Wellcome Trust and the UK Department of Health, it presented various projections about AMR's potential impact on human development if no action is taken. These projections are summarised in Chap. 1 (Fig. 1.8). The study has released multiple reports [11] and made numerous urgent recommendations to address the growing problem of AMR (see Table 4.1).

Table 4.1 Salient recommendations made under Review of AMR

Increase public awareness through massive global campaigns
Improve hygiene to prevent spread of infection
Reduce unnecessary use of antibiotics in all sectors
Enhance surveillance of AMR and antibiotics consumption in human and animal health sectors
Promote development and use of new rapid diagnostic tests
Promote development and use of vaccines to prevent infections
Increase health workforce on infectious diseases
Establish global research and innovation fund for AMR
Incentivise investment in development of new antibacterial drugs
Encourage global cooperation

The UK Review on Antimicrobial Resistance (2014–2016) had a significant and enduring influence on worldwide efforts to combat AMR, primarily by elevating it from a purely technical health concern to a major political and economic issue.

The Review redefined AMR as a global economic threat, estimating that unchecked AMR could lead to 10 million deaths annually and cause trillions of dollars in economic losses by 2050. This economic perspective resonated with finance ministries, G20 leaders, and development banks, sparking high-level political focus that extended beyond the health sector.

The Review directly shaped global governance and commitments. It played a role in the 2016 UN General Assembly High-Level Meeting on AMR, the creation of the Interagency Coordination Group (IACG) on AMR, and the enhancement of the One Health approach involving WHO, FAO, WOAH, and UNEP. Many countries also accelerated their development of National Action Plans on AMR, explicitly citing the Review's recommendations.

The Review also transformed the approach to solving the antibiotic innovation crisis. Its call for "delinked" incentive models led to the creation of new global initiatives such as the Global AMR Innovation Fund (GAMRIF), CARB-X, and later subscription-style payment models piloted in the UK and adopted elsewhere. Finally, the Review strengthened advocacy for responsible antimicrobial use, improved surveillance, and infection prevention as core pillars of AMR containment. Overall, the UK Review served as a global catalyst, aligning political will, economic arguments, and multisectoral action to sustain momentum against one of the most complex public health threats of the twenty-first century.

4.9 Antibiotic Resistance Coalition (2014)

The Antibiotic Resistance Coalition (ARC) comprises civil society organisations and stakeholders globally, spanning the health, agriculture, consumer, and development sectors [12]. Founded in May 2014, the Coalition promotes policy reforms and initiatives aimed at preventing the onset of a post-antibiotic era.

In 2014, ARC launched the "Declaration on Antibiotic Resistance" to advocate for policy change and action to prevent the post-antibiotic era from becoming a bleak reality. The Declaration calls for international leadership to take actions, including:

- Prohibit the misleading promotion and advertising of antibiotics.
- Encourage innovative, needs-driven, and transparent research and development models founded on the principle of delinkage.
- Phase out antibiotics from routine livestock disease prevention and completely end their use for growth promotion.
- Build robust systems, in all countries, to monitor and report antibiotic use and resistance trends in humans and animals.
- Improve public awareness to support an ecological understanding of the human-bacterial interaction and behaviour change around antibiotic use.

4.10 The Global AMR R&D Hub (2018)

The Global AMR R&D Hub is a collaboration between countries, non-governmental donor organisations, and intergovernmental bodies. Its goal is to tackle challenges and enhance coordination in global AMR R&D through a One Health approach. Launched in May 2018, the Hub is guided by a Board of Members, with a Secretariat managed by DZIF, the German Centre for Infection Research [13].

Since its inception in 2018, the Global AMR R&D Hub has made notable advances in enhancing international coordination on antimicrobial resistance research. It established the first comprehensive global AMR R&D database, charting funding trends, research priorities, and gaps across human, animal, and environmental health sectors. The Hub has increased transparency, minimised redundant efforts, and supported evidence-based prioritisation consistent with the One Health approach. By bringing together countries, donors, and international organisations, it has fostered strategic dialogue, encouraged innovation in overlooked areas, and influenced global policy discussions, including those involving WHO and G20.

4.11 Global Action Plan for AMR (2015)

Recognising that AMR threatens the foundation of modern medicine and the sustainability of a global public health response to infectious diseases, the World Health Assembly (WHA) highlighted that the widespread misuse and overuse of these drugs in human medicine and food production put every nation at risk. With few alternative options in development, the WHA called for immediate and coordinated global action to prevent a post-antibiotic era where common infections might once again be deadly. In response, WHO and FAO created a global action plan in 2015, which was adopted by the WHA and the FAO governing body [14].

The Global Action Plan on AMR (GAP) outlined five objectives [14]:

- To improve awareness and understanding of AMR through effective communication, education and training;
- To strengthen the knowledge and evidence base through surveillance and research;
- To reduce the incidence of infection through adequate sanitation, hygiene and infection prevention measures;
- To optimise the use of antimicrobial medicines in human and animal health; and,
- To develop the economic case for sustainable investment that takes account of the needs of all countries and to increase investment in new medicines, diagnostic tools, vaccines and other interventions.

With this approach, the WHO believed that the primary goal of ensuring treatment and prevention of infectious diseases with quality-assured, safe and effective medicines is achievable. Accordingly, it urged all countries:

1. To implement the proposed actions for Member States in the global action plan on AMR, adapted to national priorities and specific contexts;
2. To mobilise human and financial resources through domestic, bilateral and multilateral channels to implement plans and strategies in line with the global action plan on AMR;
3. To have in place, by the Seventieth WHA, national action plans on AMR that are aligned with the GAP and with standards and guidelines established by relevant intergovernmental bodies.

As of May 2025, 178 countries had created multisectoral national action plans on antimicrobial resistance. However, only 52% have a functioning multisectoral coordination mechanism, and just 68% are actively implementing their plans. Only 11% of these countries allocate dedicated funding within their national budgets for these initiatives. Meanwhile, 22% of the world's healthcare facilities lack basic water services, and at least half do not have basic hygiene services, which hampers infection prevention efforts [24].

Global health leaders acknowledge that, while the original WHO Global Action Plan on AMR (2015–2025) spurred numerous national strategies, the threat of antimicrobial resistance (AMR) continues to escalate, necessitating more robust, coordinated efforts. Member States and the Quadripartite (WHO, FAO, WOAH, UNEP) are working on a revised Global Action Plan on AMR (GAP-AMR 2.0) to build on and strengthen the existing framework beyond 2025. Ongoing consultations in 2025 aim to incorporate regional insights and practical One Health approaches. Looking ahead, there's an emphasis on turning political commitments (like the 2024 UN High-Level Meeting declaration [15, 25]) into concrete actions—covering surveillance, stewardship, equitable access to quality antimicrobials and diagnostics, infection prevention, and sustainable funding. Additionally, there's a push for specific targets—such as decreasing AMR-related deaths, expanding national action plans, enhancing diagnostic capacity, and aligning incentives for research and innovation—that are expected to be integrated into the updated plan by WHO and partners by 2026–2027. Future priorities focus on improving accountability and monitoring systems, ensuring equitable AMR response across regions, and supporting implementation at national and sub-national levels. The goal is to reduce the health and socio-economic impacts of AMR by 2030 [16].

4.12 The United Nations General Assembly, Special Session (2016)

In 2016, the United Nations General Assembly (UNGA) urged global efforts to stop the spread of AMR. It was only the fourth global health issue to be addressed by the UNGA till 2016. During an extraordinary special session that year, policymakers worldwide recognised AMR as an urgent challenge that requires an aggressive, coordinated response using the "One Health approach" [15]. The UNGA called on all countries to take appropriate actions to combat AMR [16]. The One Health approach being a straightforward, proven, and comprehensive strategy endorsed by the WHO, FAO, WOAH, and UNEP, emphasising the interconnectedness of human, animal, and environmental health, was recommended.

Recognising the scale of this global issue and the consensus on actions needed to prevent a post-antibiotic era, the UN Secretary-General established in 2016 an Interagency Coordination Group on AMR (IACG) to support the implementation of UN Resolution A/RES/71/3. The UN Deputy Secretary-General and the Director General of the WHO co-chair the Group. It includes high-level representatives from relevant UN agencies, other international organisations, and individual experts from various sectors, such as animal health, agriculture and environment. The Group's mandate is to offer practical guidance on approaches necessary to ensure sustained and effective global efforts to combat AMR, including strategies to enhance coordination, considering the Global Action Plan on AMR [14].

The IACG urged all Member States to ensure fair and affordable access to existing and new quality-assured antimicrobials, as well as alternatives, vaccines, and diagnostics. They emphasised the importance of responsible and prudent use by qualified, licenced professionals across human, animal, and plant health sectors. The report also called for active and meaningful involvement of civil society groups and organisations as key stakeholders, to systematically apply standards for assessing risks and impacts related to AMR. It requested that the Tripartite agencies (FAO, OIE, and WHO), along with UN Environment Programme (UNEP), other UN agencies, and the World Bank, enhance joint One Health actions based on established targets, country priorities, and needs. It highlighted the need for increased investment and innovation in quality-assured, new antimicrobials, diagnostics, vaccines, waste management tools, and safe, effective alternatives for human, terrestrial, aquatic animal, and plant health. The IACG promoted the strong implementation of National Action Plans and public-private partnerships within the One Health framework. Additionally, the IACG recommended the urgent formation of a One Health Global Leadership Group on AMR [16].

4.13 UN Sustainable Development Goals (SDGs) and AMR (2015)

UN Sustainable Development Goals (SDGs) clearly articulate a commitment to contain AMR [17]. At least six of the SDGs (3, 1, 2, 6, 8, 12, and 17) are influenced by AMR (Chap. 1). In 2020, two AMR indicators were included in the monitoring framework of the SDGs [18]. These indicators track the proportion of bloodstream infections (BSIs) caused by *Escherichia coli,* which is resistant to third-generation cephalosporins, and methicillin-resistant *Staphylococcus aureus* (MRSA). The World Health Organization (WHO) is the custodian agency that monitors AMR-related indicators under the Sustainable Development Goals (SDGs). WHO collects and reports these indicators primarily through the Global Antimicrobial Resistance and Use Surveillance System (GLASS). FAO, WOAH, and UNEP contribute AMR-relevant data on animal health, food systems, and the environment under the Quadripartite One Health framework, but WHO remains the official SDG monitoring agency for AMR indicators.

Data availability for these indicators has improved from 2017 to 2020. Available data indicate a slight decrease in the proportion of BSI due to *Escherichia coli* resistant to cephalosporins in Thailand and Timor-Leste. At the same time, in the remaining Asian countries, there is no change or a slight increase in the proportion of resistant pathogens.

4.14 The Global Leaders Group on AMR (2020)

The Global Leaders Group (GLG) on AMR was established in 2020, following the recommendation of the IACG, with the mission to advise on and advocate for political action to mitigate drug-resistant infections through responsible and sustainable access to and use of antimicrobials.

The GLG's recommendations [19] for the UNGA special session in September 2024 included:

(i) Engaging various stakeholders to secure sufficient, dedicated, predictable, and sustainable financing—both domestically and internationally—for addressing AMR, including research and development;
(ii) Urging existing financing mechanisms to broaden their scope to cover AMR, especially for implementing NAPs in low and middle-income countries (LMICs);
(iii) Establishing an Independent Panel on Evidence for Action against AMR by 2025, within a One Health framework, to monitor and provide regular reports to Member States on the science and evidence related to AMR;
(iv) Updating the 2015 Global Action Plan on AMR to ensure a strong, multisectoral One Health response;
(v) Requiring all countries to create a national multisectoral AMR coordination body and enhance human resources, diagnostics, laboratory, and infrastructure capacities for sustainable, sector-specific and integrated surveillance, and data-driven action;
(vi) By 2030, developing and implementing national plans to prevent environmental contamination with antimicrobials and their metabolites; and
(vii) By 2030, enforcing sector-wide strategies to prevent infections and decrease antimicrobial use. Based on these global targets, the GLG recommended that all countries should develop national, outcome-oriented, sector-specific targets with clear goals and timelines, and follow up on their implementation

4.15 G20 Leaders Declaration, New Delhi (2023)

The G20 summit in New Delhi, held in September 2023, highlighted the significance of addressing AMR in the G20 New Delhi Leaders' Declaration, Paragraph 28:iv [20]. G20 leaders pledged to implement and prioritise strategies against AMR using the One Health approach, encompassing research and development, infection prevention and control, and antimicrobial stewardship within their national action plans, supported by surveillance of AMR and antimicrobial use.

4.16 The AMR Multi-Partner Trust Fund (2004)

The AMR Multi-Partner Trust Fund is overseen by the United Nations Multi-Partner Trust Fund Office (MPTFO), which specialises in pooled funding [21]. Founded in 2004, it is the sole UN entity focused on designing and managing multi-stakeholder pooled financing mechanisms. As the UN's expert body on pooled financing, the MPTFO is a system-wide resource hosted by the United

Nations Development Programme (UNDP). It aids UN organisations and partners in swiftly translating funding into operational results, both of which are crucial for achieving the SDGs.

Addressing AMR through a collaborative 'One Health' strategy can foster the creation of strong, cost-effective, and efficient solutions. This approach also helps achieve several health security targets outlined in the SDGs. The intended outcomes include reducing and slowing the progression of AMR, preserving the ability to treat infectious diseases with effective and safe antimicrobial drugs, and mitigating the impact of AMR on humans, livestock, and animals. Key donors include the UK Government, the EU, Sweden, the Netherlands, and Germany, with recipients among the quadripartite organisations: FAO, WHO, WOAH, and UNEP.

4.17 The South Centre (1995)

The South Centre is an intergovernmental think tank representing the Global South [22]. It helps developing nations collaborate their efforts and expertise to promote their common interests worldwide. Founded through an intergovernmental agreement effective from July 31, 1995, it is headquartered in Geneva, Switzerland [23].

Achieving the SDGs, especially ending poverty, requires national policies and an international framework that bolster development rather than hinder it. The South Centre is a policy research organisation comprising and accountable to its Member States. It hosts intergovernmental meetings to discuss solutions for AMR and communicates its recommendations to developing nations.

4.18 World Health Assembly Resolution on AMR (2024)

The World Health Assembly Resolution, WHA 77.R6 [24], reiterated the importance of preventing AMR through various existing global commitments, such as the WHO's 2023 global strategy on IPC, the Immunisation Agenda 2030, and the WHO Water, Sanitation, and Hygiene Strategy (2018–2025). It also emphasised monitoring and addressing substandard and falsified antimicrobial agents. The resolution highlighted the need for targeted awareness campaigns, including communication, information efforts, and behavioural change initiatives aimed at healthcare workers and communities. It called for strengthening antimicrobial stewardship skills among healthcare professionals and supporting innovative research and development efforts for new vaccines, diagnostics, antimicrobials, therapeutics, and alternatives to traditional antibiotics.

4.19 UNGA High-Level Meeting on AMR (2024)

The High-Level Meeting of the UNGA held on 26 September 2024 [25] reiterated that AMR was one of the most urgent global health threats and development challenges and demanded immediate action to safeguard the world's ability to treat human, animal, and plant diseases, as well as to enhance food safety, food security and nutrition, foster economic development, equity and a healthy environment, and advance the 2030 Agenda for Sustainable Development Goals. It set several targets to be achieved before 2030 (Table 4.2).

Table 4.2 Salient targets set by UNGA (2024) for AMR containment

	Target	By year
1	All Member States to develop or update and implement multisectoral national action plans on AMR with national targets and to reduce the global deaths associated with bacterial AMR by 10% against the 2019 baseline of 4.95 million deaths	2030
2	Quadripartite organisations to update the Global Action Plan on AMR to ensure a robust and inclusive multisectoral response, through a One Health approach	2026
3	Quadripartite organisations to establish an Independent Panel for Evidence for Action against AMR to facilitate the generation and use of multisectoral, scientific evidence to support Member States	2025
4	All Member States to increase sustainable investments at national level for strengthening national capacities for AMR. Global community to mobilise additional US$ 100 million to catalyse the achievement of at least 60% of countries having achieved funded NAPs by 2030	2030
5	At least 90% Member States to implement IPC through WHO's global strategy on IPC (2023), the Immunization Agenda 2030, the WHO water, sanitation and hygiene strategy 2018–2025, and the WHO global patient safety action plan 2021–2030 and meet all WHO's minimum requirements for IPC programmes at national level	2030
6	All Member States to increase use of WHO Access group antibiotics to at least 70% overall human antibiotic use, through strengthening of stewardship programmes	2030
7	All Member States to report quality surveillance data on AMR and antimicrobial use to GLASS, ANIMUSE, InFARM and GISSA	2030
8	80% of Member States should have capability to test resistance in all bacterial and fungal GLASS pathogens	2030
9	95% of Member States should participate in the annual Tracking Antimicrobial Resistance Country Self-Assessment Survey (TrACSS)	2030
10	A progress report on the implementation of the Political Declaration on AMR to be presented during the eighty-first session of the General Assembly, which will serve to inform the high-level meeting to be convened in 2029	2029

4.20 WHO People-Centred Approach to Addressing AMR (2023)

In 2023, the WHO published a detailed document describing the WHO people-centred approach to tackling AMR in the human health sector [26]. This approach acknowledges the challenges and health system barriers individuals encounter when seeking health services for prevention, diagnosis, and treatment of infections. It emphasises placing people and their needs at the core of the AMR strategy.

4.21 World Antimicrobial Awareness Week (November Every Year)

Community engagement in the rational use of antimicrobial agents, particularly in preventing self-medication, is a crucial part of efforts to combat AMR.

World Antimicrobial Awareness Week (WAAW) is observed annually from 18 to 24 November to raise global awareness about AMR and promote the responsible use of antimicrobials across human health, animal health, agriculture, and the environment. The campaign is led by WHO, in collaboration with FAO, WOAH, and UNEP, reflecting the One Health approach, which recognises that AMR is a shared challenge requiring coordinated action across sectors.

The primary aim of WAAW is to influence behaviour change by improving understanding of when and how antimicrobials should be used. Through advocacy campaigns, professional training, policy dialogues, community outreach, and mass media engagement, WAAW translates complex AMR concepts into clear, actionable messages for the public, healthcare providers, veterinarians, farmers, and policymakers. Annual themes such as "Handle antibiotics with care" reinforce the importance of infection prevention, adherence to prescriptions, and avoidance of unnecessary antimicrobial use.

Importantly, WAAW has contributed to several positive outcomes. Many countries have used the week to accelerate the development and implementation of National Action Plans on AMR, strengthen laboratory capacity, and expand participation in surveillance platforms such as GLASS. WAAW has also helped institutionalise antimicrobial stewardship programmes in hospitals, improve prescribing practices, and enhance public awareness of the dangers of self-medication. By sustaining political attention and encouraging multisectoral collaboration, World Antimicrobial Awareness Week plays a vital role in preserving the effectiveness of life-saving antimicrobials and protecting global health security for future generations [27].

References

1. WHO ten threats to global health in 2019. Available at https://www.who.int/news-room/spotlight/ten-threats-to-global-health-in-2019. Accessed 20 Mar 2025.
2. WHO. https://iris.who.int/bitstream/handle/10665/66860/WHO_CDS_CSR_DRS_2001.2.pdf. Accessed 19 Mar 2025.
3. NIAID. https://www.niaid.nih.gov/research/tatfar#:~:text=TATFAR%20was%20created%20in%202009,antimicrobial%20drugs%2C%20diagnostics%20and%20alternatives. Accessed 13 Mar 2025.
4. FAO. https://www.fao.org/one-health/background/coordination/en. Accessed 12 Mar 2025.
5. FAO-OIE-WHO. The tripartite commitment providing multi-sectoral, collaborative leadership in addressing health challenges. 2017. Available at: https://www.oie.int/app/uploads/2021/03/tripartite-2017.pdf. Accessed 16 Mar 2025.
6. FAO-OIE-WHO. A tripartite guide to addressing zoonotic diseases in countries. 2019. Available at: http://www.fao.org/3/ca2942en/CA2942EN.pdf. Accessed 17 Mar 2025.
7. UNEP. https://www.unep.org/news-and-stories/press-release/unep-joins-alliance-implement-one-health-approach. Accessed 11 Mar 2025.
8. WHO. https://cdn.who.int/media/docs/default-source/searo/india/antimicrobial-resistance/rev-jaipur-declaration-2014.pdf. Accessed 20 Mar 2025.
9. WHO. https://www.who.int/news/item/07-04-2011-world-health-day-2011. Accessed 21 Mar 2025.
10. Jooma S. Executive action to combat the rise of drug-resistant bacteria: is agricultural antibiotic use sufficiently addressed? J Law Biosci. 2015;2(1):129–38. https://doi.org/10.1093/jlb/lsv005.
11. Review of Antimicrobial Resistance. Available at https://amr-review.org/sites/default/files/160525_Final%20paper_with%20cover.pdf. Accessed 3 Mar 2025.
12. Antibiotic Resistance Coalition. Available at https://www.ignitetheidea.org/about-arc. Accessed 9 Mar 2025.
13. Global AMR R&D Hub. Available at https://globalamrhub.org/. Accessed 16 Mar 2025.
14. WHO. Global action plan on AMR. Available at https://www.who.int/publications/i/item/9789241509763. Accessed 9 Mar 2025.
15. WHO. At UN, global leaders commit to act on antimicrobial resistance. Geneva: WHO. http://www.who.int/mediacentre/news/releases/2016/commitment-antimicrobial-resistance. Accessed 12 Mar 2025.
16. UN. Political declaration of the high-level meeting of the general assembly on antimicrobial resistance: resolution adopted by the general assembly. 2016. https://digitallibrary.un.org/record/845917?ln=en. Accessed 7 Mar 2025.
17. Sustainable Development Goals. 2015. https://sustainabledevelopment.un.org/sdgsummit. Accessed 9 Mar 2025.
18. WHO. https://www.who.int/data/gho/data/themes/topics/global-antimicrobial-resistance-surveillance-system-glass/sustainable-development-goals-amr-indicator. Accessed 11 Mar 2025.
19. Global Leaders Group. 2024. https://www.amrleaders.org/resources/m/item/glg-report. Accessed 12 Mar 2025.
20. G20 Leaders Declaration, New Delhi. 2003. Can be accessed at https://www.mea.gov.in/Images/CPV/G20-New-Delhi-Leaders-Declaration.pdf. Accessed 13 Mar 2025.
21. UN Multi-partner Trust Fund for AMR. Available at https://mptf.undp.org/fund/amr00. Accessed 13 Mar 2025.
22. The South Centre. https://www.southcentre.int/about-the-south-centre/. Accessed 1 Mar 2025.
23. The South Centre. Group of 77 and South Centre convening on the future of antimicrobial resistance response in developing countries. 2024. Available at https://www.southcentre.int/wp-content/uploads/2024/11/G77-AMR-Meeting-Report-FINAL-4.pdf. Accessed 1 Mar 2025.
24. WHO. WHA 77_R6 antimicrobial resistance: accelerating national and global responses. https://apps.who.int/gb/ebwha/pdf_files/WHA77/A77_ACONF1-en.pdf. Accessed 3 Mar 2025.

25. UN. Political declaration on AMR. Available at https://www.un.org/pga/wp-content/uploads/sites/108/2024/09/FINAL-Text-AMR-to-PGA.pdf. Accessed 7 Mar 2025.
26. WHO. WHO people-centred approach to addressing AMR in the human health. 2023. Available at: https://www.who.int/publications/i/item/9789240082496. Accessed 7 Mar 2025.
27. WHO. World antimicrobial awareness day. Available at https://www.who.int/campaigns/world-antimicrobial-awareness-week. Accessed 11 Mar 2025.

Chapter 5
One Health and AMR Containment

Abstract Antimicrobial resistance (AMR) is a growing global health issue that threatens humans, animals, and ecosystems. Although called a "silent pandemic," progress in implementing national and international action plans is slow, due to the complex, multisectoral nature of AMR. The One Health approach, supported by FAO, WHO, WOAH, and UNEP, offers a comprehensive framework by recognising the connections among humans, animals, plants, and ecosystems. Key components include human, animal, agricultural, and environmental health, with prerequisites such as political commitment, funding, information exchange, institutional cooperation, and community involvement. It advocates for joint efforts to promote responsible antimicrobial use, integrated surveillance, improved infection prevention, and the development of research, innovation, and public awareness. Major obstacles involve fragmented data, weak regulations, limited resources, and siloed governance. Solutions focus on multisectoral stewardship, coordinated management, sustainable policy changes, and capacity building. Moving from concept to practice, the One Health strategy presents the most promising route to controlling AMR sustainably and protecting global health security.

Keywords One Health approach · Multisectoral collaboration · Environmental contamination · Zoonotic pathogens · Policy and governance · Sustainable Development Goals (SDGs)

Antimicrobial resistance (AMR), despite being recognised worldwide as a major public health threat and a silent pandemic, remains often overlooked, underestimated, and unrecognised. Its multisectoral character has challenged developing countries from making substantial advances. There is an urgent need to clarify the complexities of AMR to enhance understanding among policymakers, prescribers, and users of antibiotics. The various aspects of AMR, combined with limited understanding, have slowed progress in tackling it, as evidenced by the slow rollout of many AMR National Action Plans (NAPs) worldwide. The One Health strategy presents the most promising way to combat AMR.

R. Bhatia, *Drug-Resistant Infections*,
https://doi.org/10.1007/978-981-92-4190-3_5

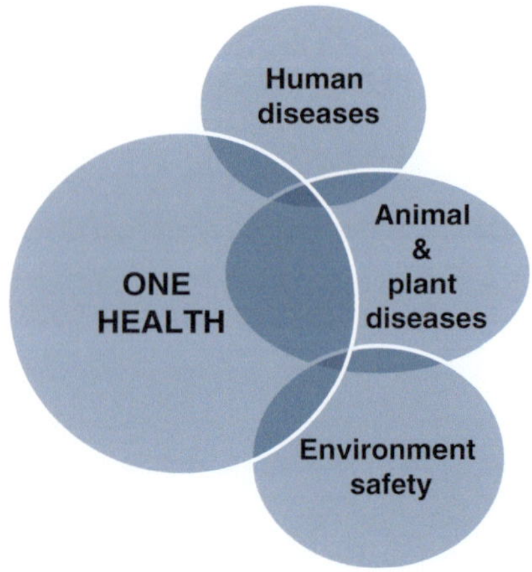

Fig. 5.1 The One Health approach is the interconnectedness of human, animal, and environmental health

AMR is one of the top public health threats of the twenty-first century, threatening human and animal health, food security, and the environment. The One Health approach, which acknowledges the links between humans, animals, and the environment, is essential for addressing AMR comprehensively and sustainably. Successfully controlling AMR demands coordinated efforts across all sectors that use antibiotics, such as healthcare, veterinary, agriculture, and environmental management.

The Wildlife Conservation Society, in a 2004 symposium, called for collective multisectoral global action to improve the health of humans, animals, and the environment through a 'One World One Health' approach [1]. Over the past two decades, One Health has attracted the attention of global agencies and leaders for addressing global health security, zoonotic infections, and AMR.

The United Nations created the "One Health High Level Expert Panel" (OHHLEP), which describes "One Health" as a comprehensive approach united in efforts to sustainably enhance the health of humans, animals, and ecosystems [2]. It emphasises that the well-being of humans, both domestic and wild animals, plants, and the environment is interconnected and depends on each other, as illustrated in Fig. 5.1. This strategy encourages collaboration across different sectors, disciplines, and communities at various societal levels to promote health and address ecological and health threats. It also aims to meet global demands for clean water, energy, and air, while ensuring access to safe, nutritious food, tackling climate change, and fostering sustainable development [3]. Several international bodies, such as the Quadripartite Agreement between the Food and Agriculture Organisation of the UN (FAO), World Organisation for Animal Health (WOAH—previously known as OIE), World Health Organisation (WHO), and United Nations Environment Programme (UNEP), viz. FAO-WHO-WOAH-UNEP, supports this concept. The core message is straightforward: working together to improve the health of humans, animals, and their shared environment.

5.1 One Health Is Complex, Multisectoral, but Efficient

One Health is a practical yet complex approach that provides solutions across multiple domains. To optimise benefits for all stakeholders and establish a comprehensive AMR control strategy in healthcare, a system facilitating seamless, interdisciplinary collaboration from planning through to monitoring is crucial. This system should leverage experiences and infrastructure from diverse sectors. Its scope can grow based on the scientific and technical insights gained via One Health. Such a strategy enhances programme robustness and promotes sector development. The knowledge gained can then be transformed into specific resources and targeted interventions.

One Health impacts all aspects of life, involving many stakeholders, including the Ministry of Health, the National Council on Veterinary Services, environmental agencies, pharmaceutical and biotech companies, research institutions, scientific organisations, science and industrial development bodies, various government branches, the private sector, civil society, and community representatives. Although this diversity offers benefits, it also makes implementation more complex.

The fundamental principle of One Health is "collaboration," emphasising that all stakeholders must work together to achieve optimal results. However, it's essential to recognise that each stakeholder is unique. The success of any project or programme relies on the unity of all parties committed to the common goal of health. The diverse interests of stakeholders can sometimes divert the project in different directions. Consequently, everyone engaged in performance monitoring and understanding should actively participate in reaching the desired outcomes.

So far, One Health remains a theoretical concept, even though it is included in several NAPs, in accordance with recommendations from the Global Action Plan on AMR [4]. The moment has arrived to transform this conceptual framework into tangible actions that make a meaningful difference. This involves elevating One Health from an exclusive government initiative to a broad, whole-of-society strategy with a multisectoral approach and coordinated intervention efforts. Clarifying the core principles of One Health and communicating them clearly is crucial for improving governance, encouraging collaboration across sectors, and enabling effective implementation. By adopting a whole-of-society approach, the world can harness the benefits of the One Health concept to combat AMR and prevent humanity from entering a bleak post-antibiotic era.

One Health is a recognized, integrated, and holistic approach supported by the WHO [5], FAO [6], WOAH, [7], and UNEP [8].

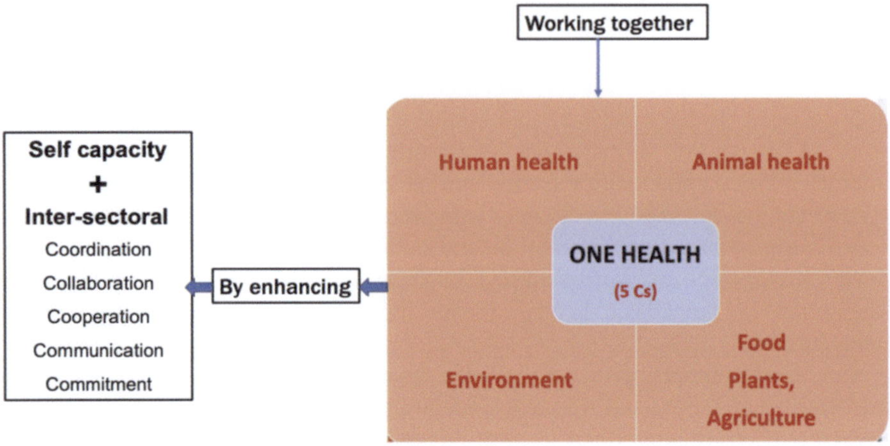

Fig. 5.2 Modalities of One Health operation

5.2 Components of One Health and Prerequisites for Implementation

Four major sectors make up the One Health approach: human health, animal health, the environment, and the agricultural industry. To effectively reduce AMR, these sectors need to enhance their respective capacity to combat AMR and collaborate, cooperate, and communicate on a continuous basis with other sectors and progress together through coordinated efforts (Fig. 5.2).

5.3 Framework for One Health Implementation for AMR Containment

The FAO has published a national framework for implementing One Health in developing countries [9, 10]. This framework highlights several key elements (Fig. 5.3) essential for effectively applying the One Health approach to contain AMR.

This framework includes political commitment, policy development, sustainable funding, programme creation, knowledge exchange, institutional collaboration, capacity building, civil society involvement, and community participation. One Health is a simple yet powerful concept that faces complex implementation challenges. Changing the national discourse on AMR and zoonoses is essential, as it will improve food security and safeguard environmental integrity. High-level political leaders must lead this shift.

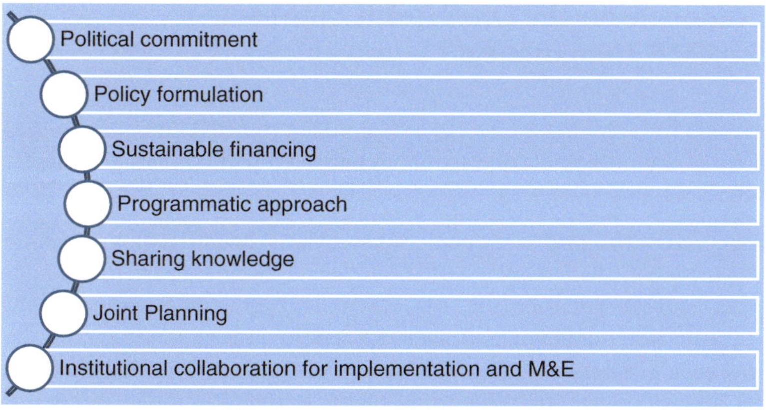

Fig. 5.3 Key elements of the One Health framework for AMR control

Consistent, strong advocacy led by international development partners, such as FAO, WOAH, WHO, and UNDP should communicate evidence-based results, anticipated economic benefits, and best global practices to high-level national leaders. With the interconnected nature of the Sustainable Development Goals, this presents a valuable chance for advocacy and implementing an integrated approach [11]. The political declaration from the United Nations General Assembly on fighting AMR [12] also strongly endorses the One Health strategy.

The success of implementing One Health relies on effective institutional collaboration, joint planning, and coordinated actions to combat AMR. These activities are based on scientific evidence and data. To quickly advance initial efforts, it is crucial to conduct rapid multisectoral capacity building across different institutions. Incorporating One Health principles and practices into educational curricula and ensuring ongoing skill development across all fields will support its long-term sustainability.

To enhance public health outcomes, supporting the faster adoption of the One Health approach can be achieved by pooling national financial resources. Transitioning from a siloed approach to one that is more integrated and interconnected between human, animal, plant, and ecosystem health requires an urgent revision of national policies. Improving coordination and governance includes incorporating knowledge integration into policy-making processes across all levels [13].

Implementing One Health effectively relies on collaboration among institutions, shared planning, and coordinated surveillance to detect and prevent zoonoses. Data and scientific research are essential for planning, executing, and overseeing these activities. Building capacity quickly and thoroughly across sectors is critical to support initial efforts. For long-term sustainability, the core principles and practices of One Health should be thoroughly integrated into educational curricula and include ongoing skills development for all relevant fields.

5.4 Rationale for the One Health Approach in AMR Containment

The rationale for applying a One Health approach to AMR containment lies in the shared use of antimicrobials and the interconnected pathways of resistance spread (Chap. 8):

- *Shared pathogens and resistance genes*: Many bacterial pathogens, such as *Escherichia coli*, *Salmonella*, and *Staphylococcus aureus*, are found in humans, animals, and the environment [14]. Resistance genes [e.g., *mcr-1*, *blaNDM-1*] can transfer horizontally across bacterial species [15].
- *Environmental contamination*: Antimicrobials and resistant bacteria enter soil, rivers, and wastewater from hospitals, pharmaceutical factories, farms, and aquaculture facilities, creating reservoirs for resistance [16].
- *Globalised food trade*: Resistant bacteria in food animals can spread internationally through meat, dairy, and seafood products [17].

The FAO-WHO-WOAH-UNEP Quadripartite Collaboration has endorsed the One Health approach as the gold standard for AMR containment [18].

5.5 Containing AMR Through a One Health Approach

AMR is an escalating worldwide health concern, complicating infection treatments and threatening medical progress. Adopting a One Health approach is essential for addressing AMR, as it recognises the interconnectedness of human, animal, plant, and environmental health, understanding that these elements influence each other and play a role in the development and dissemination of resistant microbes.

Here's how a One Health approach can effectively contain AMR:

5.5.1 Collaborative Strategies Across Diverse Sectors

A One Health approach encourages collaboration among veterinarians, healthcare professionals, environmental scientists, and policymakers to promote responsible use, surveillance, and stewardship of antimicrobials. This teamwork across disciplines helps lower the risk of resistant infections and preserves the effectiveness of treatments. Coordinated efforts to reduce antimicrobial use in both humans and animals are essential to address AMR effectively.

5.5.2 Responsible Antimicrobial Use

Promoting the careful use of antimicrobials in both human healthcare and animal farming is crucial. This means avoiding unnecessary prescriptions, sticking to proper dosages, and following guidelines for appropriate antibiotic use (see Chap. 2). Reducing antibiotic use for growth promotion in animals helps decrease the selective pressure that leads to the development of antibiotic resistance.

5.5.3 Enhanced Surveillance and Monitoring

Integrated surveillance systems that monitor AMR in humans, animals, plants, and the environment are essential for understanding how resistance develops and spreads (see Chap. 1). Data on AMR, antimicrobial use (AMU), and antimicrobial residues are exchanged across sectors to guide policies and interventions. The WHO's Global Antimicrobial Resistance and Use Surveillance System (GLASS) offers a standardised method for collecting and sharing AMR information.

5.5.4 Strengthening Infection Prevention and Control (IPC)

Effective IPC measures are essential in controlling the spread of infection, which in turn reduces the reliance on antimicrobial treatments. These measures encompass enhanced hygiene practices in healthcare settings, communities, and animal farms. Water, sanitation, and hygiene (WASH) interventions play a vital role in preventing infectious diseases and decreasing the need for antibiotics.

5.5.5 Fostering Research and Development

One Health promotes research to improve understanding of AMR and to create new therapies, diagnostics, and vaccines. Investigating the complex interactions of AMR at the human–animal–plant–environment interface is essential for forming comprehensive strategies. Additionally, developing new antibiotics and exploring alternative treatments such as phage therapy and immunotherapy are vital (also see Chaps. 18 and 19).

5.5.6 *Public Awareness and Education*

Educating the public on AMR and correct antibiotic use is crucial. Awareness efforts should focus on healthcare providers, farmers, and consumers to promote informed antimicrobial decisions (see Chap. 20). Tackling AMR also requires addressing the economic and social factors that lead to antibiotic overuse.

By adopting a One Health approach, it is possible to move from reactive measures to proactive prevention, building a healthier future for humans, animals, plants, and the environment.

5.6 Challenges in Implementing One Health AMR Containment

Despite growing recognition, the following barriers (Box 5.1) continue to hinder the implementation of One Health for AMR containment.

Box 5.1 Major Barriers in One Health Implementation for AMR Containment

- Fragmented data systems that impede cross-sector integration.
- Regulatory gaps that permit the sale of unregulated antimicrobials across sectors.
- Resource constraints in low- and middle-income countries [LMICs] that limit laboratory capacity for diagnosis and surveillance.
- Limited political will and competing priorities in major sectors, which obviate sustained and long-term investments.
- Complexity of environmental AMR monitoring due to diverse sources and a lack of standardised indicators.
- Mindset fixation on a silo approach and administrative set-ups that preclude extensive intersectoral horizontal collaboration.

5.7 Solutions Through One Health for AMR Control

The One Health approach integrates surveillance, stewardship, infection prevention, policy, and public engagement to address AMR at its root causes, recognising that resistant pathogens move freely between humans, animals, and the environment through food, water, direct contact, and trade (Table 5.1).

Table 5.1 Essential actions under the One Health approach to contain AMR

	Broad area	Major actions
1	Integrated AMR surveillance system under One Health links data from human health, animal health, and the environment	Harmonise laboratory methodologies across sectors [19]. Establish national data-sharing platforms for appropriate actions. Utilize or introduce artificial intelligence and big data analytics expand environmental monitoring to include pharmaceutical effluents [20].
2	Antimicrobial Stewardship [AMS]	Strengthen hospital-based AMS programmes to reduce inappropriate prescriptions and encourage narrow-spectrum antibiotic use [21]. Phase out routine antimicrobial use for growth promotion in healthy animals [22]. Promote vaccination, probiotics, and improved husbandry to reduce infection pressure and antimicrobial need in animals [23].
3	Infection prevention and control [IPC]	Implement IPC interventions—hand hygiene, sterilisation, isolation protocols that significantly lower hospital-acquired infection rates [24]. Establish biosecurity measures, including closed herds, vaccination, and vector control to prevent diseases [25]. Undertake environmental measures, e.g. wastewater treatment that reduces environmental dissemination of resistant organisms [20].
4	Research & development and innovations	Promote and support development of novel antimicrobials and alternatives [e.g. bacteriophages, antimicrobial peptides]. Use rapid diagnostics to guide targeted therapy. Encourage genomic surveillance to track resistance evolution. Initiate behavioural research for professionals in all sectors to improve prescribing and public engagement. Introduce incentives for innovation inform of market entry rewards for new antimicrobials and alternatives.
5	Policy, legislation, and regulations	Align National Action Plans [NAPs] with the new Global Action Plan on AMR [26] and WHO's People centered approach to control AMR [27]. Implement legislative controls on antimicrobial production, distribution, and prescription. Establish functional cross-sectoral governance bodies for coordination and oversight.
6	Public engagement and risk communication	Undertake extensive community campaigns on the pattern of WHO's *World Antimicrobial Awareness Week* to promotes responsible use of antibiotics. Integrate One Health in Curriculum of Veterinary and medical schools by incorporating One Health AMR modules. Through targeted messaging improves adherence to stewardship principles and bring about behavioural change for rational use of antibiotics [28]. Engage farmers, pharmacists, and local leaders in stewardship.

It is globally recognised that the One Health approach is essential for sustainable containment of AMR. By integrating surveillance, stewardship, IPC, research, and policy, it addresses the interconnected drivers of resistance across humans, animals, and the environment.

Box 5.2 Carry-Home Messages for One Health in AMR Containment

- One Health is a validated, holistic approach.
- One Health is a simple and powerful concept, but its implementation process is highly complex.
- One Health implementation requires a multisectoral, multi-institutional, and multidisciplinary approach.
- A strategic policy shift is required to de-sectoralise human, animal, plant, and ecosystem health in the context of AMR.
- Data and science should be made the cornerstones of programme implementation.
- Evidence-driven actions (Table 5.1), based on research and risk-benefit analyses in the local context, are essential for effectively containing AMR.
- AMR control beacons concept of "working together".

Moving forward, global and national investments must prioritise One Health capacity building, cross-sector governance, and equitable access to diagnostics and alternatives. Without such integrated action, AMR threatens to undermine decades of medical and agricultural progress. Some of the key takeaways for all stakeholders are outlined in Box 5.2.

The One Health approach is regarded as the most effective method for controlling antimicrobial resistance (AMR) because AMR arises and spreads at the intersection of humans, animals, and the environment, making actions focused on a single sector inadequate. Antibiotics are extensively used not only in human healthcare but also in livestock, aquaculture, and farming, with resistant organisms and antimicrobial residues moving through food chains, water, soil, and ecosystems. Recognising these connections, One Health advocates for coordinated, multisectoral efforts.

In human healthcare, issues like inappropriate prescriptions, self-medication, and poor infection control drive resistance. In animal health, using antimicrobials for growth and disease prevention leads to resistant pathogens that can transfer to humans via food, direct contact, or the environment. Pollution from pharmaceutical production, hospital waste, and agricultural runoff enhances resistance further. A One Health strategy addresses all these pathways collectively, not separately.

Operationally, it promotes integrated surveillance systems that compile data from humans, animals, food, and the environment, enabling early detection of new resistance and guiding evidence-based policies. It also encourages harmonised regulations, antimicrobial stewardship across sectors, and coordinated infection prevention measures such as vaccination, biosecurity, sanitation, and water safety.

Furthermore, One Health encourages shared governance and accountability among ministries of health, agriculture, environment, finance, and local authorities. This coordination boosts resource efficiency, reduces duplication, and aids the implementation of National Action Plans on AMR. By addressing root causes across different systems and fostering collaboration instead of isolated efforts, the One Health approach provides the most comprehensive, sustainable, and cost-effective way to maintain antimicrobial effectiveness and safeguard global health.

Numerous real-world examples demonstrate how the One Health approach effectively helps contain antimicrobial resistance (AMR) across human, animal, and environmental sectors. These cases are widely referenced in policy discussions and exams:

Denmark's Danish Integrated Antimicrobial Resistance Monitoring and Research Programme (DANMAP) serves as a leading example. It combines AMR and antimicrobial-use data from humans, food animals, and food products [29]. The evidence from DANMAP prompted a ban on non-therapeutic antibiotic use in livestock, leading to a sustained reduction in veterinary antibiotic consumption without affecting productivity, and a decline in resistant Salmonella and Campylobacter cases in humans.

Using a One Health framework, the Netherlands reduced antibiotic use in food animals by over 60% from 2009 to 2016 through strict regulation, farmer engagement, veterinary stewardship, and surveillance. This resulted in a decrease in livestock-associated MRSA in humans, illustrating cross-sector benefits [30].

Thailand's National Strategic Plan on AMR (2017–2021) adopted a One Health approach, connecting human health, animal health, food safety, and environmental sectors [31]. The country reported decreased antimicrobial use in humans, enhanced hospital stewardship programs, and improved multisectoral surveillance, which boosted AMR awareness and policy adherence.

Sweden's STRAMA program involves clinicians, veterinarians, public health officials, and laboratories. Through stewardship, surveillance, and infection prevention, Sweden maintains some of the lowest antibiotic usage and AMR levels in Europe, exemplifying the effectiveness of coordinated One Health governance [32].

Global efforts, such as expanding GLASS surveillance, establishing guidelines for antimicrobial use in food animals, and supporting National Action Plans on AMR, have enhanced cross-sector coordination in many low- and middle-income countries.

These examples demonstrate that success in containing AMR relies on aligning efforts across human, animal, and environmental sectors, integrating surveillance, and basing policy decisions on shared data—proving that One Health is more than just a concept, but a proven solution.

References

1. World Conservation Society One World One Health. Manhattan principles. Available from: https://oneworldonehealth.wcs.org/About-Us/Mission/The-Manhattan-Principles.aspx. Accessed 26 Mar 2025.
2. World Health Organization. One Health high level expert panel. Available from: https://www.who.int/groups/one-health-high-level-expert-panel/members. Accessed 29 Mar 2025.
3. One Health High-Level Expert Panel (OHHLEP), Adisasmito WB, Almuhairi S, Behravesh CB, Bilivogui P, Bukachi SA, et al. One Health: a new definition for a sustainable and healthy future. PLoS Pathog. 2022;18(6):e1010537. https://doi.org/10.1371/journal.ppat.1010537.
4. World Health Organization. WHO global action plan for antimicrobial resistance. Geneva: WHO; 2015. Available from: http://www.who.int/antimicrobial-resistance/globalaction-plan/en/. Accessed 28 Mar 2025.
5. World Health Organization. One Health. 2017. Available from: http://www.who.int/features/qa/one-health/en/ Accessed 27 Mar 2025.
6. Food and Agricultural Organization of the United Nations. Thoughts of FAO on One Health. Rome: FAO; 2017. Available from: http://www.fao.org/ag/againfo/home/en/news_archive/2010_one-health.html. Accessed 20 Mar 2025.
7. World Organisation for Animal Health [WOAH]. One Health "at a glance". 2017. Available from: http://www.oie.int/en/for-the-media/onehealth/ Accessed 22 Mar 2025.
8. United Nations Environment Programme. UNEP One Health. Available at https://www.unep.org/topics/chemicals-and-pollution-action/pollution-and-health/unep-one-health. Accessed 23 Mar 2025.
9. Bhatia R. Implementation framework for One Health approach. Indian J Med Res. 2019;149(3):329–31. https://doi.org/10.4103/ijmr.IJMR_1517_18.
10. Bhatia R. National framework for One Health. New Delhi: FAO; 2021. https://doi.org/10.4060/cb4072en.
11. Aslam B, Asghar R, Muzammil S, et al. AMR and sustainable development goals: at a crossroads. Glob Health. 2024;20:73. https://doi.org/10.1186/s12992-024-01046-8.
12. United Nations. General Assembly adopts political declaration on antimicrobial resistance, demanding immediate action for safeguarding ability to treat disease, enhance food security. Available at https://press.un.org/en/2024/ga12642.doc.htm. Accessed 26 Mar 2025.
13. Hitziger M, Esposito R, Canali M, Aragrande M, Häsler B, Rüegg SR, et al. Knowledge integration in One Health policy formulation, implementation and evaluation. Bull World Health Organ. 2018;96:211–8. https://doi.org/10.2471/BLT.17.202705.
14. Robinson TP, Bu DP, Carrique-Mas J, Fèvre EM, Gilbert M, Grace D, et al. Antibiotic resistance is the quintessential One Health issue. Trans R Soc Trop Med Hyg. 2016;110(7):377–80. https://doi.org/10.1093/trstmh/trw048.
15. Liu Y-Y, Wang Y, Walsh TR, Yi L-X, Zhang R, Spencer J, et al. Emergence of plasmid-mediated colistin resistance mechanism *mcr-1* in animals and human beings in China: a microbiological and molecular biological study. Lancet Infect Dis. 2016;16(2):161–8. https://doi.org/10.1016/S1473-3099(15)00424-7.
16. Karkman A, Do TT, Walsh F, Virta MPJ. Antibiotic-resistance genes in waste water. Trends Microbiol. 2018;26(3):220–8. https://doi.org/10.1016/j.tim.2017.09.005.
17. Tang KL, Caffrey NP, Nóbrega DB, Cork SC, Ronksley PE, Barkema HW, et al. Restricting the use of antibiotics in food-producing animals and its associations with antibiotic resistance in food-producing animals and human beings: a systematic review and meta-analysis. Lancet Planet Health. 2017;1(8):e31627. https://doi.org/10.1016/S2542-5196(17)30141-9.
18. WHO, FAO, OIE, UNEP. Working together to tackle antimicrobial resistance. Geneva: WHO; 2022.
19. DANMAP. Danish integrated antimicrobial resistance monitoring and research programme. Copenhagen: Statens Serum Institut; 2022.

20. Rizzo L, Manaia C, Merlin C, Schwartz T, Dagot C, Ploy M-C, et al. Urban wastewater treatment plants as hotspots for antibiotic resistant bacteria and genes spread into the environment: a review. Sci Total Environ. 2013;447:345–60. https://doi.org/10.1016/j.scitotenv.2013.01.032.
21. Barlam TF, Cosgrove SE, Abbo LM, MacDougall C, Schuetz AN, Septimus EJ, et al. Implementing an antibiotic stewardship program: guidelines by the Infectious Diseases Society of America and the Society for Healthcare Epidemiology of America. Clin Infect Dis. 2016;62(10):e51–77. https://doi.org/10.1093/cid/ciw118.
22. WHO. Guidelines on use of medically important antimicrobials in food-producing animals. Geneva: WHO; 2017. Available at https://www.who.int/publications/i/item/9789241550130. Accessed 30 Mar 2025.
23. Allen HK, Levine UY, Looft T, Bandrick M, Casey TA. Treatment, promotion, commotion: antibiotic alternatives in food-producing animals. Trends Microbiol. 2013;21(3):114–9. https://doi.org/10.1016/j.tim.2012.11.00.
24. Allegranzi B, Bagheri Nejad S, Combescure C, Graafmans W, Attar H, Donaldson L, Pittet D. Burden of endemic health-care-associated infection in developing countries: systematic review and meta-analysis. Lancet. 2011;377(9761):228–41. https://doi.org/10.1016/S0140-6736(10)61458-4.
25. Laanen M, Persoons D, Ribbens S, de Jong E, Callens B, Strubbe M, et al. Relationship between biosecurity and production/antimicrobial treatment characteristics in pig herds. Vet J. 2013;198(2):508–12. https://doi.org/10.1016/j.tvji.2013.08.029.
26. WHO. Global action plan on antimicrobial resistance. Geneva: WHO; 2015. Available at https://www.who.int/publications/i/item/9789241509763. Accessed 7 May 2025.
27. WHO. People-centred approach to addressing antimicrobial resistance in human health: WHO core package of interventions to support national action plans. Geneva: World Health Organization; 2023. Licence: CC BY-NC-SA 3.0 IGO. Available at https://www.who.int/publications/i/item/9789240082496. Accessed 10 Mar 2025.
28. Roope LSJ, Tonkin-Crine S, Butler CC, Crook D, Peto T, Peters M, et al. Reducing demand for antibiotic prescriptions: evidence from an online behavioural intervention. Health Econ. 2019;28(2):181–98. https://doi.org/10.2807/1560-7917.ES.2018.23.25.1700424.
29. Hammerum A, Heuer O, Emborg H-D, Skjøt-Rasmussen L, Jensen V, Rogues A-M, Skov R, Agersø, et al. Danish integrated antimicrobial resistance monitoring and research programme (DANMAP). Emerg Infect Dis. 2007;13:1632–9. https://doi.org/10.3201/eid1311.070421.
30. Jansen R, Gomez-Duran O. Antibiotic reduction in the Netherlands: from challenge to leading example. Pig Progress. 2025. Available at https://www.pigprogress.net/specials/antibiotic-reduction-in-the-netherlands-from-challenge-to-leading-example/. Accessed on 1 Feb 2026.
31. Sumpradit N, Wongkongkathep S, Malathum K, Janejai N, Paveenkittiporn W, Yingyong T, Chuxnum T, et al. Thailand's national strategic plan on antimicrobial resistance: progress and challenges. Bull World Health Organ. 2021;99(9):661–73. https://doi.org/10.2471/BLT.20.280644.
32. Swedish strategy to curb antimicrobial resistance 2026–2035. Government Offices of Sweden. 2026. Available at https://www.government.se/information-material/2026/01/information-material-swedens-strategy-to-curb-antimicrobial-resistance-2026-2035/#. Accessed on 3 Feb 2026.

Chapter 6
Health System and AMR

Abstract A critical relationship exists between health systems and antimicrobial resistance (AMR), which highlights how system structures and functions both drive and defend against this global health threat. AMR undermines the effectiveness of modern medicine, increasing mortality, morbidity, healthcare costs, and jeopardising essential services such as surgery and cancer care. Using the World Health Organisation's health system framework, one can analyse how governance, service delivery, financing, workforce, information systems, and access to medicines shape AMR dynamics. Key pathways include inappropriate prescribing, inadequate infection prevention and control (IPC), weak diagnostic and surveillance capacity, and perverse financial incentives. Several evidence-based interventions, such as antimicrobial stewardship programmes, IPC integration, strengthening diagnostic and surveillance capabilities, and One Health coordination, have gained importance in contributing to the control of AMR. A few innovations in stewardship metrics, digital health, and financing models to stimulate research and ensure equitable access have also become available and used. Despite demonstrated effectiveness, challenges persist in scaling and sustaining interventions, particularly in resource-limited settings with fragile laboratories, workforce shortages, and weak governance. The WHO's 2023 people-centred approach is presented as a paradigm shift, placing communities and equitable access at the core of AMR strategies. Countries need to identify and implement priority policy recommendations to embed AMR containment into routine health system strengthening and governance reforms.

Keywords Antimicrobial resistance · Health systems · Antimicrobial stewardship Infection prevention and control · Diagnostics and surveillance · Pharmaceutical governance · WHO AWaRe classification · Health system financing · People-centred approach

A health system is defined as the collective organisations, institutions, resources, and personnel responsible for enhancing health services, aimed at improving health determinants through quality care, preventive measures, and rehabilitative

R. Bhatia, *Drug-Resistant Infections*,
https://doi.org/10.1007/978-981-92-4190-3_6

interventions. It requires a workforce, funding, information networks, and overall guidance to function effectively [1].

The health system aims to promote and improve health for individuals and groups by following elements (Box 6.1), all of which are linked with containment of antimicrobial resistance (AMR).

Box 6.1 Aims of the Health System in the Context of AMR Control

- Averting dangers to health
- Protecting people against financial disasters as a consequence of ill health
- Providing equitable access to health care
- Enabling people to participate in decisions affecting their health [1]

An analytical framework used by the World Health Organisation (WHO) [2] disaggregates the health system into six core components, commonly referred to as building blocks (Fig. 6.1). These are: leadership and governance, service delivery, health system financing, health workforce, medical products, vaccines and technologies, and health information systems.

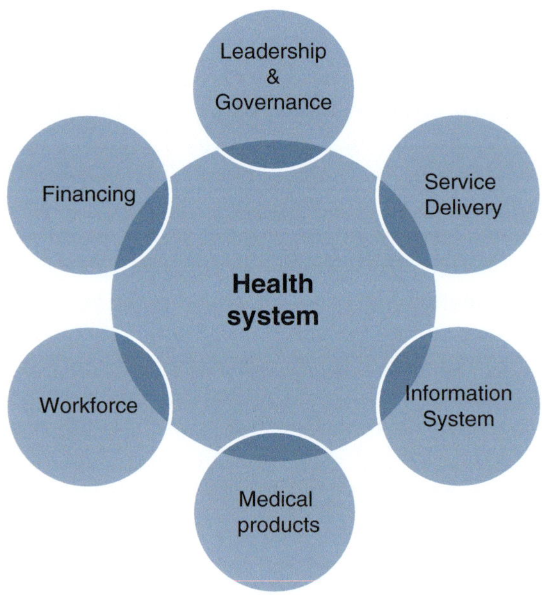

Fig. 6.1 Building blocks of the health system [2]

6.1 Health System and AMR

All building blocks of the health system influence efforts to contain AMR—a global health threat that undermines the ability of modern health systems to prevent and treat infectious diseases.

Antimicrobial resistance (AMR) is a complex challenge that cannot be effectively managed without addressing the performance of the six World Health Organization (WHO) health-system building blocks. AMR not only reflects clinical practices but also highlights underlying systemic weaknesses within healthcare systems.

Service Delivery The manner in which health services are delivered has a direct impact on AMR. Accessible, high-quality, and people-centred care helps in reducing the misuse of antibiotics. Strong primary health care, efficient referral systems, and robust infection prevention and control (IPC) practices in hospitals minimise inappropriate antibiotic use, decrease hospital-acquired infections, and reduce dependence on broad-spectrum antimicrobials.

Health Workforce A skilled and motivated health workforce is essential for containing AMR. This includes physicians, nurses, pharmacists, microbiologists, veterinarians, and community health workers. Adequate training and supervision enable rational prescribing, effective antimicrobial stewardship, precise laboratory diagnostics, proper IPC implementation, and increased community awareness. However, gaps in skills or lack of supervision often result in defensive or irrational antibiotic usage.

Health Information Systems Functional health information systems are vital for AMR control. These systems generate reliable data on antimicrobial consumption, track resistance patterns, and monitor treatment outcomes. Surveillance platforms, laboratory information systems, and reporting mechanisms like the Global Antimicrobial Resistance and Use Surveillance System (GLASS) support the creation of evidence-based guidelines, facilitate early detection of emerging resistance, and help in monitoring the impact of policies. Without timely and accurate data, AMR remains under-recognised and inadequately addressed.

Access to Essential Medicines Ensuring access to essential medicines is fundamental in combating AMR. The availability of affordable, quality-assured antibiotics prevents shortages that may lead to irrational substitutions or the growth of informal markets. Effective regulatory oversight of manufacturing, procurement, and distribution is necessary to prevent the circulation of substandard and falsified medicines, which can accelerate resistance. Medicines policies that follow standard treatment guidelines promote rational antibiotic use.

Health Financing The way health financing is structured significantly influences antibiotic usage. Reducing out-of-pocket expenses helps to discourage self-medication and over-the-counter purchases of antibiotics. Sufficient and predictable funding supports diagnostics, laboratory networks, IPC infrastructure, surveillance systems, and stewardship programmes—elements that are often overlooked in under-resourced settings.

Leadership and Governance Strong leadership and governance are critical for providing strategic direction in AMR control. This includes developing national action plans, enforcing regulations, coordinating multisectoral efforts under the One Health approach, and establishing accountability frameworks. Effective governance aligns stakeholders across human, animal, and environmental health sectors, ensuring a unified response to AMR.

It is well established now that the integrated strengthening of all six WHO health system building blocks is necessary to create a resilient health system capable of preventing, detecting, and responding to antimicrobial resistance in an effective and sustainable manner.

AMR increases mortality, morbidity, length of hospital stay, and healthcare costs, while challenging essential services such as surgery, oncology, and neonatal care that depend on effective antibiotics. Recent global burden analyses estimate over a million deaths directly attributable to bacterial AMR annually, with substantially greater indirect impacts when AMR contributes to fatal outcomes [3]; projections suggest that in future this burden will rise without coordinated action across health systems and sectors.

Health systems serve as both drivers and key defenders against AMR. Through clinical prescribing, infection prevention and control (IPC), diagnostics, surveillance, governance, financing mechanisms, and workforce practices, health systems influence patterns of antimicrobial use, the emergence and spread of resistant organisms, and the capacity to detect and respond to resistance threats. Strengthening health system functions—such as governance, service delivery, the health workforce, information systems, access to essential medicines and technologies, and financing—is therefore crucial for containing AMR.

6.2 Health System Pathways That Drive AMR

Health systems influence AMR through multiple interconnected pathways: inappropriate prescribing and overuse of antibiotics in human healthcare, inadequate IPC facilitating healthcare-associated transmission, suboptimal diagnostic capacity leading to empiric and often excessive antimicrobial use, fragmented surveillance and information systems that fail to detect and guide responses, weak regulation and pharmaceutical governance enabling over-the-counter access or poor-quality medicines, and perverse incentives in financing and service delivery [4]. The dynamics operate across primary, secondary, and tertiary health care services as well as long-term care and community settings; each setting presents unique drivers and intervention opportunities (Fig. 6.2). A few high-impact mechanisms deserve emphasis [5] (Table 6.1).

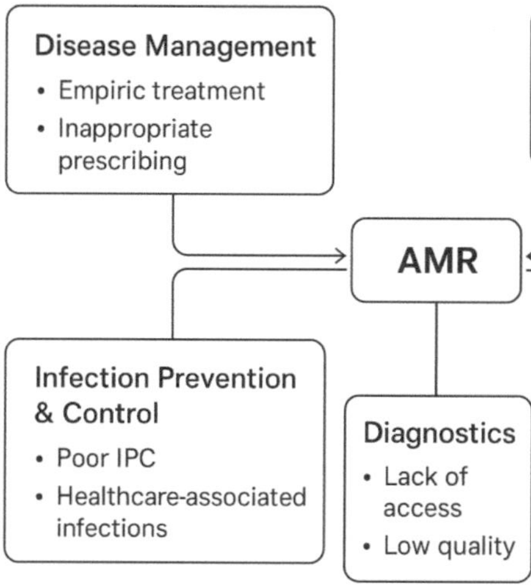

Fig. 6.2 Drivers of AMR in health systems

Table 6.1 Health system drivers of AMR and the reasons thereof

	Major influencer	Linking reasons
1	Inappropriate antibiotic prescribing	Diagnostic uncertainty Patient expectations Time pressures Lack of prescriber feedback
2	Breaks in IPC that amplify transmission of resistant organisms within facilities, converting sporadic resistance into institution outbreaks and endemicity	Hand hygiene Environmental cleaning Device care
3	Diagnostic deficits that force reliance on broad-spectrum empiric therapy	Limited access to rapid, reliable microbiology
4	Governance and financing shortfalls	Absent stewardship mandates Weak monitoring Lack of funding for laboratory networks

6.3 Core Health-System Functions for AMR Prevention and Control

6.3.1 Governance and Leadership

Strong governance ensures policy consistency, multisectoral coordination (One Health), regulatory oversight, and accountability needed to align health system efforts with national AMR strategies. Reviews of national action plans to contain AMR (NAP) show considerable variation in implementation capacity; plans without operational funding, measurable indicators, and clear coordination mechanisms often fail to produce effective results [6]. Good governance involves stakeholder participation, clear roles for public health, clinical services, veterinary, and environmental sectors, as well as legal/regulatory tools that control antimicrobial distribution and quality [7].

6.3.2 Surveillance and Information Systems

Robust surveillance—the detection, characterisation, and reporting of resistance and antimicrobial consumption—is essential for understanding AMR trends and guiding interventions. Global initiatives like WHO's Global Antimicrobial Resistance and Use Surveillance System (GLASS) have improved standardisation and reporting but still face challenges in laboratory capacity, data quality, representativeness, and integration with clinical care data. Enhancing laboratory networks, digital reporting systems, and analytics within health information systems strengthens early warning, stewardship metrics, and policy assessment [8].

6.3.3 Service Delivery, Infection Prevention and Control, and Quality of Care

Service delivery models that incorporate IPC and proper antimicrobial use help prevent both infections and resistance. Evidence indicates that IPC measures—such as hand hygiene programmes, device-associated infection prevention bundles, environmental cleaning, and staff training—reduce healthcare-associated infections (HAIs) and curb the spread of resistant organisms [9]. Embedding IPC into routine quality improvement, with metrics tied to accreditation and reimbursement, enhances long-term sustainability. Rational prescribing algorithms and clinical decision support tools—like guidelines, order sets, and stewardship rounds—further improve prescribing practices.

6.3.4 Health Workforce and Training

Physicians, pharmacists, nurses, and laboratory professionals play a crucial role in the rational use of antibiotics. Ongoing education and professional development in antimicrobial stewardship (AMS), diagnostic interpretation, IPC, and communication skills help decrease inappropriate antibiotic prescribing. Interdisciplinary stewardship teams—comprising physicians, infectious disease specialists, clinical pharmacists, microbiologists, and infection control practitioners—are linked to lower antibiotic use and better patient outcomes when properly supported [10]. However, workforce shortages, high staff turnover, and a lack of laboratory personnel hinder implementation in many settings.

6.3.5 *Diagnostics and Laboratory Capacity*

Access to timely and precise diagnostics transforms clinical decision-making from empirical to targeted therapy, reducing unnecessary use of broad-spectrum antibiotics. Evidence supports investing in high-quality microbiology services, using rapid point-of-care tests when suitable, and practising diagnostic stewardship—ensuring tests are ordered and utilised to guide therapy. Barriers include costs, supply chain issues, training needs, and integrating results into clinical workflows. Nevertheless, where these measures are adopted, diagnostics significantly improve antimicrobial targeting and enhance surveillance data [8].

6.3.6 *Access to Essential Medicines and Pharmaceutical Governance*

Health systems need to ensure access to suitable antimicrobials—covering availability, quality, and affordability—while also preventing misuse. Implementing policies that establish essential medicine lists aligned with stewardship principles, regulating dispensing practices, and taking action against substandard or falsified medicines are crucial steps. The WHO AWaRe classification (Access, Watch, Reserve) [11] offers a practical framework for monitoring and guiding national antibiotic policies, and greater adoption of it has been linked to more rational prescribing behaviours [12] (Chap. 2).

6.3.7 *Financing and Economic Incentives*

Financing influences incentives related to prescribing, procurement, and innovation. Payment models that emphasise service volume may inadvertently encourage over-prescribing, while funding that supports stewardship, laboratory investments, and IPC can benefit the entire system. Economic studies indicate that stewardship efforts often save costs or are cost-effective in many hospital environments; however, expanding financing reforms—such as support for national surveillance, laboratory networks, workforce training, and research & development (R&D)—are essential for building a resilient system [13]. Emerging pull strategies, like subscription models, are being developed to promote antibiotic R&D without boosting sales volume excessively.

6.4 Evidence-Based Health System Interventions

6.4.1 Antimicrobial Stewardship Programme

Systematic reviews and meta-analyses demonstrate that antimicrobial stewardship programmes (AMSPs) reduce antibiotic use and occasionally improve clinical outcomes without increasing mortality rates. Approaches in AMSP include prospective audit and feedback, pre-authorisation, guideline adoption, dose optimisation, and de-escalation. Successful initiatives typically involve leadership backing, dedicated staff, audit and feedback systems, locally tailored antibiogram-based guidelines, and integration with electronic health record decision support. The global evidence indicates consistent reductions in antibiotic consumption and better guideline adherence in both high- and middle-income countries, with promising signs of effectiveness in resource-limited settings when AMSPs are adapted to local contexts.

6.4.2 Infection Prevention and Control

IPC interventions reduce HAIs and limit the spread of resistant pathogens. Bundled strategies targeting central line-associated bloodstream infections and ventilator-associated pneumonia, combined with hand hygiene promotion and environmental cleaning, show significant decreases in infection rates [14]. Incorporating IPC into wider patient safety and quality initiatives enhances impact and promotes sustainability [9].

6.4.3 Diagnostic Stewardship and Laboratory Strengthening

Implementing interventions that optimise test ordering—such as reducing unnecessary cultures—can shorten turnaround times and ensure results are available at the bedside promptly. This approach enhances diagnostic accuracy and minimises unwarranted antibiotic use. Investing in laboratory personnel, supply chains, quality assurance, and connectivity—linking lab results to clinicians and national surveillance—is essential [8]. Emerging technologies like rapid molecular assays, multiplex PCR, and next-generation sequencing hold promise, but they must be strategically integrated into health systems to maximise cost-effectiveness and impact.

6.4.4 *Surveillance-Driven Policy and Feedback Loops*

Making surveillance actionable requires converting laboratory and consumption data into local antibiograms, stewardship targets, formulary guidelines, and providing feedback to prescribers. Countries that successfully connect facility, regional, and national surveillance data can develop empiric therapy guidelines and identify emerging resistance, supporting targeted interventions. However, many health systems lack the interoperability and analytical tools needed to complete these feedback loops.

6.4.5 *Multisectoral (One Health) Integration Within Health System*

AMR presents a One Health challenge involving the complex interactions among human, animal, and environmental sectors [7]. Effective health systems must work together with agriculture, veterinary services, environmental agencies, and pharmaceutical regulators. Governance models that encourage collaboration across sectors, facilitate data sharing, support joint surveillance, and align stewardship policies are associated with more efficient responses to AMR. Recent reviews emphasise key governance areas—such as coordination, accountability, equity, and sustainability—that are vital for implementing surveillance and intervention strategies within the One Health framework [15].

6.5 Innovations and Policy Mechanisms

6.5.1 *AWaRe and Stewardship Metrics*

Many countries have adopted the WHO AWaRe framework as a monitoring and stewardship tool; studies show that shifting prescribing toward Access group antibiotics and away from Watch/Reserve categories is feasible and correlates with stewardship outcomes. National reporting on AWaRe metrics helps set targets and measure progress [16].

6.5.2 R&D Incentives and Market Shaping

Weak commercial incentives for novel antibiotics have led to market failures. Innovative policy responses—pull incentives (market entry rewards, subscription models), public–private partnerships, and de-linkage strategies—aim to stimulate R&D while ensuring stewardship [17]. The UK's subscription model pilot and proposals in other jurisdictions illustrate how pay-for-availability models can reward innovation independent of sales volume. Complementary investments in rapid diagnostics and vaccines also reduce reliance on antibiotics.

6.5.3 Digital Health and Data Analytics

Digital platforms can integrate laboratory data, prescribing records, and surveillance dashboards to facilitate real-time stewardship and public health actions. While advances in machine learning for resistance prediction and prescriber decision support show promise, challenges such as data governance, interoperability, and equitable access still pose barriers.

6.6 AI and Health System Response to AMR Control

Artificial intelligence (AI) is becoming a key driver in strengthening health system responses to antimicrobial resistance (AMR), spanning prevention, detection, treatment, and governance. Its influence is most evident where data-driven decisions can improve long-standing system weaknesses.

In surveillance and information systems, AI boosts early detection of resistant pathogens by analysing large amounts of laboratory, genomic, and prescription data in real time. Machine-learning models can detect resistance patterns, forecast outbreaks, and identify unusual trends more quickly than traditional methods, enhancing platforms like GLASS and national AMR systems.

In clinical care, AI-powered decision support systems assist clinicians in selecting appropriate antibiotics, doses, and durations based on patient details, local resistance data, and guidelines. This reduces empirical overuse of broad-spectrum antibiotics and promotes antimicrobial stewardship, particularly in settings with limited specialist access.

For health workforce support, AI tools help with training and mentoring through point-of-care guidance, automated prescribing audits, and feedback to improve adherence to treatment standards. This reduces skill gaps and minimises unwarranted prescribing variations.

In medicine access and supply chains, AI enhances demand forecasting, prevents stock-outs of essential drugs, and discourages overuse of reserve antibiotics.

Improved inventory management promotes rational use and aligns procurement with stewardship objectives.

In financing and governance, AI supports policy-making by modelling the economic impact of AMR, assessing intervention cost-effectiveness, and prioritising investments in diagnostics, infection prevention, and research. Predictive analytics also assist regulators in detecting misuse, substandard medicines, and risks in informal markets.

Overall, AI does not replace core public health functions but strengthens health system capacity to respond more timely, precisely, and efficiently to AMR. Its effectiveness relies on data quality, ethical governance, interoperability, and equitable access—highlighting the need for strong health systems to enable AI' s full contribution to AMR containment.

6.7 Challenges and Limitations in Health-System Responses

Although several interventions have proven effective, their large-scale implementation and sustainability face numerous challenges. Resource-limited settings often lack the necessary laboratory facilities, trained personnel, reliable supply chains, and funding to carry out national AMR strategies. In high-income countries, behavioural factors such as prescriber independence, patient expectations, fragmented healthcare pathways, and financial incentives that discourage change further complicate efforts. Surveillance efforts are often limited by gaps in geographic and pathogen coverage, affecting data representativeness. Political focus on AMR also varies over time and may be overshadowed by immediate health concerns, impeding long-term infrastructure investments. Lastly, combating AMR requires action across multiple sectors beyond healthcare, but institutional silos and regulatory fragmentation can impede such collaboration [18].

6.8 WHO People-Centred Approach to Addressing AMR in Human Health

In 2023, the WHO introduced the *people-centred approach to addressing AMR in human health* [19]. This approach places people—their needs, challenges, and access to care—at the centre of the health system response to AMR, aligns AMR efforts with broader health system strengthening and equitable access goals. This WHO framework aims to move AMR efforts away from isolated technical measures toward a comprehensive, health system-oriented strategy that focuses on individuals and communities. It expands on the Global Action Plan for AMR, acknowledging that AMR cannot be addressed solely through narrow technical solutions. Instead, it advocates for integrated, equitable, and community-tailored responses, particularly within primary healthcare systems.

This approach prioritizes individuals, their needs, and equitable access to quality health services in the fight against AMR. It emphasises preventing infections, ensuring access to diagnosis and treatment, and building country capacity for pandemic preparedness.

It shifts the focus from seeing AMR only as a biological problem to understanding its effects on people's lives and health. It centres on people by understanding their needs and addressing them with a core set of interventions. This method guarantees that everyone can access quality prevention, diagnosis, and treatment for infections, no matter their background or location.

The approach advocates for utilising suitable diagnostic tools and strategies to determine infection causes and steer treatment choices. It guarantees patients get the correct antimicrobial, at the proper dose, and for the appropriate length, grounded in precise diagnosis and evidence-based guidelines. This method is supported by four pillars, including two foundational steps and a set of 13 interventions.

- *Four pillars*

    1. Prevention of infections through water, sanitation, hygiene (WASH), infection prevention and control (IPC) activities, and immunisation coverage.
    2. Access to essential health services, quality-assured antibiotics and diagnostics, timely diagnosis, evidence-based treatment, antimicrobial stewardship, and regulation of non-prescription antibiotic sales.
    3. Timely, accurate diagnosis.
    4. Appropriate, quality-assured treatment.

- *Two foundational steps*

    1. Effective governance, awareness, and education comprising AMR advocacy, accountability, raising awareness among the public and healthcare workers, AMR surveillance strategy, national research agenda, establishing strong leadership and governance structures to support the implementation of AMR containment strategies.
    2. Strategic information through surveillance and research by utilizing surveillance and research data to track AMR trends, inform interventions, and monitor progress.
    3. A core package of 13 people-centred interventions which aim to tackle health system and patient-level barriers across various healthcare settings.

By adopting a people-centred approach, countries can effectively address AMR, protect public health, and ensure that life-saving antimicrobial medicines remain effective for future generations.

6.9 Policy Recommendations and Way Forward

Based on the evidence, health systems should prioritise the following actions (Box 6.2):

Box 6.2 Priority Actions by the Health System to Contain AMR

- Strengthen governance and financing
- Scale up surveillance and laboratory networks
- Mainstream AMSP and IPC into clinical services
- Expand diagnostic capacity and diagnostic stewardship
- Use AWaRe and metrics for performance monitoring
- Align incentives for innovation and supply security
- Operationalise One Health
- Invest in workforce education and behaviour change

AMR presents a complex systemic challenge that both stems from and endangers health system performance. Implementing evidence-based interventions—such as surveillance, stewardship, IPC, diagnostics, governance, and financing reforms—can lower inappropriate antimicrobial use, prevent the spread of resistant organisms, and ensure continued access to effective treatments. Success depends on coordinated, ongoing investments across various system functions and sectors, guided by accurate surveillance data and accountable governance. When health systems integrate AMR prevention into everyday service delivery, quality control, and funding, they become more resilient and better equipped to safeguard public health now and in the future. There is an urgent need to empower health systems at all levels to combat AMR in human health sector.

Empowering health systems to combat antimicrobial resistance (AMR) demands deliberate, system-wide improvements rather than isolated technical solutions.

Strong primary healthcare decreases unnecessary antibiotic use by enhancing early diagnosis, maintaining continuity of care, and streamlining referral processes. Incorporating infection prevention and control (IPC), antimicrobial stewardship, and standard treatment guidelines into routine services—especially in hospitals and long- term care facilities—directly reduces inappropriate antimicrobial use.

Health workers require training and ongoing support to prescribe responsibly. This includes both pre-service and in-service education on AMR, stewardship, IPC, diagnostics, and risk communication. Empowering pharmacists, nurses, and community health workers to take on stewardship and patient education roles broadens system capacity beyond physicians alone.

Integrated surveillance of antimicrobial use and resistance across human, animal, and environmental sectors is vital. Strengthening laboratory capacity, digital reporting platforms, and feedback mechanisms enables timely detection of resistance trends and informs evidence-based policies and clinical decisions.

Ensuring reliable supply chains for essential antibiotics and rapid diagnostics minimises empirical prescribing and prevents the distribution of substandard or falsified medicines. Enforcing prescription-only policies and aligning procurement with standard treatment guidelines support rational antimicrobial use.

Reducing out-of-pocket costs discourages self-medication and informal antibiotic purchases. Dedicated funding for laboratories, IPC infrastructure, surveillance, and stewardship programmes helps sustain AMR containment efforts beyond short-term projects.

A strong political commitment is essential to implement national AMR action plans, enforce regulations on the sale and use of antimicrobials, and coordinate multisectoral efforts under a One Health framework. Clear accountability mechanisms transform policy into practical action.

Public awareness campaigns, behavioural change communications, and involvement of sectors like agriculture, animal health, and environment are critical to extending AMR containment beyond the health sector.

Collectively, these strategies foster resilient, people-centred health systems capable of preventing infections, promoting responsible antimicrobial use, and responding effectively to the growing threat of AMR.

References

1. WHO. Key components of a well-functioning health system. http://www.who.int/healthsystems/EN_HSSkeycomponents.pdf?ua=1. Accessed 29 Mar 2025.
2. WHO. Health system building blocks. Available at https://extranet.who.int/nhptool/BuildingBlock.aspx. Accessed 29 Mar 2025.
3. Naghavi M, GBD 2021 Antimicrobial Resistance Collaborators†. Global burden of bacterial antimicrobial resistance 1990–2021: a systematic analysis with forecasts to 2050. Lancet. 2024;404:1199–226. https://doi.org/10.1016/S0140-6736(24)01867-1.
4. Nguyen-Thanh L, Wernli D, Målqvist M, Graells T, Jørgensen PS. Characterising proximal and distal drivers of antimicrobial resistance: an umbrella review. J Glob Antimicrob Resist. 2024;36:50–8. https://doi.org/10.1016/j.jgar.2023.12.008.
5. Resman F. Antimicrobial stewardship programs; a two-part narrative review of step-wise design and issues of controversy Part I: step-wise design of an antimicrobial stewardship program. Ther Adv Infect Dis. 2020;7:2049936120933187. https://doi.org/10.1177/2049936120933187.
6. Patel J, Harant A, Fernandes G, Mwamelo AJ, Hein PW, Dekker D, et al. Measuring the global response to antimicrobial resistance, 2020–21: a systematic governance analysis of 114 countries. Lancet Infect Dis. 2023;23:706–18. https://doi.org/10.1016/S1473-3099(22)00796-4.
7. Ruckert A, Harris F, Aenishaenslin C, et al. One Health governance principles for AMR surveillance: a scoping review and conceptual framework. Res Dir One Health. 2024;2:e4. https://doi.org/10.1017/one.2023.13.
8. Do PC, Assefa YA, Batikawai SM, Reid SA. Strengthening antimicrobial resistance surveillance systems: a scoping review. BMC Infect Dis. 2023;23(1):593. https://doi.org/10.1186/s12879-023-08585-2.
9. Sartelli M, Marini CP, McNelis J, Coccolini F, Rizzo C, Labricciosa FM, Petrone P. Preventing and controlling healthcare-associated infections: the first principle of every antimicrobial stewardship program in hospital settings. Antibiotics (Basel). 2024;13(9):896. https://doi.org/10.3390/qntibiotics13090896.

10. Zay Ya K, Win PTN, Bielicki J, Lambiris M, Fink G. Association between antimicrobial stewardship programs and antibiotic use globally: a systematic review and meta-analysis. JAMA Netw Open. 2023;6(2):e2253806. https://doi.org/10.1001/jamanetworkopen.2022.53806.
11. WHO. The WHO 2023 AwaRe classification of antibiotics for evaluation and use. Available at https://www.who.int/southeastasia/publications/i/item/WHO-MHP-HPS-EML-2023.04. Accessed 30 Mar 2025.
12. Saleem Z, Sheikh S, Godman B, Haseeb A, Afzal S, Qamar MU, Imam MT, Abuhussain SSA, Sharland M. Increasing the use of the WHO AWaRe system in antibiotic surveillance and stewardship programmes in low- and middle-income countries. JAC Antimicrob Resist. 2025;7(2):dlaf031. https://doi.org/10.1093/jacamr/diaf031.
13. Krishnamoorthy Y, Govindan D, Karunakaran M, Parveen M, Manohar A, Al-Tawfiq JA. Global impact of antimicrobial stewardship programs in healthcare: an umbrella review of effectiveness, cost-efficiency, and implementation strategies. J Infect Chemother. 2025;31:102753. https://doi.org/10.1016/j.jiac.2025.102753.
14. Igwe U, Okolie OJ, Ismail SU, Adukwu E. Effectiveness of infection prevention and control interventions in health care facilities in Africa: a systematic review. Am J Infect Control. 2024;52:1135–43. https://doi.org/10.1016/j.ajic.2024.06.004.
15. Zhou Y, Frutos R, Bennis I, Wakimoto MD. One Health governance: theory, practice and ethics. Sci One Health. 2024;3:100089. https://doi.org/10.1016/j.soh.2024.100089.
16. Abdelsalam Elshenawy R, Umaru N, Aslanpour Z. WHO AWaRe classification for antibiotic stewardship: tackling antimicrobial resistance – a descriptive study from an English NHS Foundation Trust prior to and during the COVID-19 pandemic. Front Microbiol. 2023;14:1298858. https://doi.org/10.3389/fmicb.2023.1298858.
17. Theuretzbacher U, Jumde RP, Hennessy A, et al. Global health perspectives on antibacterial drug discovery and the preclinical pipeline. Nat Rev Microbiol. 2025;23:474–90. https://doi.org/10.1038/s41579-025-01167-w.
18. Ho CS, Wong CTH, Aung TT, Lakshminarayanan R, Mehta JS, Rauz S, McNally A, Kintses B, Peacock SJ, de la Fuente-Nunez C, Hancock REW, Ting DSJ. Antimicrobial resistance: a concise update. Lancet Microbe. 2025;6:100947. https://doi.org/10.1016/j.lanmic.2024.07.010.
19. WHO. People-centred approach to addressing antimicrobial resistance in human health: WHO core package of interventions to support national action plans. Available at https://www.who.int/publications/i/item/9789240082496. Accessed 31 Mar 2025.

Chapter 7
Veterinary Sector and AMR

Abstract The veterinary sector is a key player in the global antimicrobial resistance (AMR) crisis due to extensive antibiotic use in livestock for therapeutic, prophylactic, metaphylactic, and growth-promotion purposes. About 70% of worldwide antibiotic sales are used in animals, often surpassing human medical consumption, especially where regulatory oversight is weak. Non-therapeutic practices promote the development of resistant bacteria such as *Esch. coli*, *Salmonella*, *Campylobacter*, and methicillin-resistant *Staphylococcus aureus*, which can be transmitted to humans through food, water, the environment, or contact, jeopardising the treatment of severe infections. The emergence of plasmid-mediated colistin resistance highlights the global health dangers of the unregulated use of veterinary antibiotics. Effective AMR surveillance systems like WOAH's ANIMUSE, the EU's EARS-Vet, and national programmes (e.g. INFAAR, DANMAP, CIPARS) are essential for tracking resistance patterns, guiding stewardship efforts, and shaping policies. Strategies to reduce antibiotic use include banning growth promoters, limiting prophylaxis, improving animal husbandry, enhancing biosecurity, and adopting alternatives such as vaccines, probiotics, acidifiers, and essential oils. Public awareness, strict regulation, and international cooperation, all within a One Health approach, are vital to mitigating AMR risks. Limiting antibiotic use in animals protects animal welfare, human health, food safety, and global health security.

Keywords Veterinary medicine · Livestock · Antibiotic use · Growth promotion · Surveillance systems · One Health · Colistin resistance · Alternatives to antibiotics · Public health

Antibiotics are extensively employed in veterinary practices to achieve multiple goals, such as treating animal infections, preventing outbreaks within herds, and promoting weight gain in animals, particularly poultry (see Table 7.1). The following outlines some common uses of antibiotics:

R. Bhatia, *Drug-Resistant Infections*,
https://doi.org/10.1007/978-981-92-4190-3_7

Table 7.1 Uses of antibiotics in the veterinary sector

Therapeutics	Metaphylaxis	Prophylaxis	Growth promoters
Administration of antibiotics to animals when diagnosed with disease	Administration of antibiotics to animals when perceived to be in contact with animals diagnosed with disease	Mass administration of antibiotics to animals to prevent disease when risk is established	Administration of antibiotics to animals to boost feed efficiency and increase weight gain

7.1 Antibiotic Use in Animals

Therapeutic Use

Antibiotics are employed to combat bacterial infections in animals, similar to their use in humans. They are used to treat conditions such as pneumonia, skin infections, mastitis, and other bacterial illnesses. Providing this treatment alleviates animal suffering and supports their welfare, while also benefiting the owners' economy.

Metaphylaxis Use

When an animal in a group tests positive for an infection, antibiotics are often administered to the whole group to prevent disease spread. This practice is common in large-scale poultry and pig farming.

Prophylaxis Use

In high-risk situations, antibiotics are administered to prevent infections, especially when animals face a greater likelihood of contracting them. This practice is more prevalent in specific types of animal production and can be controversial due to its possible role in promoting antimicrobial resistance (AMR).

Growth Promotion

Historically, antibiotics have been used to enhance growth and feed efficiency in food animals. However, this practice is now decreasing in popularity, as many countries are gradually banning or limiting antibiotic use for growth promotion. The European Union led this shift by banning antibiotics for this purpose in 2006 [1].

In some countries with weak regulatory systems, especially those with large agricultural sectors, antibiotic use in animals often exceeds that in human medicine. This is mainly due to intensive farming practices where antibiotics are used for growth promotion and disease prevention, potentially leading to the development and spread of antibiotic resistance [2].

Approximately 70% of all antibiotics sold globally are used in the animal sector, particularly in intensive livestock farming, where antibiotics are often administered for disease prevention, growth promotion, and prophylactic purposes [3, 4].

7.2 Public Health Importance of Antibiotic Use in Animals

The role of farm antibiotic use in human resistance is well acknowledged. The extensive use of antibiotics in animal farming, especially for non-therapeutic reasons, significantly contributes to AMR. Resistant bacteria in animals can transfer to humans through food, water, and environmental pathways. This transfer complicates the treatment of bacterial infections in humans and presents a serious public health challenge [5, 6].

The frequent use of antibiotics in farm animals fosters ideal conditions for resistant bacteria to develop, as it kills off susceptible bacteria and allows resistant ones to thrive. These bacteria can be transferred to humans via meat handling, direct contact with animals, or environmental exposure. Occasionally, resistant bacteria from animals may colonise a human without causing immediate infection, only leading to illness years afterwards. This poses a significant risk to human health, as many antibiotics used in farming belong to the same class as those used to treat serious human infections.

A study by Van et al. [7] revealed that approximately 80% of livestock raised for food are given treatments, including antibiotics, at various stages. Only about 10% of antibiotics are used to treat infections; the majority are used for disease prevention and promoting growth [8]. In the United States, roughly half of the antibiotics used in the animal sector—mainly penicillin and tetracycline—are administered to animals. This indicates that a large portion of antibiotics given to animals is not solely for treatment but mainly aims to enhance growth and prevent diseases [9].

In certain human infections, such as those caused by *Campylobacter* or *Salmonella*, the use of antibiotics on farms is a significant factor contributing to resistance in humans. This practice has played a key role in the emergence of a new, nearly untreatable form of *E. coli*, leading to numerous deaths in the UK and other parts of Europe [10].

The widespread use of specific antibiotics in farming has led to the emergence of a new strain of methicillin-resistant *Staphylococcus aureus* (L-MRSA) in animals, which is spreading rapidly and being transmitted to humans. Several pathogens that cause human diseases are developing resistance to the "critically important" antibiotics. This trend is partly driven by the improper use of antibiotics in veterinary practice.

AMR in animals, driven by the widespread use of antibiotics, can cross borders and impact both animals in different countries and humans. In late 2015, resistance to colistin—a last-resort antibiotic—was detected in humans and pigs in China [11], mainly due to the overuse of colistin in livestock in the pig farms. This antibiotic was widely used in human medicine from the 1950s through the 1970s, but its use declined as safer alternatives became available. However, it was never completely phased out, and the rise of multidrug resistance led to its reintroduction as a critical last-resort treatment. Farmers also used colistin as a food additive, often without considering the potential for resistance development. The discovery of the *mcr*-1 gene, which confers colistin resistance on a plasmid—a mobile genetic element—has facilitated the spread of resistance among bacteria. Today, *mcr*-1 is found worldwide in the environment, animals, and humans, and it even causes infections in humans [12]. Colistin resistance has also been observed alongside other resistance elements, resulting in infections that are unresponsive to antibiotics. Consequently, colistin-resistant bacteria were quickly identified in numerous countries globally [13].

7.3 Increasing Use of Antibiotics in Animals

Since the early 1950s, antibiotics have been used in livestock rearing. In Europe, they were first used to promote growth in animals, but this practice was banned across the EU in 2006. Meanwhile, in Asia and Oceania, farm antibiotic sales per livestock unit are nearly four times higher than those in Europe [14].

Antibiotics classified by the WHO as "highest-priority critically important" for humans [15] are also frequently used in animals, which can contribute to the development of resistance against these vital medicines for treating serious human diseases.

In human medicine, antibiotics are primarily used to treat the ill. However, in the farming industry, these valuable drugs are frequently administered to groups of healthy animals. In the UK, 75% of farm antibiotic use is for mass treatments, and in Europe, this proportion rises to 86% [3]. This practice of widespread medication helps prevent diseases in environments that are often prone to disease outbreaks. The extensive use of antibiotics supports the continuation of intensive farming practices and contributes to the growing problem of antibiotic resistance in humans.

7.4 AMR Surveillance in Animals

AMR surveillance system in the animal sector involves tracking the levels and trends of AMR in animal populations, usually alongside antimicrobial use. This information is vital for shaping policies and interventions to reduce the impact of AMR on animal health, human health, and the environment.

Surveillance systems play a crucial role in detecting and monitoring the emergence and spread of AMR across different animal species, including livestock, pets, and wildlife. Data collected from these systems is vital for devising and applying effective strategies to manage and prevent AMR, such as implementing proper antimicrobial use protocols and infection control practices.

AMR in animals can threaten human health, particularly through zoonotic diseases or the food chain. Surveillance is essential. AMR in food-producing animals may lead to antimicrobial residues in food products, creating risks for consumers. Surveillance helps ensure the safety and quality of food.

Surveillance data can inform decisions about which antimicrobials are most effective for treating infections in animals, promoting responsible and judicious use.

An effective AMR surveillance system should aim for

(a) *Data collection*: This involves gathering samples from clinical cases, food products, or the environment, along with data on antimicrobial usage, susceptibility testing results, and other relevant information;
(b) *Laboratory testing*: Conducting antimicrobial susceptibility testing (AST) on bacterial isolates to determine resistance patterns;
(c) *Data analysis and reporting*: Analysing the collected data to identify trends, patterns, and risk factors linked to AMR; and
(d) *Dissemination of information*: Sharing surveillance findings with stakeholders such as veterinarians, farmers, policymakers and the public to inform decisions and enhance awareness.

Aligning national surveillance systems with global initiatives like the WHO GLASS and WOAH's *ANI*mal Anti*M*icrobial *Use* Global Database (ANIMUSE) is important for international monitoring and response. The ANIMUSE is a critical instrument for international monitoring and response to antimicrobial resistance (AMR). ANIMUSE systematically collects, standardises, and analyses country-reported data on antimicrobial use in animals, enabling global and regional comparisons over time. This evidence helps identify high-risk usage patterns, informs risk-based stewardship policies, and supports implementation of the One Health approach linking human, animal, and environmental health. By improving transparency and accountability, ANIMUSE strengthens global surveillance, guides regulatory action, and supports coordinated international responses to reduce inappropriate antimicrobial use and slow the emergence and spread of AMR [25].

Implementing strong and comprehensive AMR surveillance systems in the animal sector enables countries to gauge the scope of the issue better, develop targeted strategies, and safeguard both animal and human health against the escalating threat of AMR.

Currently, multiple AMR surveillance systems operate worldwide within the animal sector, each with different levels of integration across countries and regions. These systems tend to focus on particular pathogens, antimicrobial agents, and animal populations, with some being part of larger One Health initiatives. They include national, regional, and global surveillance networks.

7.4.1 National Surveillance Systems

Many countries have established national surveillance programmes to monitor AMR in animals. These systems can vary significantly in their scope, methodologies, and data reporting practices. Among Asian countries, India has established a surveillance network called Indian Network for Fishery and Animal AMR (INFAAR) [16], while other examples include CIPARS (Canada) [17], DANMAP (Denmark)

[18], MARAN (Netherlands) [19], GERM-Vet (Germany) [20], and CZ NMTP (Czech Republic) [21]. These are national surveillance systems that also integrate AMR data from both human and animal sectors.

7.4.1.1 European Union Surveillance Programmes

The European Union (EU) runs several programmes aimed at monitoring antimicrobial resistance (AMR) in animals. A key initiative, the European Antimicrobial Resistance Surveillance Network in Veterinary Medicine (EARS-Vet), continues under EU-JAMRAI2. EARS-Vet was launched during the EU Joint Action on Antimicrobial Resistance and Healthcare-Associated Infections (EU-JAMRAI) from 2017 to 2021 and remains ongoing as part of EU-JAMRAI2, funded by the EU4Health programme for 2024–2027. The network includes 38 partners across 18 countries and collaborates closely with European and global organisations such as FAO, WHO, and WOAH [22].

ESAC-Net concentrates on antimicrobial use in both human and animal sectors, as outlined by the European Centre for Disease Prevention and Control [22]. These initiatives are designed to track, analyse, and report data to address AMR.

7.4.2 InFARM

The Food and Agriculture Organisation's InFARM system [23] is designed to assist countries in sharing data on AMR and antimicrobial usage (AMU), supporting global surveillance efforts. It contributes to the Quadripartite Global Integrated System for Surveillance of Antimicrobial Resistance and Antimicrobial Usage (GISSA) [24].

The inFARM initiative has significantly contributed to global efforts to combat antimicrobial resistance (AMR) in the food and agriculture sectors. One of its key successes is strengthening national capabilities to produce, analyse, and apply data on AMR and antimicrobial use (AMU) in animals and food systems, especially in low- and middle-income countries. By providing technical guidance, standardised methods, and country support, inFARM has improved data comparability and integration across regions. The initiative also promotes a One Health approach, fostering collaboration among the veterinary, public health, and environmental sectors. Countries supported by inFARM have used the evidence generated to shape national AMR action plans, revise regulations on veterinary antimicrobial use, and adopt responsible livestock practices. By linking surveillance data with policy and practice, inFARM has helped turn data into actionable steps, supporting more sustainable food systems and global AMR containment.

Numerous AMR surveillance systems are present in the animal sector worldwide, each with varying levels of integration and focus. More efforts are needed to standardise data, enhance data sharing and accessibility, and better link human and animal surveillance data for a more effective One Health approach.

Surveillance programmes are vital for detecting new antibiotic-resistant bacteria and formulating strategies to manage their dissemination. Monitoring antibiotic consumption and resistance in animal farming enables the identification of regions that require intervention to reduce antibiotic use and curb the development of AMR. Furthermore, these programmes support policymaking and public health efforts to control the proliferation of resistant bacteria.

7.5 Surveillance on Use of Antibiotics in Animals

Since 2015, WOAH has monitored antimicrobial use in food-producing animals to help prevent the rise of drug-resistant bacteria. Excessive use of antimicrobials that are medically important in these animals is seen as a significant factor driving increased AMR.

Recognising that measuring the amount of antimicrobials given to animals is crucial for understanding usage patterns, ensuring compliance with international standards, and preventing health issues, deaths, and economic losses, WOAH employs an online platform called ANIMUSE [25]. This interactive, automated database enables countries to report, access, analyse, and share data on antimicrobials used in animals with various stakeholders. It offers simplified reporting, error detection, and data visualisation features. Ultimately, ANIMUSE aims to enhance the practises of veterinary and aquatic animal health services related to antimicrobial use. The platform is open to all countries, whether WOAH Members or non-members. National Veterinary Services can submit general information, and if quantitative data is available, they can choose from different options based on the level of detail of their data.

Every year, WOAH releases a report outlining global and regional trends in antimicrobial use in animals. This report is based on data collected annually between September and May.

The latest WOAH report, issued in May 2025, details the global use of antimicrobial agents relative to animal biomass for 2022 and summarises the eighth annual data collection on antimicrobial usage in animals. It reveals that 34 of 157 responding countries (22%) still report using antibiotics for growth promotion, predominantly in the Americas and Asia-Pacific regions. Meanwhile, almost three-quarters of these countries (112 out of 157; 71%) say this non-veterinary use is no longer authorised, regardless of legislation or regulations [26]. Notably, eight countries still report using colistin—an antimicrobial of highest priority for human health—despite the commitment by all WOAH Members 10 years ago to eliminate this practice.

WOAH estimates that the total adjusted amount of AMU could reach up to 74,035 t. Tetracyclines and penicillin together make up nearly half of the global usage—28.29% and 17.75%, respectively [26]. Although both are classified as veterinary critically important antimicrobials (VCIAs) in the WOAH List of Antimicrobials of Veterinary Importance [27], they are not among the highest-priority critically important antimicrobials for human health, according to the WHO [28]. In that list, WHO includes fluoroquinolones (3.7%), polymyxins (1.8%), and third- and fourth-generation cephalosporins (0.9%).

WOAH estimates that in 2022, AMU was between 89 and 93 mg/kg of animal biomass. A global decline of 5% in antibiotic use was observed across 81 countries in Europe, Africa, the Americas, and Asia, whereas Middle East countries experienced a 43% increase during the same period [26].

Recent years have seen notable changes in Europe regarding antibiotic use in livestock. Between 2011 and 2022, antibiotic sales for animals decreased by 53%. In 2022, the EU implemented regulations to eliminate routine antibiotic use on farms [29]. Meanwhile, in the UK, antibiotic use in livestock has decreased by approximately 59% since 2014. New UK regulations, effective from 17 July 2024, align with EU standards and prohibit the routine use of antibiotics; however, they do not ban prophylactic group treatments or require mandatory antibiotic-use data collection, unlike the EU.

7.6 Why Is It Important to Reduce the Use of Antibiotics in Animals?

The antibiotics used in animals are either the same as or similar to those used in human medicine. As antibiotic use selects for resistance in bacteria, overuse in animals increases resistance levels in bacteria in the animal's environment, including among farmers. These resistant pathogens or genes can then spread throughout the community via humans, manure, or animals, often facilitated by abattoirs, ultimately leading to the development of severe antibiotic-resistant diseases in people [3].

Using antibiotics excessively in animals fosters an environment where resistant bacteria can flourish and multiply, which may lead to the transfer of resistance genes to other bacteria and eventually to humans [3].

Resistant bacteria or resistance genes can spread from animals to humans through multiple routes, including direct contact, consuming contaminated food (such as meat, milk, or eggs), and via environmental sources like manure and water.

Globally, about 70% of antibiotics are used in farm animals rather than humans [4]. Much of this usage is routine, allowing farm animals—primarily pigs and poultry, and sometimes cattle—to be kept in unsuitable conditions where diseases spread rapidly. Authorities like the European Medicines Agency and the WHO highlight that the overuse of antibiotics in agriculture plays a role in increasing antibiotic resistance in some human infections.

There are solid evidence-based outcomes especially from Denmark [17], Netherlands [30] and Sweden [31] where concerted efforts have resulted in substantial reduction in use of antibiotics in animals.

7.7 How to Reduce Antibiotic Use in Farm Animals?

To curb the development of resistance in animal agriculture, measures need to be taken to reduce the use of antibiotics. Such measures include [3, 32]:

- Stop using antibiotics for growth promotion.
- Minimise antibiotic use for prevention of infection.
- Implement infection prevention measures, including vaccines, to reduce the incidence of disease.

The U.S. Department of Agriculture recommends several approaches to reduce antibiotic use in livestock [32]. These include employing immunomodulators to boost animals' immune systems and resistance, quickly diagnosing and treating sick animals to stop disease transmission, maintaining a clean and healthy environment, and using laboratory tests to detect animals at risk of disease.

Strategies to decrease therapeutic antibiotic use fall into two main categories: preventing disease and infection, and accurately diagnosing the presence of a pathogen to select an effective antibiotic that thoroughly eliminates the infection.

Reducing antibiotic use in subtherapeutic disease prevention and growth promotion could be the most significant opportunity to decrease antibiotics in food animals. Alternative approaches will mainly involve implementing suitable management strategies and practices (see Box 7.1).

Box 7.1 Management Strategies and Practices to Reduce Antibiotic Use in Animals

Provide stringent controls on hygiene, population dynamics, feed quality, and environmental conditions to prevent or reduce stress

Eradicate/control specific diseases

Optimise nutrition to enhance natural immunity

Breed genetically disease-resistant livestock

Use alternative growth promoters such as cattle anabolics

Another practical approach involves reducing antibiotic use in animal feed and instead promoting good husbandry practices, such as maintaining proper hygiene and nutrition, to prevent disease.

7.8 Alternative Options to Antibiotics in Food-Producing Animals

It is now scientifically proven that animals don't require routine antibiotics to stay healthy. Organic and higher-welfare systems administer antibiotics sparingly, only when animals genuinely need them. Livestock can and should be kept healthy through proper animal husbandry and welfare, rather than relying on "bought-in" immunity.

Probiotics are beneficial bacteria that enhance gut health and immune function, offering an alternative to antibiotics. They can be added to animal feed or water and have been shown to promote growth and decrease infectious diseases in livestock. For instance, a study on dairy calves demonstrated that a probiotic containing *Lactobacillus acidophilus* and *Bifidobacterium lactis* lowered the rates of diarrhoea and respiratory infections [33].

Acidifiers constitute another alternative that can be used as feed additives to lower the pH in the gastrointestinal tract, creating an environment that inhibits the growth of harmful bacteria. Essential oils can be added to food to enhance immune function and reduce the risk of infections.

Reducing antibiotic use in animals is essential for global efforts to combat antimicrobial resistance (AMR). Importantly, no antibiotic alone decreases overall antibiotic use; instead, a systematic approach replaces routine, preventive, and inappropriate antibiotic use with effective non-antibiotic measures, supported by targeted therapy when necessary. Policies should prioritise prevention, management, and stewardship over just switching to other antimicrobials.

Vaccination is a highly effective tool for lowering antibiotic demand in animal agriculture. By preventing common infectious diseases in livestock and poultry, vaccines greatly reduce morbidity and mortality, decreasing the need for therapeutic antibiotics. Strengthening national animal vaccination programmes and improving access to quality vaccines should be policy priorities. Likewise, biosecurity and hygiene improvements—such as better housing, sanitation, controlled animal movement, and all-in/all-out systems—help prevent disease spread and reliance on antibiotics.

Nutrition and gut health management are also crucial. Balanced diets, micronutrient supplementation, and optimised feed formulations boost immune function. The use of probiotics, prebiotics, and synbiotics can stabilise gut microbiota, especially in poultry and pigs, reducing enteric infections and antibiotic use. Phytogenic feed additives and organic acids further enhance health by lowering pathogen load and improving feed efficiency.

When antibiotics are necessary, policies must promote rational use under veterinary supervision, accurate diagnosis, and antimicrobial susceptibility testing. Preference should be given to narrow- spectrum, first- line antibiotics, while critically important antimicrobials for human medicine should be restricted. These strategies—centred on prevention, management, and stewardship—offer a sustainable way to reduce antibiotic use in animals, protect animal health, food security, and public health within a One Health approach.

Multiple studies indicate that these alternatives effectively improve animal health and productivity without affecting food safety or quality. They offer environmental advantages by decreasing the release of antibiotics and chemicals into the environment via animal waste. It is essential to emphasise that strict biosecurity and hygiene protocols on farms are vital to prevent infectious diseases and AMR.

Reducing antibiotic use in animals plays a key role in preventing the development and spread of AMR. Limiting antibiotics' selective pressure decreases the likelihood of resistant bacteria arising and being transferred to humans. Since AMR is a major threat to both animal and human health, affecting disease management and risking economic losses, implementing alternative measures is vital. These include enhanced biosecurity, vaccination, proper nutrition, and good animal husbandry practices to lower infectious disease rates.

Raising awareness among the public, industry, and animal farming communities about the risks of AMR and the significance of responsible antibiotic use can lead to significant shifts in consumer behaviour. It also encourages producers to implement more sustainable practices to reduce AMR, addressing it as a pressing global public health issue.

References

1. Alliance to Save our Antibiotics. Ending routine farm use of antibiotics. Available at https://saveourantibiotics.org/media/2035/report-ending-routine-farm-antibiotic-use-in-europe.pdf. Accessed 5 Apr 2025.
2. Alhassan MY, Kabara MK, Ahmad AA, et al. Revisiting antibiotic stewardship: veterinary contributions to combating antimicrobial resistance globally. Bull Natl Res Cent. 2025;49:25. https://doi.org/10.1186/s42269-025-01317-3.
3. Baudoin F, Hogeveen H, Wauters E. Reducing antimicrobial use and dependence in livestock production systems. Front Vet Sci. 2021;8:584593. https://doi.org/10.3389/fvets.2021.584593.
4. Van Boeckel TP, Brower C, Gilbert M, Grenfell BT, Levin SA, Robinson TP, Teillant A, Laxminarayan R. Global trends in antimicrobial use in food animals. Proc Natl Acad Sci USA. 2015;112(18):5649–54. https://doi.org/10.1073/pnas.1503141112.
5. Uddin TM, Chakraborty AJ, Ameer Khusro BM, Zidan RM, Mitra S, Emran TB, et al. Antibiotic resistance in microbes: history, mechanisms, therapeutic strategies and future prospects. J Infect and Public Health. 2021;14(12):1750–66. https://doi.org/10.1016/j.jiph.2021.10.020.
6. Manyi-Loh C, Mamphweli S, Meyer E, Okoh A. Antibiotic use in agriculture and its consequential resistance in environmental sources: potential public health implications. Molecules. 2018;23(4):795. https://doi.org/10.3390/molecules23040795.
7. Van TTH, Yidana Z, Smooker PM, Coloe PJ. Antibiotic use in food animals worldwide, with a focus on Africa: pluses and minuses. J Glob Antimicrob Resist. 2020;20:170–7. https://doi.org/10.1016/j.jgar.2019.07.031.
8. D'Atri F, Arthur J, Blix HS, Hicks LA, Plachouras D, Monnet DL. Targets for the reduction of antibiotic use in humans in the Transatlantic Taskforce on Antimicrobial Resistance [TATFAR] partner countries. Euro Surveill Bull Eur Sur Les Mal Transm Eur Commun Dis Bull. 2019;24:1800339. https://doi.org/10.2807/1560-7917.ES.2029.24.28.1800339.

9. Martin MJ, Thottathil SE, Newman TB. Antibiotics overuse in animal agriculture: a call to action for health care providers. Am J Public Health. 2015;105:2409–10. https://doi.org/10.2105/AJPH.2015.302870.
10. Bennani H, Mateus A, Mays N, Eastmure E, Stärk KDC, Häsler B. Overview of evidence of antimicrobial use and antimicrobial resistance in the food chain. Antibiotics [Basel]. 2020;9(2):49. https://doi.org/10.3390/antibiotics9020049.
11. Peng Z, Zhang X, Li X, et al. Characteristics of colistin-resistant *Escherichia coli* from pig farms in Central China. Anim Dis. 2021;1:9. https://doi.org/10.1186/s44149-021-00009-5.
12. Reardon S. Resistance to last-ditch antibiotic has spread farther than anticipated. Nature. 2017. https://doi.org/10.1038/nature.2017.22140.
13. Dadashi M, Sameni F, Bostanshirin N, Yaslianifard S, Khosravi-Dehaghi N, Nasiri MJ, et al. Global prevalence and molecular epidemiology of *mcr*-mediated colistin resistance in *Escherichia coli* clinical isolates: a systematic review. J Glob Antimicrob Resist. 2022;29:444–61. https://doi.org/10.1016/j.jgar.2021.10.022.
14. OIE Report. 2019. Available at http://www.oie.int/fileadmin/Home/eng/Our_scientific_expertise/docs/pdf/AMR/Annual_Report_AMR_3.pdf. Accessed 7 Aug 2025.
15. World Health Organization Advisory Group. Ranking of antimicrobials according to their importance in human medicine: a critical step for developing risk management strategies to control antimicrobial resistance from food animal production. Clin Infect Dis. 2016;63:1087–93. https://doi.org/10.1093/cid/ciw475.
16. Public Health Agency of Canada. CIPARS. Available at https://publications.gc.ca/site/fra/9.923025/publication.html. Accessed 6 Apr 2025.
17. Hammerum AM, Heuer OE, Emborg HD, Bagger-Skjøt L, Jensen VF, Rogues AM, Skov RL, Agersø Y, Brandt CT, Seyfarth AM, Muller A, Hovgaard K, Ajufo J, Bager F, Aarestrup FM, Frimodt-Møller N, Wegener HC, Monnet DL. Danish integrated antimicrobial resistance monitoring and research program. Emerg Infect Dis. 2007;13(11):1632–9. https://doi.org/10.3201/eid1311.070421.
18. NethMap. Consumption of antimicrobial agents and antimicrobial resistance among medically important bacteria in the Netherlands in 2023/MARAN 2024. Monitoring of antimicrobial resistance and antibiotic usage in animals in the Netherlands in 2023. 2024. Available at https://www.rivm.nl/publicaties/nethmap-2024-consumption-of-antimicrobial-agents-and-antimicrobial-resistance. Accessed 7 Apr 2025.
19. GE RM-Vet. The national resistance monitoring of animal pathogenic bacteria. Available at https://www.bvl.bund.de/DE/Arbeitsbereiche/05_Tierarzneimittel/01_Aufgaben/05_AufgAntibiotikaResistenz/05_GERMvet/GERMvet_node.html#:~:text. Accessed 8 Apr 2025.
20. Mader R, Muñoz Madero C, Aasmäe B, Bourély C, Broens EM, Busani L, Callens B, et al. Review and analysis of national monitoring systems for antimicrobial resistance in animal bacterial pathogens in Europe: a basis for the development of the European Antimicrobial Resistance Surveillance Network in Veterinary Medicine [EARS-Vet]. Front Microbiol. 2022;13:838490. https://doi.org/10.3389/fmicb.2022.838490.
21. European Antimicrobial Resistance Surveillance Network-Veterinary Medicine. Available at https://eu-jamrai.eu/surveillance/ears-vet/#:~. Accessed 9 Apr 2025.
22. European Centre for Disease Prevention and Control. European Surveillance of Antimicrobial Consumption Network [ESAC-Net]. Available at https://www.ecdc.europa.eu/en/about-us/partnerships-and-networks/disease-and-laboratory-networks/esac-net. Accessed 9 Apr 2025.
23. FAO. InFarm System. Available at https://www.fao.org/antimicrobial-resistance/resources/infarm-system/en/. Accessed 9 Apr 2025.
24. Quadripartite global integrated system for surveillance of antimicrobial resistance and antimicrobial usage (GISSA). Available at https://www.qjsamr.org/docs/librariesprovider25/default-document-library/qjs-report-vf0571b0c0-8193-4612-b54e-f972a4f5d962.pdf?sfvrsn=7f91d0cf_1. Accessed 5 July 2025.
25. World Organization for Animal Health. ANIMUSE. Available at https://amu.woah.org/amu-system-portal/home. Accessed 11 Apr 2025.

26. World Organisation for Animal Health. Annual report on antimicrobial agents intended for use in animals, 9th report. Paris; 2025, 49 pp. https://doi.org/10.20506/woah.3584. Licence: CC BYSA 3.0 IGO.
27. World Organisation for Animal Health [WOAH]. List of antimicrobial agents of veterinary importance. Paris: WOAH; 2024. Available at: https://www.woah.org/en/document/list-of-antimicrobial-agents-of-veterinary-importance/. Accessed 28 Mar 2025.
28. World Health Organization [WHO]. WHO medically important antimicrobial list. Geneva: WHO; 2024. Available at: https://www.who.int/news/item/08-02-2024-who-medically-important-antimicrobial-list-2024. Accessed 10 Apr 2025.
29. World Animal Protection. European Union bans the routine use of antibiotics in animal farms. Available at https://www.worldanimalprotection.org/latest/news/eu-bans-antibiotic-overuse-farmed-animals/. Accessed 6 Apr 2025.
30. Jansen R, Gomez-Duran O. Antibiotic reduction in the Netherlands: from challenge to leading example. Pig Progress. 2025. Available at https://www.pigprogress.net/specials/antibiotic-reduction-in-the-netherlands-from-challenge-to-leading-example/. Accessed on 1 Feb 2026.
31. Swedish Strategy to Curb Antimicrobial Resistance 2026–2035. Government Offices of Sweden. 2026. Available at https://www.government.se/information-material/2026/01/information-material-swedens-strategy-to-curb-antimicrobial-resistance-2026-2035/#. Accessed on 3 Feb 2026.
32. National Research Council [US] Committee on Drug Use in Food Animals. The use of drugs in food animals: benefits and risks. Washington, DC: National Academies Press [US]; 1999. 8. Approaches to minimizing antibiotic use in food-animal production. Available from: https://www.ncbi.nlm.nih.gov/books/NBK232568/. Accessed 7 Apr 2025.
33. Frizzo LS, Zbrun MV, Soto LP, Signorini ML. Effects of probiotics on growth performance in young calves: a meta-analysis of randomized controlled trials. Anim Feed Sci Technol. 2011;169(3–4):147–56. https://doi.org/10.1016/j.anifeedsci.2011.06.009.

Chapter 8
Environment and AMR

Abstract Antimicrobial resistance (AMR) poses a significant global health threat, with the environment playing a vital yet often underestimated role in its development and dissemination. In addition to the misuse of antibiotics in humans and animals, environmental routes—such as soil, water, air, and waste—act as reservoirs and transmission pathways for resistant bacteria and resistance genes. Sources like untreated sewage, hospital effluents, pharmaceutical waste, agricultural runoff, and livestock practices significantly contribute to environmental contamination, fostering resistance hotspots. Sub-inhibitory levels of antibiotics in soil and water apply selective pressure, while mobile genetic elements support horizontal gene transfer among microbes. People face exposure through contaminated water, food products, direct contact, or inhaling bioaerosols, which increases serious health risks for both humans and animals. Despite limited surveillance and monitoring of environmental AMR, these efforts are crucial within the One Health framework. Global and national strategies, including initiatives by UNEP and WHO, expose regulatory gaps, especially in wastewater treatment and pharmaceutical waste control. Effective mitigation requires improved wastewater treatment, proper waste disposal, responsible antibiotic use, collaboration between the public and private sectors, and heightened public awareness. Recognising the environment as a key factor in AMR is essential for sustainable management and for preserving the efficacy of antimicrobials for future generations.

Keywords Antimicrobial resistance · One Health · Environmental reservoirs · Wastewater and sewage · Pharmaceutical effluents · Agriculture and livestock · Soil and water contamination · Resistance genes · Mitigation strategies

Antimicrobial resistance (AMR) has become one of the most urgent global health issues of the twenty-first century. Once considered miracle drugs, antibiotics and other antimicrobials are quickly losing their ability to fight infections because resistant pathogens are evolving and spreading. While the overuse and misuse of antibiotics in human health and the animal industry are well-known causes, the environment—including soil, water, and waste—is increasingly recognised as a

R. Bhatia, *Drug-Resistant Infections*,
https://doi.org/10.1007/978-981-92-4190-3_8

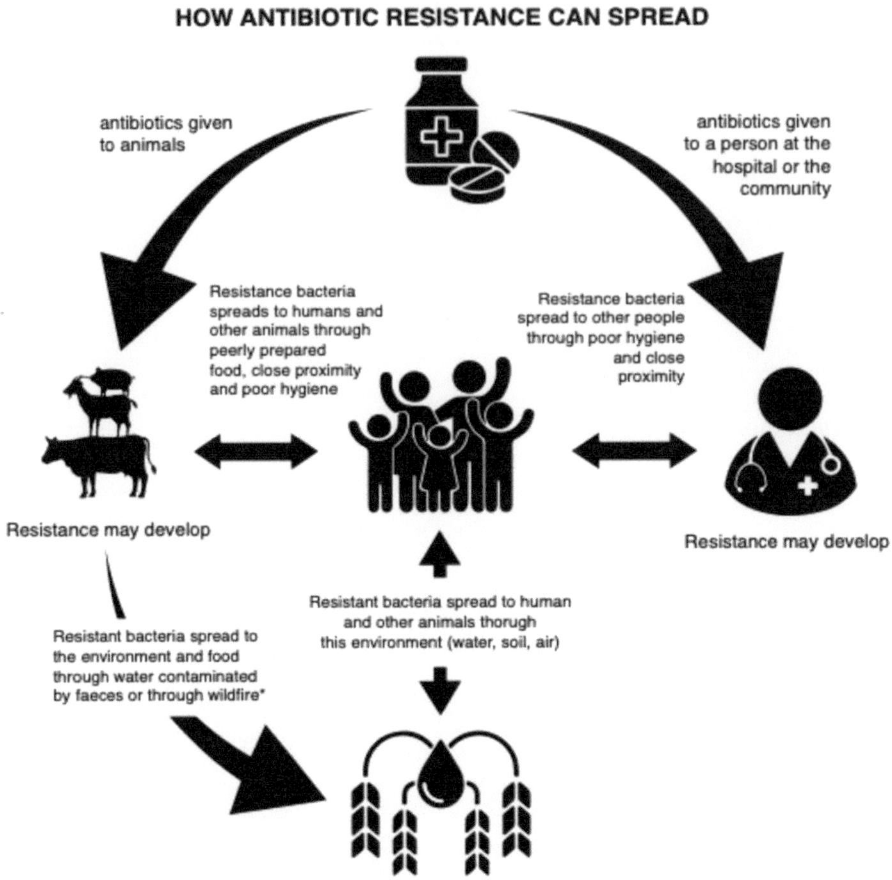

Fig. 8.1 How antibiotic resistance can spread between humans, animals, and environment

significant factor. These three interconnected sectors form an ecosystem that facilitates the transmission of resistant pathogens (Fig. 8.1). The environment can encourage the transfer of resistance and support the development of resistant strains, influenced by the presence of antibiotics and the pressure they exert. While some AMR arises naturally, the accelerated pace at which it is now occurring is largely due to anthropogenic activities—many of which intersect with the environment.

Resistance in bacteria arises naturally through genetic changes that cannot be stopped. Antibiotics, when not used properly, tend to eliminate susceptible bacteria, allowing resistant strains—if environmental conditions favour them—to become dominant. Resistance can develop wherever antibiotics interact with pathogens, not only within humans and animals, or in hospitals and veterinary settings, but also in external environments such as water and soil. Humans, animals, agriculture, and the environment are interconnected, enabling resistant bacteria or resistance genes to circulate freely across sectors within the One Health framework [1]. Environmental health, including water, sanitation, hygiene (WASH), waste management, and food safety, plays a crucial role in preventing the spread of AMR, especially in developing countries, and has the potential to mitigate this global threat.

Multiple routes of resistance spreading in the environment are well established [2, 3]. The environment—including soil, water, air, and ecosystems—plays a crucial role in the emergence, development, and spread of AMR [4]. Contaminated rivers, polluted wastewater, agricultural runoff, and unmanaged industrial discharges act as reservoirs and transmission channels for resistant bacteria and resistance genes. The interactions between the environment and AMR are complex. Several major environmental sources and pathways have been identified, and their impacts on human and animal health are thoroughly studied. Various strategies have been suggested to combat this increasing issue.

8.1 The Environment as a Reservoir and Pathway for AMR

8.1.1 Water Systems

Wastewater, which includes domestic sewage, hospital effluents, and industrial discharges, serves as a major environmental reservoir for antimicrobial-resistant bacteria (ARB) and resistance genes (ARGs) [5]. While wastewater treatment plants (WWTPs) aim to eliminate pathogens and pollutants, they frequently fail to remove resistant bacteria or resistance genes entirely. In many low- and middle-income countries, untreated or inadequately treated sewage is often discharged into rivers and lakes, contaminating natural water sources used for drinking, bathing, irrigation, and recreation [6].

Surface waters contaminated with ARBs present both direct and indirect health risks [7]. People may be exposed to this substance through recreational activities or by consuming crops that have been irrigated with it. Aquatic life, such as fish and shellfish, can serve as carriers for resistant pathogens [8].

8.1.2 Soil and Agriculture

The *agricultural use of antimicrobials*, especially in livestock farming, is a major driver of AMR. Manure from treated animals, which contains unmetabolised antibiotics and resistant bacteria, is often used as fertiliser [9]. This practice introduces antibiotics and ARGs into the soil environment.

In soil, bacteria naturally compete for survival, and the antibiotics produced by them intensify selective pressures. Soil is rich in microbial diversity and provides an ideal environment for horizontal gene transfer, promoting the spread of resistance among bacteria—including zoonotic and environmental strains that can potentially infect humans [10].

The use of pesticides and heavy metals in agriculture can also co-select for resistance [11]. Some metals, like copper and zinc, support the continued presence of resistance genes even without antibiotics, because resistance to metals and antibiotics is often genetically linked.

8.1.3 Air and Bioaerosols

Although it's less explored, airborne transmission of AMR is gaining attention as an emerging issue [12]. Bioaerosols—tiny airborne particles containing bacteria and resistance genes—may be present in the air around livestock farms, wastewater plants, and hospitals. These particles can be inhaled or settle on surfaces, offering another exposure pathway. Dust and wind can transport ARBs from farms and manure-treated land to neighbouring areas, expanding the environmental reach of AMR.

8.2 Sources of Environmental AMR Contamination

8.2.1 Human Waste and Healthcare Facilities

Hospitals and healthcare facilities use a wide range of antibiotics, and their waste often contains high concentrations of antibiotics and multidrug-resistant organisms (MDROs). Improper disposal of hospital wastewater, especially in countries with limited wastewater treatment infrastructure, significantly contributes to environmental AMR [13].

8.2.2 Pharmaceutical Manufacturing

An often overlooked but vital contributor is the pharmaceutical industry. Facilities in countries like India and China, which produce much of the world's antibiotics, have been found to release very high levels of antibiotic residues into rivers. This leads to hotspots for the development and spread of resistant bacteria [14].

Research has shown that river sediments close to these factories contain antibiotic levels that are thousands of times higher than safe environmental limits, resulting in the spread of MDROs or superbugs in these regions [15].

8.2.3 *Animal Husbandry*

Antibiotics are commonly and extensively used in animal husbandry, not just for treating infections but also to promote growth and prevent disease (Chap. 7). In countries with lax regulations, subtherapeutic doses are added to animal feed and water, thus increasing the chances of the development of resistance.

Animals release a large part of the antibiotics they consume, along with resistant bacteria, into the environment. Intensive livestock farms produce significant amounts of waste that, if not properly managed, can contaminate nearby water sources and soil [16].

The environmental aspects of AMR are diverse and interrelated. To grasp how AMR develops, transmits, and spreads in the environment, it is crucial to examine it from multiple perspectives.

According to the United Nations Environment Programme (UNEP), AMR challenges are closely linked to the triple planetary crisis of climate change, biodiversity loss and pollution and waste, all of which are driven by human activity, including unsustainable consumption and production patterns.

This broad range of environments plays a crucial role in the development, dissemination, and evolution of AMR (Fig. 8.2). Waste, sewage, and effluents containing diverse bacteria and antibiotic residues originate from numerous sources, with limited knowledge about effective treatment methods. Managing this diversity presents a significant challenge.

8.3 Environmental Persistence and Evolution of AMR

Once in the environment, antibiotics and resistance genes can persist for long periods, especially in sediments, soils, and biofilms. Sub-inhibitory concentrations of antibiotics—which are too low to kill bacteria but still apply selective pressure—are especially concerning because they promote the development of resistance without eradicating pathogens [17].

The environmental microbiome, made up of a diverse range of bacterial species, offers many chances for gene transfer. Mobile genetic elements such as plasmids can transfer ARGs between environmental bacteria and pathogens, potentially leading to new resistant strains [18]. This exchange of genes links ecological and evolutionary boundaries, affecting environmental, animal, and human health.

8.3.1 *Impacts on Human and Animal Health*

The environmental spread of AMR poses significant risks to public and animal health (Chap. 1). Environmental transmission can occur through:

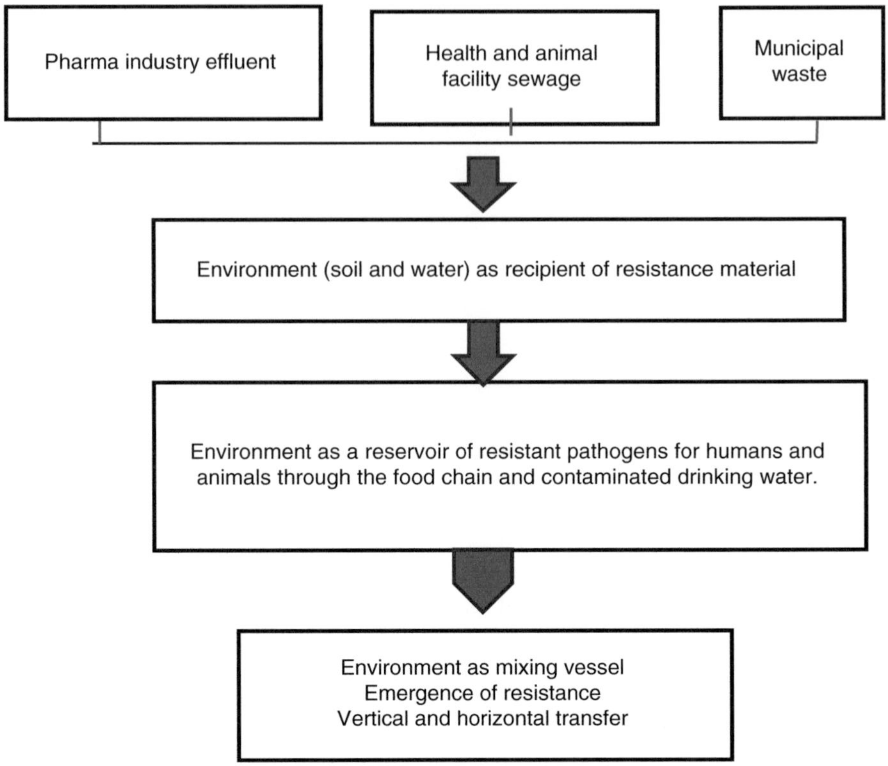

Fig. 8.2 Dynamics of AMR in environment

- Contaminated drinking water.
- Consumption of contaminated food.
- Direct contact with contaminated soil or surfaces.
- Inhalation of bioaerosols.

Communities close to polluted water sources or large-scale animal farms face especially high risks. Infections caused by resistant pathogens are more difficult and expensive to treat, tend to last longer, and have higher mortality rates. AMR also endangers the safety of surgeries, cancer treatments, organ transplants, and other advanced medical procedures that rely on effective antibiotics.

8.4 Surveillance and Monitoring

Effective environmental surveillance of AMR remains limited but is crucial. Conventional methods mainly target clinical settings and often ignore environmental factors. Adopting a "One Health" approach—which emphasises the link between human, animal, and environmental health—is essential for thorough AMR monitoring. Environmental surveillance involves [19] measuring:

- Antibiotic concentrations in water and soil.
- Prevalence of ARBs and ARGs in environmental samples.
- Genetic sequencing to identify and track resistance genes.

Advanced methods like metagenomics and quantitative polymerase chain reaction (qPCR) are increasingly utilised to analyse complex microbial communities and identify resistance genes in environmental samples [20].

8.5 Policy and Regulatory Responses on Environment and AMR

Several international organisations and national frameworks are addressing the environmental aspects of AMR. These are

The Global Action Plan on AMR [21] emphasises the importance of the environment and encourages multisectoral collaboration. The Quadripartite Alliance (FAO, WHO, WOAH, UNEP) promotes coordinated One Health strategies to tackle AMR [22]. This quadripartite arrangement between FAO, WHO, WOAH, and UNEP, through their joint action plan, has been collectively advocating and supporting acceleration of national efforts in building capacity and undertaking actions that minimise the emergence and spread of resistant pathogens.

The Stockholm Convention and Basel Convention [23] regulate hazardous waste management, indirectly supporting AMR control by addressing pharmaceutical pollution.

UN agencies, especially UNEP, have been undertaking a global advocacy, awareness, and evidence dissemination role. During the past 5 years, the United Nations Environment Assembly has advocated the impact of climate change, biodiversity loss and pollution on AMR through its resolutions (UNEP/EA.3/R4 [24]: 2018 and UNEP/EA.5/R6: 2022 [25]) calling upon countries and UN agencies to accelerate activities on environmental aspects of AMR.

Countries are increasingly incorporating environmental aspects into their National Action Plans (NAPs) on AMR, though the degree of implementation differs. These plans recognise the environmental factor and suggest measures such as surveillance, regulations on pharmaceutical effluents, and research into environmental transmission.

However, challenges remain in enforcement, inter-agency coordination, and technical capacity to monitor environmental contamination.

8.5.1 *Regulatory Gaps*

Many countries lack enforceable standards for antibiotic residues in the environment. Wastewater discharge regulations seldom specify limits for antimicrobial substances. The absence of legal policies on how to dispose of unused antibiotics and treat pharmaceutical waste continues to contribute to environmental contamination.

8.6 Mitigation Strategies

Although the link between environmental pollution, AMR, and the reservoir of resistance genes in the environment has been established, the overall significance and contribution of these factors to global AMR remain unclear. Nonetheless, enough knowledge is available to implement strategies that mitigate environmental influences on AMR. Effectively combating environmental AMR necessitates a combined approach involving regulatory, technological, and behavioural strategies.

8.6.1 *Strengthening Wastewater Treatment*

Investing in advanced treatment technologies like membrane filtration, ozonation, and activated carbon adsorption can considerably lower antimicrobial residues and resistant bacteria in wastewater.

8.6.2 *Regulating Pharmaceutical Effluents*

Establishing enforceable limits for antibiotic levels in industrial discharge is essential. In 2020, India released draft standards for antibiotic residues in pharmaceutical industry effluents, which was seen as a significant advancement, but the proposal was later withdrawn.

In August 2024, the UK National Health Service announced that pharmaceutical companies seeking contracts through its antibiotic subscription model must demonstrate compliance with responsible antibiotic manufacturing standards, as certified by BSI, in accordance with the AMRIA Antibiotic Manufacturing Standard [26].

In 2024, the WHO issued its first guidance on antibiotic pollution from manufacturing [27]. This new guidance addresses wastewater and solid waste management for antibiotic production, setting human health-based targets to lower the risk of AMR and protecting aquatic life from all antibiotics used in humans, animals, or plants. It covers each stage, from manufacturing active pharmaceutical ingredients and formulations to producing finished products, including primary packaging. In the future, countries might develop their own standards based on this guidance.

8.7 Responsible Use of Antibiotics in the Environment

Phasing out non-therapeutic antibiotic use in agriculture, promoting antimicrobial stewardship in healthcare, and limiting the sale of over-the-counter antibiotics are essential steps to reduce environmental contamination.

8.7.1 Safe Manure and Sludge Management

Composting, anaerobic digestion, and various other treatment methods can lower microbial loads and antibiotic residues in animal waste and sewage sludge prior to land application.

8.7.2 Public–Private Partnership

Private companies have the ability to develop and deploy innovative technologies to address environmental issues, including renewable energy, carbon capture, and waste management. Collaboration between governments and private entities through public–private partnerships can facilitate the implementation of environmental projects and help achieve common sustainability objectives.

8.7.3 Public Awareness and Research

Raising awareness among the public and stakeholders about how AMR spreads through environmental pathways can encourage safer practices. Additional research is necessary to understand the fate of resistance genes in various ecological matrices and to evaluate the effectiveness of mitigation strategies.

AMR is not just a medical concern but a complex environmental crisis. The environment acts as both a reservoir and a pathway for resistant bacteria and genes. Human activities, especially from the healthcare, agriculture, and pharmaceutical sectors, contribute to the faster spread of AMR in nature.

8.8 Emerging Perspectives on Impact of Environment on AMR

The environmental aspects of AMR are diverse and interrelated. To grasp how AMR develops, transmits, and spreads in the environment, it is crucial to examine it from multiple perspectives.

Environmental contamination with antibiotics and co-selective agents, along with active horizontal gene transfer and ecological dissemination mechanisms, collectively provide strong evidence linking environmental factors to the emergence and spread of AMR. Therefore, addressing AMR requires integrated surveillance and mitigation across clinical, agricultural, and environmental domains.

AMR is becoming more prominent as both an environmental and clinical issue. Environmental reservoirs—such as soil, water, air, and living organisms—are essential in the development, persistence, and spread of antimicrobial resistance genes (ARGs).[1] The connection between environmental influences and the rise of AMR is supported by multiple mechanistic and ecological evidence.

Environmental matrices are influenced by antimicrobial selection pressure, leading to the proliferation of resistant organisms. Antibiotics and biocides contaminate the environment through effluent from wastewater treatment plants, agricultural runoff, aquaculture discharge, and improper pharmaceutical disposal. Surface waters often contain antibiotic concentrations—such as sulfamethoxazole and ciprofloxacin—that surpass minimal selective concentrations, which are the thresholds where resistant subpopulations begin to dominate. Even small levels can promote resistance in environmental bacterial communities by inducing de novo mutations and horizontal gene transfer. Research indicates that environmental antibiotic pollution correlates with higher levels of ARGs in sediments and biofilms, irrespective of clinical antibiotic use [28].

Horizontal gene transfer mechanisms like transformation,[2] transduction,[3] and especially conjugation[4] are highly active in the environment. Mobile genetic

---

[1] ARG: ARGs are specific segments of DNA that enable bacteria, to withstand the effects of antibiotics and other antimicrobial agents. These genetic elements encode proteins that protect microbes—such as enzymes that degrade drugs or efflux pumps that remove them—allowing bacteria to survive and flourish despite treatment. ARGs work by directing the synthesis of enzymes that break down drugs, modifying the drug's target site, or exporting the drug out of the cell. These genes can be transmitted between bacteria.

[2] Transformation: Bacterial transformation is a form of horizontal gene transfer where competent bacteria uptake naked, foreign DNA from their environment and incorporate it into their own genome, often resulting in new phenotypic traits which may be resistant to antibiotics.

[3] Transduction: Transduction in bacteria is a form of horizontal gene transfer where foreign DNA is introduced into a bacterial cell via a virus, specifically a bacteriophage, without direct cell-to-cell contact.

[4] Conjugation: Bacterial conjugation is a mechanism of horizontal gene transfer where genetic material (usually a plasmid) is transferred from a donor bacterium to a recipient cell through direct physical contact, often via a structure called a pilus.

elements (MGEs), such as plasmids, integrons, and transposons, act as vectors for transferring antibiotic resistance genes (ARGs) among phylogenetically diverse bacteria. Environmental hotspots, like river sediments downstream of wastewater treatment plant (WWTP) effluent, contain high densities of MGEs and ARGs. One study found that class 1 integrons—key drivers of multidrug resistance—were 100 to 1000 times more abundant in impacted areas than in upstream reference sites, indicating human influence on horizontal gene transfer potential [29].

Furthermore, soil microbiomes exposed to manure fertilization show increased levels of plasmid-borne ARGs, linking agricultural practices to environmental gene transfer networks. Third, ecological co-selection pressures enhance AMR reservoirs. Heavy metals, pesticides, and other toxicants in soils and waters can co-select for resistance, as many resistance determinants (such as efflux pumps) provide cross-protection. Environments contaminated with copper, zinc, or arsenic—common in mining and intensive agriculture areas—display higher ARG frequencies [30].

Microcosm experiments reveal that co-exposure to metals and sub-inhibitory antibiotics accelerates the fixation of multidrug resistance traits relative to exposure to antibiotics alone.

Environmental dissemination pathways enable the widespread distribution of resistance. Aerosols from farms, irrigation return flows, and flooding can transport resistant bacteria and ARGs across regions. Wildlife, such as migratory birds and insects, serve as vectors, spreading environmental AMR beyond borders. Metagenomic studies of air particles downwind of concentrated animal feeding operations reveal a variety of ARG profiles similar to those in manure lagoons, indicating that aerosolisation contributes to the spread of AMR.

The climate and hydrological changes affect the spread of AMR. Higher temperatures can boost microbial growth and mutation rates [31]. Heavy rainfall events cause contaminants to run off into water bodies, while drought conditions lead to higher concentrations of pollutants and microbes. Seasonal variations impact community makeup and gene transfer rates. These environmental factors interact with human activities to influence the timing and location of AMR prevalence.

UNEP [1] states that AMR challenges are strongly connected to the triple planetary crisis—comprising climate change, biodiversity loss, and pollution and waste—all of which are caused by human activities such as unsustainable consumption and production.

Ignoring the environmental aspect of AMR can weaken global efforts to tackle it. A coordinated, multisectoral, and worldwide response—based on the One Health approach—is crucial. This involves enhancing wastewater management, controlling industrial emissions, improving surveillance, and promoting responsible antimicrobial use across various sectors.

Only by recognising and tackling the environmental origins of AMR can we ensure the continued effectiveness of antimicrobials for future generations and safeguard global health.

References

1. United Nations Environment Programme. Bracing for superbugs: strengthening environmental action in the One Health response to antimicrobial resistance. Geneva; 2023. Available at: https://www.unep.org/resources/superbugs/environmental-action. Accessed 9 Apr 2025.
2. Musoke D, Namata C, Lubega GB, et al. The role of Environmental Health in preventing antimicrobial resistance in low- and middle-income countries. Environ Health Prev Med. 2021;26:100. https://doi.org/10.1186/s12199-021-01023-2.
3. Larsson DGJ, Flach CF. Antibiotic resistance in the environment. Nat Rev Microbiol. 2022;20:257–69. https://doi.org/10.1038/s41579-021-00649-x.
4. Sassi A, Basher NS, Kirat H, Meradji S, Ibrahim NA, Idres T, Touati A. The role of the environment (water, air, soil) in the emergence and dissemination of antimicrobial resistance: a one health perspective. Antibiotics. 2025;14(8):764. https://doi.org/10.3390/antibiotics14080764.
5. La Rosa MC, Maugeri A, Favara G, La Mastra C, Magnano San Lio R, Barchitta M, Agodi A. The impact of wastewater on antimicrobial resistance: a scoping review of transmission pathways and contributing factors. Antibiotics (Basel). 2025;14(2):131. https://doi.org/10.3390/antibiotics14020131.
6. Flach KA, Bones UA, Wolff DB, Silveira A d O, da Rosa GM, Carissimi E, Silvestri S. Antibiotic resistant bacteria and genes (ARB and ARG) in water and sewage treatment units: a review. Environ Nanotechnol Monit Manag. 2024;21:100941. https://doi.org/10.1016/j.enmm.2024.100941.
7. Singh AK, Kaur R, Verma S, Singh S. Antimicrobials and antibiotic resistance genes in water bodies: pollution, risk, and control. Front Environ Sci. 2022;10:1. https://doi.org/10.3389/fenvs.2022.830861.
8. Thibodeau AJ, Barret M, Mouchet F, Nguyen VX, Pinelli E. The potential contribution of aquatic wildlife to antibiotic resistance dissemination in freshwater ecosystems: a review. Environ Pollut. 2024;350:123894. https://doi.org/10.1016/j.envpol.2024.123894.
9. Fu Y, Hu F, Wang F, Xu M, Jia Z, Amelung W, Mei Z, Han X, Virta M, Jiang X, Tiedje JM. Field-based evidence for the prevalence of soil antibiotic resistomes under long-term antibiotic-free fertilization. Environ Int. 2025;195:109202. https://doi.org/10.1016/j.envint.2024.109202.
10. Gentile A, Di Stasio L, Oliva G, Vigliotta G, Cicatelli A, Guarino F, Guidi Nissim W, Labra M, Castiglione S. Antibiotic resistance in urban soils: dynamics and mitigation strategies. Environ Res. 2024;263:120120. https://doi.org/10.1016/j.envint.2024.109202.
11. Zhang Y, Wang H, Hu M, Cai R, Miao Y, Zhu X. Heavy metals potentially drive co-selection of antibiotic resistance genes by shifting soil bacterial communities in paddy soils along the middle and lower Yangtze River. Pedosphere. 2024;34:606–19. https://doi.org/10.1016/j.pedsph.2023.01.012.
12. Chen ZY, Gao FZ, Bai H, Zhang M, He LY, Liu YS, Ying GG. Key contribution and risk of airborne antibiotic resistance: total suspended particles or settled dust? Environ Sci Technol. 2025;10:10788–98. https://doi.org/10.1021/acs.est.4c11038.
13. Hounmanou YMG, Houefonde A, I-CRECT Consortium, Nguyen TT, Dalsgaard A. Mitigating antimicrobial resistance through effective hospital wastewater management in low- and middle-income countries. Front Public Health. 2025;12:1525873. https://doi.org/10.3389/fpubh.2024.1525873.
14. Macedo H E, Lehner B, Nicell JA, Khan U, Klein EY. Antibiotics in the global river system arising from human consumption. PNAS Nexus. 2025;4(4):pgaf096. https://doi.org/10.1093/pnasnexus/pgaf096.
15. Pharmaceutical effluent evokes superbugs in the environment: a call to action. Biosaf Health. 2023;05(06):363–71. Available at https://mednexus.org/doi/abs/10.1016/j.bsheal.2023.10.005. Accessed 9 Apr 2025.

16. Zhang T, Nickerson R, Zhang W, Peng X, Shang Y, Zhou Y, Luo Q, Wen G, Cheng Z. The impacts of animal agriculture on One Health—bacterial zoonosis, antimicrobial resistance, and beyond. One Health. 2024;18:100748. https://doi.org/10.1016/j.onehlt.2024.100748.
17. Rajendra S, Kim K. Environmental occurrence of antibiotic resistance, control measures and challenges in finding therapeutic management. Emerging Contam. 2025;11:100440. https://doi.org/10.1016/j.emcon.2024.100440.
18. Rana C, Vikas V, Awasthi S, Gautam D, Vats A, Rajput S, Behera M, Ludri A, Berwal A, Singh D, De S. Antimicrobial resistance genes and associated mobile genetic elements in Escherichia coli from human, animal and environment. Chemosphere. 2024;369:143808. https://doi.org/10.1016/j.chemosphere.2024.143808.
19. Hart A, Warren J, Wilkinson H, Schmidt W. Environmental surveillance of antimicrobial resistance (AMR), perspectives from a national environmental regulator in 2023. Euro Surveill. 2023;28(11):2200367. https://doi.org/10.2807/1560-7917.ES.2023.28.11.2200367.
20. Mao Y, Shisler JL, Nguyen TH. Enhanced detection for antibiotic resistance genes in wastewater samples using a CRISPR-enriched metagenomic method. Water Res. 2025;274:123056. https://doi.org/10.1016/j.watres.2024.123056.
21. WHO. Global action plan on AMR. 2015. Available at https://www.who.int/publications/i/item/9789241509763. Accessed 5 Apr 2025.
22. UNEP. Quadripartite One Health joint action plan (2022–2026). Available at https://www.unep.org/resources/publication/one-health-joint-plan-action-2022-2026. Accessed 4 Apr 2025.
23. UNEP/POPS/. SC-5/9: measures to reduce or eliminate releases from wastes. Available at https://www.pops.int/implementation/wastestockpiles/overview/tabid/446/default.aspx. Accessed 6 Apr 2025.
24. United Nations Environment Assembly of UNEP. Resolution ¾. 2018. Available at https://wedocs.unep.org/bitstream/handle/20.500.11822/30795/UNEA3_4EN.pdf?sequence=1&isAllowed=y. Accessed 7 Apr 2025.
25. United Nations Environment Assembly of UNEP. Resolution 5/6. 2022–2023. Available at https://wedocsuneporg/bitstream/handle/. Accessed 1 Apr 2025.
26. AMR Industry Alliance. UK's NHS to require companies to meet responsible antibiotic manufacturing standards. Available at https://www.amrindustryalliance.org/mediaroom/uks-nhs-to-require-companies-to-meet-responsible-antibiotic-manufacturing-standard/#. Accessed 2 Apr 2025.
27. WHO. New global guidance aims to curb antibiotic pollution from manufacturing. Available at https://www.who.int/news/item/03-09-2024-new-global-guidance-aims-to-curb-antibiotic-pollution-from-manufacturing. Accessed 3 Apr 2025.
28. Li Z, Tang J, Wang X, Ma X, Yuan H, Gao C, Guo Q, Guo X, Wan J, Dagot C. The environmental lifecycle of antibiotics and resistance genes: transmission mechanisms, challenges, and control strategies. Microorganisms. 2025;13(9):2113. https://doi.org/10.3390/microorganisms13092113.
29. Berglund B. Environmental dissemination of antibiotic resistance genes and correlation to anthropogenic contamination with antibiotics. Infect Ecol Epidemiol. 2015;5(1):28564. https://doi.org/10.3402/iee.v5.28564.
30. Zou H-Y, Gao F-Z, He L-Y, Zhang M, Liu Y-S, Qi J, Ying G-G. Prevalence of antibiotic resistance genes in mining-impacted farmland environments. Ecotoxicol Environ Saf. 2025;289:117651. https://doi.org/10.1016/j.ecoenv.2024.117651.
31. Dutta SS. Climate change is accelerating antibiotic resistance across the Western Pacific. News-Medical. 2026. Available at https://www.news-medical.net/news/20260206/Climate-change-is-accelerating-antibiotic-resistance-across-the-Western-Pacific.aspx. Accessed on 5 Feb 2026.

Chapter 9
Private Sector and AMR Containment

Abstract The private sector plays a pivotal role in global health systems, contributing significantly to healthcare delivery, innovation, and economic development. Its involvement in combating antimicrobial resistance (AMR) is particularly crucial in low- and middle-income countries where private providers, laboratories, and pharmaceutical companies dominate service delivery. The sector supports infrastructure development, research, diagnostics, and awareness generation, while also complementing public sector gaps through public–private partnerships. In human health, private clinics influence antibiotic prescribing practices, and laboratories generate valuable surveillance data. In veterinary health, private practitioners, drug manufacturers, and service providers ensure animal care, herd management, and vaccine delivery, while also shaping antimicrobial use practices that are central to AMR containment. Environmentally, private industries can mitigate resistance risks by adopting sustainable manufacturing standards and reducing antibiotic discharge. Global initiatives, such as the Davos Compact on AMR, UCARE, the AMR Industry Alliance, and Investor Action on AMR, demonstrate structured private engagement. Despite challenges—such as profit orientation, weak regulation, and limited incentives—strengthening partnerships, harmonising policies, and fostering innovation are essential for leveraging the private sector's strengths in safeguarding human, animal, and environmental health against AMR.

Keywords Private sector · Antimicrobial resistance · Public–private partnerships · Antimicrobial stewardship · Veterinary services · Sustainable manufacturing · Global AMR initiatives

The private sector plays a significant role in human health, particularly in healthcare delivery, innovation, and economic development. Although its involvement can be complex and raise questions about equity and quality [1], it contributes to the national health system in the following ways:

Healthcare Delivery The private sector provides a substantial amount of healthcare services globally, including specialised treatments, diagnostics, and primary

R. Bhatia, *Drug-Resistant Infections*,
https://doi.org/10.1007/978-981-92-4190-3_9

care. In some developing countries, the role played by the private sector is greater than that of the public sector in providing curative services [2].

Infrastructure Development Private investment in healthcare facilities, equipment, and technology can improve access to care and enhance the overall healthcare infrastructure in a given geographical area or the entire country. Private companies are developing mobile health (mHealth) technologies to improve access to healthcare information, diagnostics, and remote patient monitoring.

Innovation and Research The private sector drives innovation in medical technologies, pharmaceuticals, and healthcare delivery models, resulting in advancements in treatment and care. Countries like India are recognised as global pharmacies because of the significant contribution of the private sector. The private sector is essential in developing, producing, and distributing vaccines, supporting global health security.

Economic Growth The private healthcare industry generates employment, stimulates economic activity, and can contribute to a country's GDP.

Medical Tourism In certain countries, the private sector serves as a hub for medical tourism [3], attracting patients who seek specialised treatments and procedures, which in turn increases revenue and stimulates local economic growth.

Flexibility and Responsiveness Private healthcare providers can be more adaptable to changing needs and offer more personalised, patient-centric care.

Addressing Public Sector Gaps In many settings, the private sector fills gaps in public healthcare services, particularly in areas where public resources are limited or access is restricted.

Public–Private Partnerships Many countries have leveraged collaborations between public and private entities to harness the strengths of both sectors, improving healthcare outcomes, especially in several national health programmes of importance [4].

Despite the significant contribution of the private health sector in various domains of the healthcare system, given its fundamental tenet of being a profit-making entity, several challenges and considerations are faced in all countries. These issues pertain to unequal access, high cost, and, in some places, provision of services of questionable quality. The private sector's long-term sustainability and its contribution to universal health coverage depend on factors like financial viability, quality of care, and equitable access.

Nevertheless, the private sector remains a vital player in the global healthcare landscape, making significant contributions to healthcare delivery, innovation, and economic development. Addressing the challenges related to equity, quality, and affordability is crucial to ensure that the private sector's potential benefits are realised by all segments of society [5].

9.1 Potential Role of Private Health Sector in Containing AMR

The private sector plays a vital role in combating antimicrobial resistance (AMR), particularly in low- and middle-income countries, where it often constitutes a significant portion of healthcare services. Private healthcare providers, drug sellers, and laboratories all contribute to AMR through antibiotic use, sales, and data collection. Engaging the private sector through public–private partnerships, encouraging antimicrobial stewardship, and setting up regulatory frameworks are critical actions to reduce AMR. Private clinics and doctors frequently prescribe and dispense antibiotics, which can lead to AMR if not managed responsibly.

Private laboratories generate valuable antimicrobial susceptibility data, which can be crucial for surveillance and informing treatment decisions. Private laboratories can contribute to national AMR surveillance systems by sharing data on antibiotic susceptibility patterns.

Private sector stakeholders can play a key role in raising awareness about AMR, promoting responsible antibiotic use, and educating patients and employees. Private healthcare providers can implement internal antimicrobial stewardship programmes (AMSP) to reduce unnecessary antibiotic use within their workforce and supply chains. Encouraging the adoption of best practices, such as infection prevention and control (IPC) measures, can help minimise the spread of AMR. The private pharmaceutical industry must also move away from sales incentives that encourage the over-prescription or over-selling of antibiotics.

The private sector can advocate for stronger policies and regulations to combat AMR at national and international levels. Companies can play a role in raising public awareness about AMR through various communication channels, including social media, workshops, and seminars. Private sector entities can support community-based initiatives that educate the public about AMR and promote responsible antibiotic use. By actively engaging in these strategies, the private sector has the potential to play a vital role in containing the spread of AMR and safeguarding global health.

9.1.1 Role of Private Corporate Sector in Containing AMR

The private corporate health sector has a crucial role in fighting AMR, especially in developing countries such as India, where many outpatient and inpatient services are provided by private facilities. Due to its size, resources, and impact on prescribing, diagnostics, and pharmaceutical markets, the corporate health sector can notably influence the progress of AMR management.

Private hospitals play a key role in antimicrobial stewardship (AMS). Corporate hospital chains generally have superior infrastructure, including microbiology laboratories, infection control teams, and electronic medical records. These resources support the development of evidence-based antibiotic policies, formulary restrictions, prospective audits, feedback mechanisms, and antibiotic usage surveillance. Through establishing stewardship committees and connecting prescription audits to clinician accountability, private hospitals can decrease the misuse of antibiotics, especially broad-spectrum and last-resort options.

Private laboratories and diagnostic companies play a vital role in enhancing access to quick, reliable diagnostics. Prompt microbiological confirmation helps minimise unnecessary antibiotic use and supports appropriate de-escalation. Investment by companies in automated blood culture systems, molecular diagnostics, and antimicrobial susceptibility testing improves early detection of resistant pathogens. Incorporating diagnostic stewardship into clinical pathways ensures antibiotics are prescribed based on solid evidence rather than guesswork.

The private sector plays a role in infection prevention and control (IPC). Corporate hospitals frequently adhere to international accreditation standards like Joint Commission International or India's National Accreditation Board for Hospitals & Healthcare Providers. These standards require comprehensive IPC practices, hand hygiene adherence, infection surveillance, and antimicrobial policy enforcement. Effective IPC efforts lessen resistant infections and decrease transmission within healthcare facilities.

Pharmaceutical companies play a vital role in combating AMR by promoting responsible marketing and investing in research. Ethical promotion of antibiotics, discouraging incentives that lead to over-prescription, and supporting prescriber education are critical. The global AMR Industry Alliance exemplifies industry commitment through responsible manufacturing, controlling effluents to minimise environmental impact, and maintaining transparency in antibiotic promotion. Additionally, private sector investments in R&D for new antimicrobials, vaccines, and diagnostics help fill the innovation gap in the AMR pipeline.

Corporate hospitals have the capability to generate and share surveillance data. Engaging in national and international surveillance platforms, like the Global Antimicrobial Resistance and Use Surveillance System, improves data representativeness and quality. Data from the private sector are especially crucial in countries where the majority of antibiotic use happens outside public health systems. Transparent reporting underpins evidence-based policies and treatment guidelines at the national level.

Furthermore, the private corporate sector bears a responsibility to tackle community-level factors contributing to AMR. By implementing outpatient stewardship, telemedicine protocols, and standardised treatment guidelines, private providers can curb unnecessary antibiotic prescriptions for viral illnesses. Additionally, corporate chains can run patient awareness campaigns in line with national initiatives like World Antimicrobial Awareness Week, reinforcing messages about rational antibiotic use among their extensive patient populations.

The private sector faces several challenges in managing AMR. Financial motivations linked to service volume, patient expectations for fast results, and competitive pressures can encourage overprescribing. Therefore, establishing regulatory frameworks, reforming insurance reimbursement systems, and aligning quality metrics with stewardship objectives are essential to encourage responsible prescribing. Furthermore, public–private partnerships can support standardisation and unified reporting.

National authorities need to recognise that the private corporate health sector is not just a stakeholder but a key player in combating AMR. Engaging in stewardship, diagnostics, infection control, responsible pharmaceutical practices, surveillance, and public engagement can significantly decrease inappropriate antimicrobial use and hinder the development and spread of resistance. Aligning corporate incentives with public health objectives is essential to unlock this potential.

9.2 Role of Private Veterinary Sector in Containing AMR

Antibiotics are used in animals to treat infections, prevent disease outbreaks, and, in some cases, promote growth (Chap. 7). While antibiotics are crucial for animal health and welfare, their use, particularly in food production, is under scrutiny due to concerns about the development and spread of AMR.

The private sector plays a crucial role in delivering veterinary services, complementing the public sector by providing a wider range of services, including clinical diagnosis and treatment, the production and distribution of drugs and vaccines, artificial insemination, and herd health management. Private practitioners are often the first point of contact for individual animal owners and can contribute significantly to disease surveillance, workforce capacity building, vaccine production and containment of AMR.

Private veterinarians provide essential clinical diagnosis and treatment services for individual animals, addressing a wide range of health issues, including infectious diseases that require the administration of antibiotics to the sick animal. They also offer preventive care, including vaccinations and parasite control, and promote best practices for animal health and welfare.

The private sector is involved in the production and distribution of veterinary drugs and vaccines, ensuring their availability to animal owners. They offer artificial insemination services, contributing to improved animal breeding and productivity. Private veterinarians play a vital role in managing herd health, helping farmers optimise animal production and minimise disease outbreaks. These activities also require judicious use of antibiotics, thus play a role in the prevention and control of AMR.

Private veterinary practitioners have the potential to undertake tasks traditionally carried out by the public sector, supporting national disease control programmes and other initiatives. Efficient public–private partnership (PPP) policies facilitate structured engagement between the public and private sectors, ensuring long-term investment and participation in veterinary services.

The private pharmaceutical organisations are engaged in the production and distribution of veterinary products, contribute to research and development, and provide specialised services.

By fostering a strong and collaborative relationship between the public and private sectors, countries can ensure a robust and effective veterinary service system that supports animal health, public health, and the overall livestock sector. Judicious use of antibiotics in animals is critical for any national initiative to control AMR [6].

9.3 Private Sector and Environmental Aspects of AMR

The private sector is vital for environmental protection, as it fosters innovation, offers resources, and shapes policy. Although it can cause environmental damage, its capacity to bring about positive change is substantial. This involves creating green technologies, adopting sustainable practices, and supporting stricter environmental regulations.

The private sector can significantly contribute to global efforts in containing AMR by engaging in responsible manufacturing practices, investing in research and development (R&D) for new antibiotics and diagnostics, promoting AMSP, and collaborating with governments and other stakeholders in maintaining freedom of the environment from a milieu that encourages the development of resistance in pathogens.

The private sector can minimise the release of antibiotics into the environment during manufacturing by implementing best practices, establishing discharge targets, and developing monitoring frameworks. Collaboration with suppliers is crucial for assessing and mitigating AMR risks throughout the entire supply chain, thereby preventing the spread of resistant bacteria.

The private sector should keep in consideration the interconnectedness of human, animal, and environmental health when developing new solutions and focus on addressing AMR across all sectors.

At a micro level, the companies can educate their employees and the public about AMR and the importance of responsible antibiotic use. Engaging with civil society organisations (CSOs) can help raise awareness, promote responsible use, and ensure accountability in AMR efforts.

9.4 Private Sector Initiatives to Contain AMR

Private sector initiatives have the potential to play a crucial role in combating AMR by focusing on R&D, promoting the responsible use of antibiotics, ensuring access to quality medicines, setting manufacturing standards, and minimising environmental impact from manufacturing [7]. Examples of these initiatives are presented in Box 9.1.

Box 9.1 Private Sector Initiatives in the AMR Ecosystem

- Davos Compact on AMR
- United Coalition for AMR Response (UCARE)
- Corporate AMR Responsibility (CARE) for the future
- AMR Industry Alliance against AMR (AMRIA)
- Multistakeholder Partnership Platform (MSPP)
- Investor Action on AMR (IAAMR)

9.4.1 Davos Compact on AMR

Following the UNGA High-Level meeting on AMR (2024) (Chap. 3) and the adoption of its political declaration, the World Economic Forum's Global Future Council on the Future of Tackling AMR developed the Davos Compact on AMR [8]. The compact has received inputs and support from the Quadripartite Joint Secretariat on AMR. It was launched on January 23, 2025, at the World Economic Forum's annual meeting in Davos.

The *Davos Compact on AMR* is now turning political commitments from the 2024 UN High-Level Meeting on AMR into actionable private-sector efforts. A significant milestone has been rallying corporate leaders from healthcare, pharmaceuticals, diagnostics, insurance, and finance around a shared accountability framework aligned with the Unified Coalition for AMR Response (UCARE). Several multinational firms have publicly pledged to boost antimicrobial stewardship in hospitals, increase transparency in antibiotic marketing, and strengthen environmental protections within manufacturing supply chains.

The compact has fostered organised dialogue among industry, governments, and multilateral agencies, aligning corporate efforts with national AMR strategies. Early achievements include creating standardised metrics for private-sector reporting, encouraging responsible antibiotic procurement, and supporting innovations in diagnostics and new antimicrobials. Additionally, it has raised the profile of AMR in boardroom risk and sustainability conversations, framing antimicrobial resistance as a key global health and economic priority instead of just a public health concern.

The compact outlines the key areas of need for private sector engagement and collaboration in response to the UN political Declaration on AMR. In doing so, it highlights the key areas of focus and impact for the Forum's future work in tackling AMR with the Unified Coalition for the AMR Response (UCARE).

9.4.2 United Coalition for AMR Response (UCARE)

Under the auspices of the Unified Coalition for the AMR Response (UCARE) [9], several governments and philanthropic organisations have agreed to collaborate to create an environment that incentivises private sector investment in tackling AMR. This collaborative effort aims to attract significant financial resources by fostering partnerships and leveraging the strengths of various stakeholders from both global and local businesses to fund and deploy innovative solutions for combating drug-resistant infections.

Governments and philanthropic organisations propose working together to establish the necessary conditions, such as policy frameworks and financial incentives, to attract private sector investment. In return, businesses are expected to commit substantial financial resources to develop and implement solutions for AMR.

UCARE collaborates with other international initiatives, such as the Global Leaders Group on AMR and shall do so with the upcoming Independent Panel for Evidence for Action against AMR,[1] to maximise the impact of their work. The ultimate goal is to unlock sustainable financing from both public and private sources for reducing global deaths associated with AMR and saving millions of lives.

UCARE recognises that collaborative efforts between the public and private sectors to address AMR will ensure sustainable financing for a healthier, safer, and more resilient world for future generations. Together, the members of UCARE are committed to applying a One Health, multisectoral approach. This will help to mobilise the financial resources required to achieve the global goal of reducing the deaths associated with AMR, saving more than 100 million lives by 2050 [10].

9.4.3 Corporate AMR Responsibility (CARE) for the Future

Responsible manufacturing practices play a pivotal role in addressing the global challenge of AMR. This involves not only adopting environmentally friendly processes and minimising waste but also ensuring that the production of antibiotics aligns with international guidelines for responsible use. To contribute effectively to the fight against AMR, businesses can integrate these practices into their operations and transparently disclose their efforts to promote transparency and accountability.

9.4.4 AMR Industry Alliance Against AMR (AMRIA)

The AMR Industry Alliance (AMRIA) is a major private-sector coalition focused on delivering sustainable solutions to AMR [11]. It includes over 100 biotech, diagnostic, generic, and research-based pharmaceutical companies, as well as associations. The alliance encompasses the commercial production of antibiotic active

[1] Likely to be operational in 2026.

ingredients and drug products, accounting for approximately 30% of global human antibiotic manufacturing. In 2018, AMRIA introduced the Common Antibiotic Manufacturing Framework, which employs a risk-based approach to assess and manage antibiotic manufacturing waste streams. In 2022, to formalise this framework, AMRIA published its Antibiotic Manufacturing Standard, establishing numerical emission standards at the production site to mitigate the development of antibiotic resistance and aquatic ecotoxicity in the environment caused by antibiotics intended for human use. In 2023, the British Standards Institution (BSI) established a certification scheme to ensure antibiotics are produced in accordance with AMRIA standards. This scheme helps global manufacturers verify responsible antibiotic production and reduce environmental AMR risks [12].

The AMR Industry Alliance was established in May 2017, building on two key industry pledges to combat AMR: the January 2016 "Declaration by the Pharmaceutical, Biotechnology, and Diagnostics Industries on Combating Antimicrobial Resistance" [11] and, during the first UN High-level Meeting on AMR in September 2016, the "Industry Roadmap for Progress on Combating Antimicrobial Resistance" [13]. The Alliance ensures that members from the biotech, diagnostics, generics, and research-based pharmaceutical sectors collectively fulfil the commitments outlined in these documents and track progress in combating AMR. It aligns its efforts around four key pillars: manufacturing, R&D, access, and responsible use [14] (Fig. 9.1).

Since launching in 2017, the AMR Industry Alliance has consistently met its commitments and continues to do so. In 2018, the Alliance introduced the Common Antibiotic Manufacturing Framework and published its initial list of discharge targets for antibiotics, including the predicted no-effect concentration (PNEC), with updates to these targets planned over time. Building on this Framework, the Alliance released a manufacturing standard in 2022. Since 2023, it has partnered with the independent, non-profit British Standards Institution to offer a certification programme for both member and non-member manufacturers who adhere to this Standard [15].

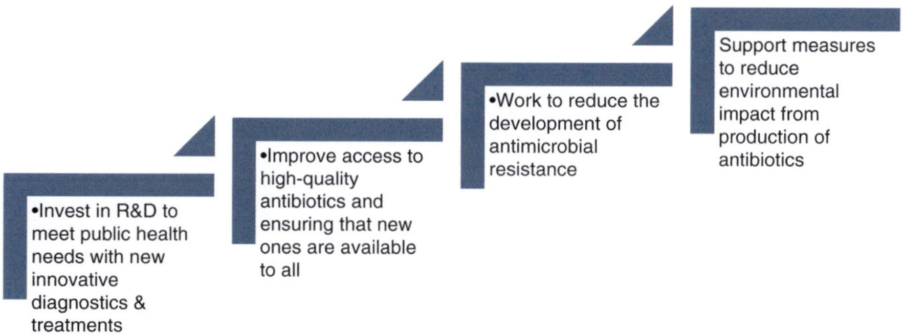

Fig. 9.1 Four major areas of work by AMRIA

9.4.5 *Multistakeholder Partnership Platform*

The AMR Multistakeholder Partnership Platform (MSPP) is part of global governance structures on AMR, including the AMR Global Leaders Group. Facilitated by the Quadripartite, composed of the Food and Agriculture Organisation of the UN (FAO), the World Health Organisation (WHO), the World Organisation for Animal Health (WOAH, previously known as OIE), and the United Nations Environment Programme (UNEP), the platform serves as a voluntary, collaborative mechanism for coordination. It aims to be an inclusive, international, multistakeholder forum that brings together stakeholders from human, animal, plant, and environmental sectors to help preserve antimicrobials as lifesaving medicines and promote their responsible use within a One Health framework [16].

The MSPP remains a vital platform for engaging the private sector. It enables industries to collaborate internally and with other sectors, such as those related to human and environmental health. Additionally, it fosters meaningful dialogue and public–private partnerships with key stakeholders, including governments, research institutions, academia, and civil society. This private sector cluster now includes 11 members, including industry networks and federations focused on AMR across the One Health spectrum within the Platform.

To fulfil the Political Declaration from the high-level UNGA meeting on AMR (2024), several MSPP members, including Health for Animals, the International Poultry Council, the International Feed Industry Federation, the International Meat Secretariat, and the World Farmer's Organization, along with FAO, agreed [17] to support the implementation of various commitments made by the UNGA, including addressing specific needs (Box 9.2).

Box 9.2 Possible Contribution of MSPP in Contributing to UNGA Commitments

- Significantly reducing the global use of antibiotics in agrifood systems by 2030 from current levels.
- Ensuring that antibiotics use in animals and agriculture is prudent and responsible.
- Developing further global guidance to prevent and reduce the use of antibiotics in plants and agriculture.
- Establishing defined animal vaccination strategies with implementation plans by 2030, including international cooperation.
- Investing in animal health systems to support equitable access to essential veterinary services, improve animal health, and promote appropriate management practices.

MSPP continues to involve industries and other stakeholders in the fight against AMR, utilising the influence of the AMR Partnership Platform. This includes deepening ties with FAO's RENOFARM initiative, which focuses on reducing antimicrobial use on farms and promoting sustainable agrifood systems, along with other existing programmes and organisations to encourage tangible collaborations, public–private partnerships, and practical measures on AMR within the One Health framework [18]. As a key FAO program, RENOFARM is designed to be action-driven, country-specific, and led by the countries themselves, aligning with the global goal of transforming agrifood systems. It involves the entire supply chain, from farm to table, and aims to enhance partnerships across the public and private sectors. Additionally, it comprises regional and global components to support countries in implementing their national action plans on AMR.

9.4.6 Investor Action on AMR (IAAMR)

The Investor Action on AMR (IAAMR) was established in 2020 [19] as a joint effort by the Access to Medicine Foundation, the Farm Animal Investment Risk and Return (FAIRR) Initiative, and the UK Department of Health and Social Care. Its goal is to mobilise investor actions against drug-resistant infections. Backed by 22 investors with over US$14 trillion in total assets, IAAMR seeks to reduce excessive antibiotic use in the food industry and healthcare. To protect society, economies, and the long-term value of investments, it promotes investors' regular assessment and integration of AMR risks and containment opportunities. It impacts through the comprehensive, multisectoral One Health approach. It stresses the importance of global collaboration, ongoing funding, and innovative solutions.

Ahead of the UNGA-HLM on AMR in 2024, IAAMR issued a public investor statement, endorsed by 80 investors, calling on global leaders to take decisive and coordinated action to curb AMR to safeguard global health, economic stability, and financial markets.

9.4.7 Alliance to Save Our Antibiotics

The Alliance to Save Our Antibiotics comprises 70 supporting members, as well as over 500 affiliated organisations. These members come from diverse sectors, including medicine, health, agriculture, environment, consumer rights, and animal welfare, across the European Union [20].

Joining the Alliance provides a multidisciplinary platform to enhance the visibility of AMR in human and animal health, influencing policy at both government and industry levels. Members can participate in outreach efforts, briefings, consultations, and support media activities and policy advocacy led by the Alliance.

In the recent past, the Alliance has played a key role in raising awareness about the connection between antibiotic use in livestock and AMR. It has effectively campaigned for stricter regulations on routine and prophylactic antibiotic use in farm animals, especially within UK and EU policy discussions. The Alliance provided evidence supporting limits on medically important antibiotics used for growth promotion and disease prevention. Additionally, it launched public campaigns, encouraged retailers to follow responsible sourcing practices, and enhanced collaboration among health, veterinary, and environmental groups, promoting a One Health approach to preserve antibiotic effectiveness.

9.5 Challenges in Engaging the Private Sector in AMR Control

Engaging the private sector in controlling global AMR is crucial but difficult. Main challenges include lack of financial incentives, low awareness of AMR's impact, and weak public–private partnerships. Inconsistent collection and reporting of AMR surveillance data across countries, along with varying regulatory frameworks, further hinder effective cooperation and coordination.

Pharmaceutical companies and the private sector may not find sufficient financial incentives to develop new antibiotics or fund AMR containment, especially in resource-limited areas.

Implementing robust surveillance systems, developing new diagnostics, and adopting stewardship programmes requires significant financial investment, which can be a barrier for some private sector entities unless assured returns on investment are guaranteed.

Some private organisations may prioritise profits over public health objectives, potentially leading to the overuse or misuse of antibiotics or the development of new products that are inaccessible or unaffordable for everyone.

For surveillance of AMR, the private sector has varying levels of capacity and infrastructure for collecting and reporting AMR data, making it difficult to track trends and implement targeted interventions.

Even if some private institutions have functional surveillance systems, these may not be compatible with other or official national surveillance systems, hindering the ability to share data and collaborate effectively. At the same time, many private sector facilities may not have access to the necessary AMR data to inform their decision-making or participate in collaborative efforts.

In many countries with antibiotic regulations, the private sector faces challenges in implementing these regulations. Poor enforcement often results in ongoing misuse and overuse of antibiotics, promoting the development and spread of AMR. Successful private sector engagement depends on robust public–private partnerships, which are frequently lacking or insufficiently supported.

Inadequate awareness and education are significant hindrances in the private sector's understanding of the severity of AMR and the need for an urgent, robust response. Some private sector actors may not fully grasp the severity of the AMR threat or the importance of their role in containment efforts. Insufficient training and capacity building in AMR management can hinder private sector engagement.

The development of new antibiotics and alternative therapies has been slow, and the private sector may be hesitant to invest in this area due to high costs and low returns on investment. There is a need for increased collaboration between public and private research institutions to accelerate the development and deployment of new AMR solutions [21].

9.6 Possible Solutions for Efficient Collaboration with Private Sector

Addressing challenges described above requires several actions by the global community (Box 9.3). A strong public–private partnership is crucial for effective AMR containment. This involves collaboration between governments, healthcare providers, pharmaceutical companies, research institutions, and the public to implement comprehensive strategies. These strategies include public awareness campaigns, antibiotic stewardship programmes, regulation of antibiotic sales, expanded AMR surveillance, and investment in new technologies [22].

Box 9.3 Enhancing the Contribution of the Private Sector in Containing AMR

Strengthening public–private partnerships:

- Creating platforms for collaboration and knowledge sharing between the public and private sectors.

Developing sustainable financing mechanisms:

- Providing financial incentives for private sector investment in AMR containment.

Improving data collection and surveillance systems:

- Establishing standardised systems for collecting and sharing AMR data.

Harmonising regulations and strengthening enforcement:

- Creating a level playing field for all actors.

Promoting awareness and education:

- Raising awareness about AMR and the role of the private sector in its containment.

Fostering innovation and research:

- Supporting research and development of new antibiotics and alternative therapies.

The private sector's involvement in the containment of AMR is critical because it has the resources and expertise to drive innovation in diagnostics and therapeutics, can play a key role in promoting responsible antibiotic use across various sectors, and can leverage its influence to encourage sustainable manufacturing practices. Private sector engagement shall certainly help build a more robust and comprehensive response to the global AMR challenge.

Innovative strategies to strengthen public–private partnerships (PPPs) for AMR control include outcome-based financing, which ties incentives to actual reductions in inappropriate antibiotic use and infection rates. Blended finance can lower the risks for private investments in diagnostics, vaccines, and antimicrobial research and development. Digital platforms for surveillance facilitate real-time data sharing between government agencies and private hospitals and labs. Advance market commitments can boost antibiotic innovation while promoting stewardship. Standardised accreditation and pooled procurement systems help align quality standards. Furthermore, multistakeholder innovation hubs and regulatory sandboxes support the rapid testing of stewardship tools, diagnostics, and AI-enabled prescribing systems.

References

1. Liverani M, Oliveira Hashiguchi L, Khan M, Coker R. Antimicrobial resistance and the private sector in Southeast Asia. In: Jamrozik E, Selgelid M, editors. Ethics and drug resistance: collective responsibility for global public health. Public health ethics analysis, vol. 5. Cham: Springer; 2020. https://doi.org/10.1007/978-3-030-27874-8_5.
2. USAID. Private delivery care in developing countries. Available at https://www.dhsprogram.com/pubs/pdf/WP76/WP76.pdf. Accessed 11 Apr 2025.
3. Medical tourism. Available at https://www.medicaltourism.com/#:~. Accessed 11 Apr 2025.
4. Unnikrishnan B, Prabhu GGL, Rao PLG, Kumar N. Public-private partnership model in delivering quality health care and medical education - an enduring success story for the past seven decades. Indian J Community Med. 2024;49(6):786–90. https://doi.org/10.4103/ijcm.ijcm_430_24.
5. Rao KS. Public health and the role of the private sector. Prev Med Res Rev. 2024;1(1):8–9. https://doi.org/10.4103/PMRR.PMRR_45_23.
6. FAO. https://www.fao.org/4/w4338e/w4338e04.htm#:~:text. Accessed 12 Apr 2025.
7. European Bank of Reconstruction and Development. EBRD engagement in global efforts to curb antimicrobial resistance (AMR). Private sector initiatives. Available at https://www.ebrd.com/home/news-and-events/publications/economics/special-reports/ebrd-engagement-in-global-efforts-to-curb-antimicrobial-resistance-amr.html. January 2025.
8. Davos Compact on Antimicrobial Resistance. Available at https://reports.weforum.org/docs/WEF_AMR_Davos_Compact_2025.pdf. Accessed 13 Apr 2025.
9. WEF: how global collaboration is addressing the growing threat of antimicrobial resistance. Available at https://www.weforum.org/stories/2025/01/global-collaboration-antimicrobial-resistance-AMR. Accessed 11 Apr 2025.
10. WEF. https://www.weforum.org/stories/2025/01/global-collaboration-antimicrobial-resistance-amr/. Accessed 11 Apr 2025.

11. AMR Industry Alliance. Declaration by the pharmaceutical biotechnology and diagnostics industries on combating antimicrobial resistance. AMR Industry Declaration. 2016. Available at https://www.amrindustryalliance.org/mediaroom/launch-of-the-declaration/ Accessed 11 Apr 2025.
12. BSI. New certification aims to mitigate antimicrobial resistance risk in antibiotic manufacturing. Available at https://www.bsigroup.com/en-US/insights-and-media/media-center/press-releases/2023/june/new-certification-aims-to-mitigate-antimicrobial-resistance-risk-in-antibiotic-manufacturing/. Accessed 14 Apr 2025.
13. AMR Industry Alliance. Industry roadmap for progress on combating antimicrobial resistance. AMR Industry Alliance. 2016. https://www.amrindustryallianceorg/industry-roadmap-for-progress-on-combating-antimicrobial-resistance/. Accessed 10 Apr 2025.
14. AMR Industry Alliance. Shared goals | The AMR Industry Alliance's commitments. AMR Industry Alliance. 2016. https://www.amrindustryalliance.org/%20shared-goals/. Accessed 11 Apr 2025.
15. AMR Industry Alliance. New certification aims to mitigate antimicrobial resistance risk in antibiotic manufacturing. 2023. https://www.amrindustryallianceorg/mediaroom/amr-industry-allianceannounces-certification/. Accessed 12 Apr 2025.
16. AMR Multi-Stakeholder Partnership Platform. Available at https://openknowledge.fao.org/server/api/core/bitstreams/2dffcc21-f3ac-4a88-bcf1-c91bebba022d/content. Accessed 9 Apr 2025.
17. FAO: FAO and Private Sector collaborate to address Antimicrobial Resistance in agrifood sector. The role of the private sector in delivering on UNGA commitments in the agrifood sector. Available at: https://www.qjsamr.org/news-and-events/news/qjs-news-item/20-03-2025-fao-and-private-sector-collaborate-to-address-antimicrobial-resistance-in-agrifood-sector#. Accessed 3 Apr 2025.
18. FAO. RENOFORM. Reduce the need for antimicrobials on farms for sustainable agrifood systems transformation. Available at https://www.fao.org/antimicrobial-resistance/background/fao-role/renofarm/en/#. Accessed 5 Apr 2025.
19. Investor Action on AMR. Available at https://amrinvestoraction.org/. Accessed 7 Apr 2025.
20. Alliance to Save our Antibiotics. Available at https://www.saveourantibiotics.org/alliance-members/. Accessed 14 Apr 2025.
21. WHO. WHO outlines 40 research priorities on antimicrobial resistance. Available at https://www.who.int/news/item/22-06-2023-who-outlines-40-research-priorities-on-antimicrobial-resistance. Accessed 11 Apr 2025.
22. Singh S, Charani E, Devi S, Sharma A, Edathadathil F, Kumar A, Warrier A, Shareek PS, Jaykrishnan AV, Ellangovan K. A road-map for addressing antimicrobial resistance in low- and middle-income countries: lessons learnt from the public private participation and co-designed antimicrobial stewardship programme in the State of Kerala, India. Antimicrob Resist Infect Control. 2021;10(1):32. https://doi.org/10.1186/s13756-020-00873-9.

Chapter 10
Civil Society Role in Containment of AMR

Abstract Civil society organisations (CSOs) are vital for strengthening health systems and tackling public health issues like antimicrobial resistance (AMR). Operating independently of governments and the private sector, CSOs connect communities and healthcare providers through advocacy, service delivery, awareness-raising, and the empowerment of marginalised groups. Their roles in AMR containment are varied—ranging from educational campaigns and community outreach to policy influence, promoting responsible antibiotic use, supporting operational research, and fostering multisector collaborations. Groups such as ReAct, the Antibiotic Resistance Coalition, and the South Centre have had significant impacts on global policy, while others, such as CHAI, GARDP, and REACH, focus on diagnostics, research, and community engagement. The WHO collaborates with CSOs via its Civil Society Task Force on AMR, amplifying the voices of survivors and communities. However, CSOs face challenges like limited funding, regulatory hurdles, capacity gaps, and fragmented efforts. Strengthening partnerships, improving training, fostering accountability, and integrating CSOs into national action plans are essential steps to harness their potential in fighting AMR and achieving sustainable health outcomes.

Keywords Civil society organisations (CSOs) · Community engagement · Advocacy and policy influence · Awareness and behaviour change · Partnerships and collaboration

According to the World Bank [1], civil society encompasses a diverse set of organisations: community groups, NGOs, labour unions, indigenous communities, charitable and faith-based organisations, professional associations, and foundations. Civil society organisations (CSOs) are non-governmental, not-for-profit entities operating in the public domain, advocating for the interests and values of their members or other stakeholders. Civil society is defined by the voluntary and autonomous involvement of individuals and groups.

When mobilised, civil society—often referred to as the "third sector" (after government and commerce)—can influence the decisions of elected policymakers and

R. Bhatia, *Drug-Resistant Infections*,
https://doi.org/10.1007/978-981-92-4190-3_10

businesses. Its scope, focus areas, and extent of engagement are continually evolving alongside technological advances and shifting societal needs.

Civil society basically encompasses the social space outside government and private sectors where individuals organise around issues they find important. It frequently functions as a watchdog for government actions, amplifies voices, and offers support to those who lack it. CSOs work independently of the government and private businesses, focusing on social, cultural, and political issues, including health [2].

10.1 Civil Society and Health

CSOs are crucial in the health sector by complementing government initiatives, delivering vital services, advocating for health rights, and encouraging community involvement. They serve as a link between communities and healthcare providers, ensuring that health services are accessible, responsive, and equitable. CSOs are key partners in the health field, working with governments to enhance health outcomes, advance health equity, and empower communities to manage their own health. An outline of the potential roles CSOs can play in health is presented in Box 10.1.

Box 10.1: Possible Roles of CSOs in Health Sector

- Advocacy with health policymakers and administrators.
- Complementing governments' service delivery and health system strengthening actions.
- Improving access to health services in underserved areas and for marginalised populations, especially women, children, people with disabilities, and ethnic minorities.
- Acting as a bridge between the health provider and the community, creating trust in services and communication, especially health messages.
- Championing health rights.
- Catalysing community engagement and empowerment through advocacy and capacity enhancement.
- Undertaking health promotion and countering social stigmas.
- Providing an independent appraisal of the services provided by providers.
- Facilitating partnerships between communities with various stakeholders in the health sector.

Civil society is crucial in strengthening health systems by ensuring services are accessible, equitable, and responsive to community needs. They serve as a vital bridge between communities and formal healthcare, empowering individuals and local groups to take charge of their own health.

10.2 CSOs Role and Impact on AMR

Among the various functions of CSOs and NGOs in the health sector, addressing antimicrobial resistance (AMR) is a key aspect. These organisations can help contain AMR by raising awareness, encouraging responsible antibiotic use, advocating for policy reforms, and supporting research efforts. They serve as essential links between communities and policymakers, facilitating the translation of scientific knowledge into practical actions [3]. Table 10.1 summarises some activities undertaken by several CSOs and NGOs, aligning with their general roles in health (Box 10.1) but with a specific focus on AMR.

Table 10.1 Role of CSOs and NGOs in containing AMR and their impact

	Activity	Impact
1	To conduct educational campaigns, workshops, and community outreach programmes to inform the public about the dangers of antibiotic misuse and the importance of appropriate antibiotic use (a) Targeted tailor-made campaigns for different subsets of population appropriate to the local culture and language (b) Participating in the World Antimicrobial Awareness Week [3] amplifying key messages and promoting responsible antibiotic use	Raises Awareness and Promotes Responsible Use of antibiotics with the objective of bringing about change in behaviour towards rational use of antibiotics and avoiding self-medication
2	To engage with policymakers at local, national, and international levels to influence policy decisions and ensure that AMR remains a priority To advocate for policies that support AMR mitigation efforts, including promoting access to antibiotics, advocating against irrational antibiotic use, and pushing for research and development of new antibiotics	Influences policy and programme improvement through advocacy

(continued)

Table 10.1 (continued)

	Activity	Impact
3	To contribute to research efforts by generating/contributing to data collection, conducting studies, and disseminating research findings to relevant stakeholders. To assist in planning and implementation of AMR-related operational research and field studies that improve programmatic interventions and community engagement To play a role in influencing research priorities and ensuring that research efforts are aligned with the needs of communities and policymakers	Supports research and data generation and assists in operational research to improve programmatic approach of AMR containment
4	To work in collaboration with governments, healthcare providers, and other stakeholders to implement AMR interventions To facilitate partnerships between different sectors and ensure that interventions are aligned with national priorities	Enhances Collaboration and Partnerships between various stakeholders in public and private sectors
5	To identify and address specific gaps in the AMR response, such as the need for better access to antibiotics, the promotion of infection prevention and control measures, or the need for improved surveillance systems and share these with relevant health officials	Addresses specific gaps in AMR containment programmes
6	To create awareness on infection prevention and control amongst communities with guidance/support from local health functionaries	Reduces infections and factors propagating it
7	To promote use of vaccines, safe water, hygiene and nutrition with focus on marginalised and vulnerable sections of society	Reduces disease burden and facilitates reduction in use of antibiotics.

10.3 Major NGOs and CSOs

Several NGOs and CSOs are actively involved in tackling AMR. Key organisations include ReAct, Antibiotic Resistance Coalition (ARC), and The South Centre, along with global health initiatives like the Global Fund and organisations working on specific issues such as HIV, TB, and malaria. These have been mentioned earlier (Chap. 3), and many are also listed in Box 10.2.

Box 10.2: Few Prominent CSOs and NGOs Engaged in Controlling AMR

- ReAct [4]
- Antibiotic Resistance Coalition (ARC) [5]
- The South Centre [6]
- The Global Fund for HIV, TB and Malaria [7]
- Clinton Health Access Initiative (CHAI) [8]
- International Union Against Tuberculosis and Lung Disease [9] (The Union)
- KNCV Tuberculosis Foundation [10]
- Global Antibiotic Research and Development Partnership (GARDP) [11]
- Medical and veterinary professional associations
- Family Health International 360 (FHI 360) [12]
- Resource Group for Education and Advocacy for Community Health (REACH) [13]
- One Health Poultry Hub [14]
- SHARE India
- The Foundation for Innovative New Diagnostics (FIND) [15]

ReAct is a prominent international network committed to increasing awareness of antibiotic resistance and its root causes. They are recognised for their efforts in mobilising civil society to build movements.

The Antibiotic Resistance Coalition (ARC) is a global CSO network that advocates for policy changes and action on AMR across various sectors. They have been instrumental in influencing global AMR policies.

The South Centre, an intergovernmental organisation of developing nations, supports these countries in international AMR collaborations, including facilitating dialogue between governments and CSOs.

The Global Fund for HIV, TB, and Malaria primarily targets these diseases but also addresses AMR through activities like surveillance, funding grants, and market shaping.

The Global Antibiotic Research and Development Partnership (GARDP) focuses on developing new antibiotics and advancing AMR research.

The Resource Group for Education and Advocacy for Community Health (REACH) addresses community health and development topics, including AMR.

The One Health Poultry Hub focuses on poultry health, which is connected to the AMR issue due to antibiotic use in animal farming.

The Foundation for Innovative New Diagnostics (FIND) is another global health organisation that emphasises diagnostics and contributes to AMR efforts.

Several CSOs have documented their work on AMR-related activities in Africa [16], showing a notable contribution to enhancing surveillance, delaying the emergence of resistance, limiting transmission, and reducing harm from infections caused by AMR microorganisms. Their efforts primarily involve advocacy, with additional focus on accountability and service delivery.

10.3.1 World Health Organisation

The World Health Organisation (WHO), despite being an intergovernmental organisation, encourages active civil society involvement in all public health initiatives. It remains vital in coordinating worldwide efforts on AMR, creating frameworks and guidance through numerous CSOs operating at different levels—from international policy to community involvement—and tackling various facets of the AMR issue.

WHO Civil Society Task Force on AMR [17] brings together various CSOs and NGOs to coordinate activities and ensure a unified approach to tackling AMR.

The WHO Civil Society Task Force on AMR
The WHO Civil Society Task Force on AMR [17] is a group dedicated to amplifying the voices of those impacted by drug-resistant infections and advocating for change. Its members include survivors of AMR infections and caregivers for those with severe drug-resistant infections, acting as "champions" to shape AMR policy and raise awareness.

The Task Force highlights the human impact of AMR by sharing personal stories of those affected by drug-resistant infections, aiming to make the issue more relatable and urgent.

The members of this Task Force actively engage in advocacy efforts to promote policy changes, increased funding, and improved messaging around AMR, thereby enhancing awareness of this subject.

The Task Force emphasises a patient-centred approach, underscoring the value of incorporating patients' perspectives and experiences into the global fight against AMR. This strategy aligns with WHO's latest (2023) guidance on a Patient-Centred Approach to Controlling AMR [18]. The Task Force leverages multiple platforms, including social media, to share survivor stories and engage a worldwide audience. It collaborates with other WHO initiatives and stakeholders to promote a unified and impactful response to AMR.

The WHO Civil Society Task Force on AMR serves as a crucial bridge between the technical aspects of AMR and the human experience, working to ensure that the voices of those most impacted by drug-resistant infections are heard and acted upon.

10.4 Why Civil Society Engagement Has Been Suboptimal

Despite recognising the critical role and potential of civil society in making a significant contribution to the control of AMR at the grassroots level, there has not been much success. Several contributions that CSOs can make in the efficient implementation of respective national action plans on AMR (Box 10.3) have been consistently ignored.

Box 10.3: Potential Contribution Pathways for Civil Society to AMR Control

- Community education and behaviour change
- Accountability and transparency in antibiotic regulation
- Advocacy for responsible pharmaceutical marketing practices
- Monitoring implementation of national action plans
- Bridging local realities with national policy
- Without civil society, AMR control risks becoming a technical exercise detached from everyday antibiotic use behaviours.

Some of the salient reasons for this neglect have been described below:

10.4.1 Technical Framing and Limited Public Visibility

AMR is frequently perceived as a laboratory, surveillance, or pharmaceutical policy matter instead of a social and community issue. Discussions at the national level are led mainly by clinicians, microbiologists, and policymakers, resulting in a technocratic atmosphere that marginalises grassroots participants. Unlike HIV/AIDS or maternal health, AMR does not have prominent, emotionally resonant stories that inspire civil society to act.

10.4.2 Weak Institutional Inclusion in NAP Governance

In many countries, civil society organisations are not officially part of national AMR coordinating committees. Even when they are included in documentation, their participation often remains symbolic rather than meaningful. Without defined roles in areas like monitoring, awareness-raising, or ensuring accountability, civil society stays on the fringe of the implementation process.

10.4.3 Funding and Capacity Constraints

Most AMR funding in developing countries prioritises technical aspects of AMR, e.g. surveillance systems, laboratory strengthening, and clinical stewardship programmes. Few resources are earmarked for civil society capacity building, public education, or community advocacy. Many CSOs lack technical understanding of AMR, limiting their ability to engage in policy dialogue or generate evidence-informed advocacy.

10.4.4 Competing Development Priorities

In resource-constrained settings, civil society organisations often focus on urgent and visible issues such as malnutrition, maternal health, sanitation, infectious disease outbreaks, and livelihoods. Because AMR develops slowly and is complex, it is frequently viewed as a secondary concern.

10.4.5 Fragmentation Across Sectors

AMR demands cooperation among sectors such as health, agriculture, veterinary, environmental, and consumer protection. Nonetheless, in many developing countries, civil society tends to operate in silos. Health NGOs infrequently collaborate with agricultural advocacy groups, and environmental organisations rarely participate in antimicrobial policy discussions.

10.4.6 Limited Rights-Based Framing

AMR is seldom viewed as a matter of rights or equity. However, drug resistance mainly impacts vulnerable groups that depend on public health services and have few antibiotic choices. Failing to connect AMR to the right to effective treatment and fair access to medicines has hindered broader civil society efforts.

10.4.7 Political and Commercial Sensitivities

AMR impacts key sectors such as pharmaceuticals, private healthcare, and agriculture. CSOs dependent on government or donor funding may hesitate to challenge antibiotic overuse or insufficient regulatory enforcement.

10.5 Challenges Faced by CSOs in Control of AMR

CSOs encounter significant challenges in executing measures to combat AMR. These include limited funding, complex regulations, capacity limitations, and barriers to accessing information and data. Furthermore, fragmented efforts, poor coordination, and insufficient diagnostic tools further hinder their effectiveness.

Specific challenges include the following:

Funding and Resources: CSOs often face limited financial resources, which hinder their ability to implement large-scale projects and maintain long-term initiatives.

Complex Regulatory Environments: Navigating the complicated regulatory systems in various countries can be difficult for CSOs, especially those working internationally.

Capacity Constraints: Many CSOs do not have enough expertise, training, or personnel to effectively handle AMR, especially in areas like surveillance and data analysis.

Barriers to accessing relevant information and data on AMR prevalence, resistance patterns, and best practices impede the development of targeted interventions.

Coordination and Fragmentation: The lack of coordination and collaboration among different CSOs can lead to duplication of efforts and an inefficient use of resources.

In many countries, fragile health systems and insufficient healthcare infrastructure hinder efforts to control AMR. CSOs frequently encounter difficulties in elevating AMR on national health agendas and in obtaining essential political and financial commitments from governments.

Despite these challenges, CSOs are a critical community of volunteers who must be tapped, trained, and actively engaged in all initiatives aimed at containing AMR.

10.6 Way Forward to Promote Engagement of CSOs in AMR Control

To effectively engage CSOs in AMR control, a comprehensive strategy must be employed. This encompasses building CSO capacity, encouraging collaboration, and securing their active involvement in policy creation and execution. It includes explicitly improving communication and awareness efforts, advocating for policy reforms, promoting responsible antibiotic consumption, and ensuring stakeholder accountability.

Institutionalise civil society involvement in national AMR governance by formally including civil society representatives in key bodies such as national AMR steering committees, technical working groups, and monitoring and evaluation platforms. Their participation should be meaningful, with explicit mandates outlining

CSOs' roles in awareness campaigns, accountability, and community engagement. Furthermore, NAP governance frameworks should be updated to guarantee sufficient civil society representation across various sectors.

Establish Dedicated Funding Windows for CSO Engagement International development partners and governments should allocate earmarked funding for CSO-led public awareness-raising campaigns, their capacity-building workshops, policy advocacy initiatives and community monitoring mechanisms. Even small grants programmes can enable grassroots organisations to integrate AMR messaging into existing health or agricultural programmes. These must be facilitated and ensured. National authorities must include civil society funding lines in national AMR budgets and donor-supported programmes.

Build Technical Capacity of CSOs on AMR Civil society actors require simplified, policy-relevant training in antibiotic stewardship principles, regulatory frameworks, interpretation of surveillance data, and One Health approaches. To this end, partnerships among academic institutions, public health agencies, and CSOs can build sustained expertise. The AMR programme manager must develop national AMR training toolkits tailored for non-technical audiences.

Promote Cross-Sector Civil Society Coalitions Creating and sustaining national AMR civil society coalitions can overcome fragmentation. Such platforms should include: health NGOs/CSOs, *f*armer associations, *v*eterinary groups, *c*onsumer protection organisations and *e*nvironmental advocacy groups. These coalitions can amplify advocacy, align messaging, and engage policymakers more effectively, and authorities must foster this collaboration.

Reframe AMR as a Social Justice and Development Issue Civil society mobilisation is strongest when issues are linked to rights and equity. AMR should be framed as a threat to universal health coverage, a barrier to poverty reduction, a food safety concern and a risk to future generations. This reframing can expand engagement beyond health-focused organisations.

Leverage Community Platforms for Behaviour Change CSOs are well-positioned to influence antibiotic use behaviours through community health worker networks, *f*armer training programmes, *y*outh engagement initiatives and *m*edia campaigns. CSOs may need an orientation in developing and disseminating right public messages which emphasise *c*ompleting prescribed antibiotic courses, *a*voiding self-medication, *d*iscouraging over-the-counter misuse and *r*educing unnecessary use in livestock. CSOs may be advised to integrate AMR awareness into existing community outreach platforms rather than creating standalone programmes.

Strengthen Accountability and Transparency Mechanisms Civil society can serve as a watchdog by tracking antibiotic procurement and stockouts, monitoring the enforcement of prescription-only policies, and advocating against unethical pharmaceutical promotion. Transparency tools like public dashboards and annual AMR implementation reports can strengthen advocacy efforts. Action step: Require public reporting on NAP implementation progress.

Align Global Support with Civil Society Strengthening International development partners should combine technical assistance with social mobilisation tactics. Programmes funded by global agencies must clearly incorporate activities to strengthen civil society. Technical and funding support proposals should, as a condition of funding, include civil society engagement strategies.

To make best use of CSOs in supporting national efforts to contain AMR, especially at the community level, the national authorities should endorse inclusive CSOs governance structures and ensure sustained engagement. CSOs may be supported in devising and implementing strategies that are tailored to local antibiotic use, regulations, and cultural norms. Monitoring indicators linked to contributions of CSOs must be part of national M&E framework.

In summary, the limited involvement of civil society in AMR efforts in developing nations results from structural exclusion, capacity limitations, funding issues, and weak public understanding, not from disinterest or irrelevance. Enhancing civil society participation is crucial for turning technical AMR policies into real community behaviour change, accountability, and ongoing political support.

Without active civil society, national action plans may just stay as policies rather than becoming transformative tools. By formalising inclusion, boosting capacity, and viewing AMR as a development and equity concern, governments and partners can tap into civil society's full potential to fight antimicrobial resistance.

Strengthening CSO capacity can be achieved through regular training focused on making CSOs understand AMR in simple terms, the critical role that communities can play through CSOs' advocacy, and ongoing interactions with the public. CSOs' training should include a component on communication. AMR, being a complex subject, requires effective communication skills to help communities grasp its impact and the actions everyone can take to reduce it. The ultimate goal of developing communication skills is to encourage positive behavioural changes towards the rational use of antibiotics [19].

AMR programme managers should actively promote the development of CSO networks and partnerships, both domestically and internationally, to facilitate knowledge sharing and exchange of best practices. They need to be continuously involved in planning and implementing different AMR-related campaigns, with support (financial and technical) provided to CSOs to help execute these initiatives effectively.

Empowering CSOs to contribute to the development and execution of national action plans at the local level is beneficial, especially when these plans are aligned with local needs and priorities. CSOs should be encouraged to advocate with the governments and stakeholders to implement AMR policies and programmes effectively. Implementing these strategies enables CSOs to make a significant contribution to addressing the AMR challenge and promoting a healthier future.

References

1. The World Bank. Working together – World Bank Civil Society relationship. 2003. Published by the World Bank, Washington. Available at https://documents1.worldbank.org/curated/en/339011468779979043/pdf/292760PAPER0Wo1er0WB10civil0society.pdf. Accessed 11 Apr 2025.
2. Schurmann AT, Mahmud S. Civil society, health, and social exclusion in Bangladesh. J Health Popul Nutr. 2009;27(4):536–44. https://doi.org/10.3329/jhpn.v27i4.3400.
3. WHO. World antimicrobial awareness week (18–24 Nov). https://www.who.int/campaigns/world-amr-awareness-week. Accessed 11 Apr 2025.
4. ReAct. Available at https://www.reactgroup.org/. Accessed 11 Apr 2025.
5. The Antibiotic Resistance Coalition (ARC). Available at https://www.ignitetheidea.org/arc. Accessed 12 Apr 2025.
6. The South Centre. Available at https://www.southcentre.int/about-the-south-centre/.
7. The Global Fund for HIV, TB and Malaria. Available at https://www.theglobalfund.org/en/. Accessed 13 Apr 2025.
8. Clinton Health Access Initiative. Available at https://www.clintonhealthaccess.org/about-us/. Accessed 14 Apr 2025.
9. International Union Against Tuberculosis and Lung Disease (The Union). Available at https://theunion.org/. Accessed 14 Apr 2025.
10. KNCV Tuberculosis Foundation. Available at https://www.kncvtbplus.com/. Accessed 11 Apr 2025.
11. Global Antibiotic Research and Development Partnership (GARDP). Available at https://gardp.org/?gad_. Accessed 15 Apr 2025.
12. Family Health International 360. Available at https://www.fhi360.org/. Accessed 11 Apr 2025.
13. Resource Group for Education and Advocacy for Community Health (REACH). Available at https://reachindia.org.in/. Accessed 10 Apr 2025.
14. One Health Poultry Hub. Available at https://www.onehealthpoultry.org/. Accessed 11 Apr 2025.
15. The Foundation for Innovative New Diagnostics (FIND). Available at https://www.finddx.org/. Accessed 7 Apr 2025.
16. Fraser JL, Alimi YH, Varma JK, Muraya T, Kujinga T, Carter VK, Schultsz C, Del Rio Vilas VJ. Antimicrobial resistance control efforts in Africa: a survey of the role of Civil Society Organisations. Glob Health Action. 2021;14(1):1868055. https://doi.org/10.1080/16549716.2020.1868055.
17. WHO. The WHO Civil Society Task Force on antimicrobial resistance. Available at https://www.who.int/news-room/articles-detail/apply-to-be-a-member-of-the-who-civil-society-task-force-on-antimicrobial-resistance-(amr)-call-for-expressions-of-interest. Accessed 7 Apr 2025.
18. WHO. People-centred approach to addressing antimicrobial resistance in human health: WHO core package of interventions to support national action plans. Geneva: World Health Organization; 2023. Licence: CC BY-NC-SA 3.0 IGO.
19. Nair MM, Mahajan R, Burza S, Zeegers MP. Behavioural interventions to address rational use of antibiotics in outpatient settings of low-income and lower-middle-income countries. Trop Med Int Health. 2021;26(5):504–17. https://doi.org/10.1111/tmi.13550.

Part III
Surveillance, Monitoring, and Stewardship

Chapter 11
AMR Surveillance in Health Sector

Abstract Antimicrobial resistance (AMR) surveillance in the health sector is vital to global efforts to combat drug-resistant pathogens. It involves systematically collecting, analysing, and sharing data to guide treatment, inform policy, and improve infection prevention and control. Surveillance enables early detection of emerging resistance patterns, quantifies the disease burden, and assesses the success of interventions. Key components of national AMR systems include a National Coordinating Centre, a National Reference Laboratory, and sentinel surveillance sites, which collectively ensure the accurate generation and reporting of data. WHO's GLASS provides standardised methods to harmonise reporting internationally. Regional and multicountry networks such as EARS-Net, ReLAVRA+, and CAESAR also facilitate coordinated responses. Countries such as the US and India have developed national networks for resistance monitoring and public health guidance. Despite these advances, challenges such as limited funding, weak laboratory capacity, fragmented systems, poor data quality, and uneven global coverage persist. Overcoming these requires political will, adoption of One Health strategies, investment in laboratory and workforce infrastructure, and implementation of standardised reporting. Effective AMR surveillance is essential to safeguard antimicrobial effectiveness and ensure global health security.

Keywords Antimicrobial resistance · Surveillance systems, GLASS, One Health approach · National AMR networks · Public health policy

Surveillance involves the continuous collection, compilation, and analysis of data, along with timely sharing of information with relevant stakeholders, especially those who can respond. AMR surveillance and monitoring identify and track trends and changes in microbial populations, including drug-resistant microorganisms and resistance factors like genes and mechanisms [1].

Monitoring AMR across the health, animal, and environmental sectors is essential for understanding, controlling, and combating the spread of drug-resistant pathogens [2]. It provides critical data that inform treatment decisions, influence policies, and assess the effectiveness of efforts to reduce AMR.

R. Bhatia, *Drug-Resistant Infections*,
https://doi.org/10.1007/978-981-92-4190-3_11

Within the scope of AMR, the World Health Organisation (WHO) highlights that surveillance is crucial for developing policies and infection prevention and control strategies. It acts as the foundation for tracking the dissemination of AMR and assessing the effectiveness of measures at local, national, and global levels [3].

11.1 Guiding Principles for AMR Surveillance

Collecting specific surveillance data is mandatory for global efforts to combat AMR. The guiding principles are outlined in Box 11.1.

Box 11.1 Guiding Principles for AMR Surveillance

Define the scope of the resistance problem

Develop interventions that improve the appropriate application of antibiotics

Decrease resistance selection pressure [4, 5]

Understand the mechanisms of resistance whereby microorganisms avoid the effects of antibiotics and

Apply information to discover/develop new compounds, or modify older agents, that preserve the potent activity of antibiotics against key target pathogens

Following key principles for effective AMR surveillance must be adopted under any national, regional, or local AMR surveillance activity.

One Health Approach AMR surveillance should adopt a One Health model, integrating data from human health, animal health, food systems, and the environment. Resistance trends in hospitals, livestock, and wastewater are interconnected, and a coordinated approach helps detect transmission early and guides cross-sector policies.

Standardisation and Data Quality Consistent laboratory methods, harmonised case definitions, and standardised antimicrobial testing are vital for reliable data. Participation in external quality assurance is necessary, and expanding sentinel sites should not compromise data quality; accuracy is more important than quantity.

Inclusivity and Fairness Networks should include not just urban hospitals but also district, rural, and private health facilities. Data must accurately reflect antibiotic use and resistance patterns, including among vulnerable groups.

Timeliness and Alerts Surveillance should serve as a real-time warning system. Digital platforms, interoperable lab data systems, and rapid alert mechanisms are crucial for detecting threats such as carbapenem-resistant organisms and enabling rapid response through infection control.

Data-driven action Surveillance results must inform policies. Data should shape treatment guidelines, stewardship programmes, procurement, and national plans. Regular feedback to clinicians and policymakers promotes accountability.

Linking AMR and AMU Resistance data should connect with antimicrobial use patterns in humans and animals. Monitoring prescriptions, sales, and veterinary use helps create targeted interventions.

Transparency and Sharing Open reporting, global participation (like GLASS), and publishing national reports build trust, improve credibility, and encourage collaboration, research, and public confidence.

Sustainable Ownership Surveillance systems must be part of routine health services, with reliable domestic funding. Overdependence on external donors risks fragmentation. Building long- term capacity—labs, workforce, digital tools—is essential.

Ethics and Data Security Clear policies on patient confidentiality, genomic data, and information sharing are vital to maintain trust and meet legal standards.

Robust AMR surveillance needs political backing, multisector coordination, and ongoing investment. Countries should focus on integrating surveillance into existing health systems, expanding equitable coverage, and ensuring that data informs effective policies. Following these principles, AMR surveillance can shift from mere reporting to a strategic tool for health security and global cooperation.

11.2 Importance of AMR Surveillance in Health Sector

AMR surveillance in healthcare is essential [6] for tracking the emergence and spread of drug-resistant pathogens, aiding treatment decisions, and guiding public health policies to combat AMR effectively. It enables understanding the extent of the problem, identifying new resistance patterns, and assessing intervention outcomes.

AMR surveillance data is crucial for countries to effectively respond to the challenge of AMR, enabling the early detection of risks before they escalate into major crises. It plays a key role in developing, monitoring, and assessing AMR control strategies and interventions [7].

AMR surveillance is essential for understanding and measuring the burden of drug-resistant pathogens in any region, along with their epidemiological characteristics, to grasp their dynamics [7]. It enables early detection of emerging and spreading resistant infections, facilitating timely interventions to curb further dissemination. By offering real-time data on resistance trends, surveillance guides clinicians in selecting effective antibiotics, thereby optimising treatments and enhancing patient outcomes. Additionally, surveillance data support the formulation of evidence-based regulations [8] on antimicrobial use across healthcare, veterinary, agriculture, and other sectors, encouraging responsible practices and helping to combat resistance.

AMR surveillance plays a crucial role in evaluating the success of antibiotic stewardship initiatives, infection control measures, and other strategies aimed at combating resistance [9]. Surveillance data improve our ability to tackle AMR-related public health challenges by providing insights into circulating pathogens and resistance patterns within specific regions. Additionally, it helps identify the most common pathogens and resistance mechanisms, guiding the development of new antimicrobial treatments targeted at these issues.

AMR surveillance data is important for understanding how human, animal, and environmental health are interconnected, supporting a holistic strategy to fight resistance [10, 11]. It also aids in tracking the appearance and spread of resistant bacteria, viruses, fungi, and parasites in humans.

Surveillance data helps clinicians determine which drugs remain effective against specific pathogens, supporting better treatment decisions.

Surveillance systems can help detect and respond to outbreaks of drug-resistant infections quickly, preventing further spread.

Surveillance data can be used to evaluate the effectiveness of infection control measures and other interventions aimed at reducing AMR.

Many countries, particularly low- and middle-income nations, require assistance in developing their capacity for AMR surveillance and monitoring. This support will enable countries to effectively generate, collect, analyse, and interpret data regarding AMR, antimicrobial usage, levels of antimicrobial residues in the food supply, and AMR presence in the environment.

11.2.1 Potential Support from Development Partners to Strengthen AMR Surveillance

AMR disproportionately impacts developing countries due to high infectious disease rates, unregulated antibiotic use, limited laboratory facilities, and fragmented health systems. Although many nations have adopted national action plans aligned with the WHO Global Action Plan and participate in GLASS, surveillance capacity remains uneven. In the animal and food sectors, collaboration with organisations such as the World Organisation for Animal Health and the Food and Agriculture Organisation has improved reporting, but significant technical and financial gaps remain.

To establish effective, integrated AMR surveillance, developing countries require strategic, long-term support from international development partners in several areas, some of which are outlined below:

Long-Term and Predictable Funding Sustainable AMR surveillance depends on continuous investments in labs, equipment, reagents, digital tools, and personnel. Countries seek multiyear, predictable funding instead of short-term projects, flexible funding aligned with national priorities, mixed financing models combining grants, concessional loans, and domestic contributions, and support for comprehensive system strengthening, not isolated projects. Stable funding is essential to embed surveillance in routine health services in developing countries.

Laboratory Infrastructure and Support Many countries have gaps in microbiology laboratories at district and peripheral levels. Support should include upgrading laboratory infrastructure and biosafety, procurement of quality diagnostics, supply chain enhancements for media, reagents, and consumables, participation in external quality assurance and accreditation. International investments should focus on decentralisation and equitable geographic coverage of efficient laboratory support.

Workforce Development Shortages of skilled professionals are a key barrier to AMR surveillance. Countries need training of microbiologists, laboratory technologists, epidemiologists, veterinarians, and data scientists; field epidemiology programmes with AMR modules, knowledge exchange and regional training hubs and mentorships or linkages with advanced laboratories.

Digital Infrastructure and Data Integration Effective AMR surveillance depends on interoperable systems. Countries expect help with laboratory information systems (LIMS), integrating AMR and antimicrobial use data, real-time dashboards and early warning tools and cross-sector data sharing. Support to the countries must include cybersecurity and long-term system maintenance.

One Health Coordination Success in AMR surveillance requires cross-sector collaboration. It requires joint human–animal–environment surveillance frameworks, harmonised standards, coordination mechanisms and regional data-sharing platforms. Support from international development partners should strengthen national ownership without creating parallel systems.

Research and Innovation *Developing* countries expect assistance with local resistance research, genomic surveillance and molecular studies, cost-effectiveness analyses, implementation research for stewardship and building research ecosystems for evidence-based policies.

Policy and Regulatory Frameworks The development partners can help by developing surveillance laws and mandates, regulating antibiotic sales and prescriptions, integrating AMR into health system reforms, incorporating AMR indicators into monitoring frameworks. It is well known that legal backing enhances sustainability.

Equity and Access Support should ensure coverage of rural areas, informal providers, and private sectors. Prioritising inclusivity and reducing urban bias is essential for an efficient surveillance system.

Developing countries now seek a shift from fragmented, short-term projects towards systemic, long-term, integrated support. Focus areas include domestic ownership, One Health coordination, digital systems, workforce capacity, and sustainable financing. With coordinated global efforts, AMR surveillance can become a key pillar of health security, economic resilience, and sustainable development.

11.3 Components of AMR Surveillance System in Health Sector

WHO has outlined detailed guidelines on the key elements of a national AMR surveillance system and how they interconnect [12]. Typically, a national AMR surveillance system within the health sector includes three main components:

- A National Coordinating Centre (NCC),
- A National Reference Laboratory (NRL),
- Surveillance Sites.

These components work together to monitor and manage AMR within a country.

1. *The National Coordinating Centre (NCC)* serves as the main authority overseeing and coordinating the national AMR surveillance system. It is responsible for establishing the system, setting its objectives, and ensuring smooth operation. The NCC gathers and analyses AMR data from multiple sources, such as surveillance sites and the NRL, and shares this information with relevant stakeholders, including the WHO-managed GLASS. The NCC offers expertise in epidemiology, laboratory procedures, and data management to support the system's effectiveness.
2. *The National Reference Laboratory (NRL)* is essential in fostering and upholding high standards of laboratory practices within the surveillance system. It supports other laboratories through guidance, standardisation, and quality assurance processes. The NRL may conduct advanced testing and analysis of AMR samples. It guarantees that the data generated by laboratories is both accurate and reliable.
3. *Surveillance Sites* are healthcare facilities like hospitals and clinics that collect data on AMR from patients. They gather essential information from patients, including demographics, clinical details, epidemiological data, and microbiological results such as pathogen identification and susceptibility tests. These

sites serve as the core data sources, supplying the raw information to the NCC. The number of surveillance sites may differ based on the country's size and available resources.

In essence, the NCC provides the overall direction and management, the NRL ensures data quality, and the surveillance sites are the data collection points, all working together to create a comprehensive AMR surveillance system.

11.4 Global, Regional, and National AMR Surveillance Systems

Some examples of existing AMR surveillance systems are:

11.4.1 WHO Global Antimicrobial Resistance and Use Surveillance System (GLASS)

The WHO plays a crucial role in global AMR monitoring through the Global Antimicrobial Resistance and Use Surveillance System (GLASS). GLASS is a global partnership coordinated by WHO aimed at standardising AMR surveillance and enhancing AMR knowledge.

GLASS is a standardised system designed for collecting, analysing, interpreting, and sharing AMR data from countries, territories, and regions. Its goal is to inform strategies for containing AMR by tracking the spread of resistance and evaluating the effectiveness of interventions.

GLASS was established in 2015 to streamline AMR surveillance, address knowledge gaps, and guide strategies across all levels. GLASS includes monitoring of AMR in bacteria responsible for common human infections, antimicrobial consumption (AMC), invasive fungal infections, and adopts a One Health approach that integrates human health, the food chain, and the environment. It offers a standardised method for data collection, analysis, and sharing.

Key objectives of GLASS are:

- To assess the burden of AMR.
- To monitor the spread of resistance.
- To evaluate the impact of local, national, and global strategies to combat AMR.

GLASS has made substantial progress in enhancing global AMR surveillance over recent years. A key milestone has been its rapid increase in country participation, expanding from a core group of early adopters to include most WHO Member States, with many low- and middle-income nations regularly submitting data on priority pathogens. This growth reflects heightened political commitment and better technical capacity worldwide.

Additionally, GLASS has improved the standardisation of AMR reporting by encouraging harmonised case definitions, uniform antimicrobial susceptibility testing (AST) methods, and structured reporting formats. This has boosted the comparability of resistance data across different regions and countries. The creation of guidance documents and training tools has helped laboratories enhance data quality and reliability.

A notable advancement is the integration of antimicrobial consumption (AMC) surveillance. More countries now report both antimicrobial use and resistance data, allowing for a deeper understanding of the link between antibiotic consumption and resistance trends. This development signifies a move towards more actionable surveillance.

In recent cycles, GLASS has increased data detail and transparency by providing publicly accessible dashboards and comprehensive global reports. These resources offer vital insights into resistance patterns of key pathogens like Escherichia coli, Klebsiella pneumoniae, and Staphylococcus aureus, guiding treatment strategies and stewardship efforts.

Moreover, GLASS has adopted a One Health approach by fostering connections with animal and environmental surveillance systems. Through capacity building, technical support, and data sharing, GLASS has transitioned from a simple reporting platform to a vital component of global AMR intelligence, promoting evidence-based policies and international cooperation.

11.4.2 WHO Support to National AMR Surveillance Systems

WHO assists countries in creating, executing, and overseeing multisectoral national action plans for AMR, with surveillance as a key element [13].

WHO provides technical support to countries, particularly low- and middle-income nations, to improve data collection and its use for policy-making. It also conducts training sessions and workshops that focus on national action plans, leadership skills, and AMR surveillance.

WHO emphasises the importance of data quality and representativeness in surveillance systems. WHO releases reports and guidance on AMR and its monitoring. These include yearly AMR data summaries, national action plan updates, and country-specific guidance. The annual GLASS reports are key resources offering a global perspective on AMR trends [14].

WHO Collaborating Centres on AMR

WHO currently recognises 38 designated collaborating centres [15] working on AMR worldwide, each offering 4-year renewable support to WHO and all countries in areas such as surveillance (Table 11.1). These centres are essential for executing the WHO's GLASS framework and assisting low- and middle-income countries in building capacity and improving data quality and comparability.

Table 11.1 WHO Collaborating Centres for AMR-linked activities in 2025

Country	Location	Name of Collaborating Centre
Argentina	La Plata	WHO Collaborating Centre for Rational Use of Medicines
Argentina	Buenos Aires	WHO Collaborating Centre for AMR Surveillance
Australia	Sydney	WHO Collaborating Centre for sexually transmitted infections and AMR
Australia	Melbourne	WHO Collaborating Centre for AMR
Canada	Toronto	WHO Collaborating Centre for Global Governance of AMR
China	Hong Kong	WHO Collaborating Centre for Infectious Diseases Epidemiology and Control
Costa Rica	Tres Rios	WHO Collaborating Centre for AMR Surveillance
Germany	Berlin	WHO Collaborating Centre for AMR, AMC and healthcare associated infections
Germany	Hanover	WHO Collaborating Centre for health at human-animal-environment interface
Denmark	Copenhagen	WHO Collaborating Centre for AMR in food-borne pathogens and genomics
India	Chandigarh	WHO Collaborating Centre for reference and research on fungi of medical importance
India	Bengaluru	WHO Collaborating Centre for AMR
Japan	Tokyo	WHO Collaborating Centre for AMR surveillance and research
Japan	Tokyo	WHO Collaborating Centre for prevention, preparedness, & response to AMR
Mexico	Ciudad de Mexico	WHO Collaborating Centre for AMR in food borne and environmental bacteria
Netherlans	Bilthoven	WHO Collaborating Centre for risk assessment of pathogens in food and water
Netherlands	Urecht	WHO Collaborating Centre for Reference and Research on Campylobacter and AMR from a One Health perspective
Netherlands	Bilthoven	WHO Collaborating Centre for AMR Epidemiology and Surveillance
Norway	Oslo	WHO Collaborating Centre for drug statistics methodology
Russia	Smolensk	WHO Collaborating Centre for capacity building in AMR surveillance and research
South Korea	Cheongju-si	WHO Collaborating Centre for AMR Reference and One Health Research
Saudi Arabia	Riyadh	WHO Collaborating Centre for Infection Prevention, Control and AMR
South Africa	Johannesberg	WHO Collaborating Centre for AMR
Sweden	Stockhom	WHO Collaborating Centre for AMR containment
Sweden	Orebro	WHO Collaborating Centre for gonorrhoea and other STIs
Sweden	Vaxjo	WHO Collaborating Centre for standardisation of antimicrobial susceptibility testing of bacteria
Switzerland	Geneva	WHO Collaborating Centre for IPC and AMR
Thailand	Bangkok	WHO Collaborating Centre for AMR prevention and containment
Thailand	Nonthaburi	WHO Collaborating Centre for AMR surveillance and training

(Continued)

Table 11.1 (Continued)

Country	Location	Name of Collaborating Centre
United Kingdom	London	WHO Collaborating Centre for Reference and Research on AMR & HAI
United Kingdom	Oxford	WHO Collaborating Centre for genomic surveillance of AMR
USA	Boston	WHO Collaborating Centre for pharmaceutical policy
USA	Atlanta	WHO Collaborating Centre for surveillance, epidemiology and control of food-borne diseases and fungal diseases
USA	Raleigh	WHO Collaborating Centre for Global One Health and AMR
USA	Stanford	WHO Collaborating Centre for antimicrobial stewardship and AMR
USA	Atlanta	WHO Collaborating Centre for international monitoring of bacterial resistance to antimicrobial agents
USA	Boston	WHO Collaborating Centre for surveillance of AMR

11.4.2.1 WHONET

WHONET is a free Windows-based desktop application designed for managing and analysing microbiology laboratory data, with a special emphasis on AMR surveillance. It is developed and supported by the WHO Collaborating Centre for Surveillance of Antimicrobial Resistance at Brigham and Women's Hospital in Boston, Massachusetts. Available in 45 languages, WHONET assists with local, national, regional, and global surveillance efforts across more than 2300 hospitals, public health, animal health, and food laboratories in over 130 countries worldwide [16]. The software is particularly valuable in hospitals for quickly identifying antibiograms, thereby enhancing patient care [17].

11.5 Regional and Multicountry AMR Surveillance Networks

Regional and multicountry AMR surveillance networks in the health sector are essential for tracking and managing AMR. They coordinate data collection and analysis across different countries or regions. These networks (Table 11.2), often backed by global initiatives like the WHO's GLASS, are crucial for detecting resistance patterns, shaping treatment guidelines, and directing public health actions [25].

11.6 National AMR Surveillance Network (NARS-Net)

Multiple countries have set up national AMR surveillance networks to monitor and address the increasing threat of drug-resistant infections. Notable examples include the United States' National Antimicrobial Resistance Monitoring System (NARMS)

Table 11.2 Regional and multicountry AMR surveillance networks

	Network	Region/countries covered
1	*EARS-Net* (European Antimicrobial Resistance Surveillance Network) [18]	Western Europe
2	*ReLAVRA+* (Latin American and Carribean Network for Antimicrobial Resistance Surveillance) [19]	Latin America and Caribbean countries
3	*CAESAR* (Central Asian and Eastern European Surveillance of Antimicrobial Resistance) [20]	Central Asia and Eastern Europe
4	*WPRACSS* (Western Pacific Regional Antimicrobial Surveillance System) [21]	Western Pacific Region
5	*ECOWAS* (Economic Community of West African States) [22]	West Africa
6	*CAPTURA* (Capturing Data on Antimicrobial Resistance Patterns and Trends in Use in Regions of Asia) [23]	South and South-East Asia
7	*SMART* (Study for Monitoring Antimicrobial Resistance Trends) [24]	200 sites in more than 60 countries

and two networks in India, among others. These networks are vital for monitoring AMR trends, shaping public health policies, and guiding efforts to curb the spread of resistance.

11.6.1 National Antimicrobial Resistance Monitoring System (NARMS), USA

NARMS is a joint initiative involving the US FDA, US CDC, and USDA that monitors antibiotic resistance in bacteria from retail meats, human illnesses, and food-producing animals. It delivers data on emerging AMR, mechanisms of resistance spread, and distinctions between resistant and susceptible infections [26].

11.6.2 Indian and Thailand AMR Surveillance Networks

India has established a comprehensive, multilayered AMR surveillance system over the past decade, led by the National AMR Surveillance Network [27] managed by the Indian Council of Medical Research (ICMR). This network connects select tertiary hospitals and reference labs nationwide to produce standardised data on key pathogens and resistance trends, with annual publications. Key findings include high resistance rates to third-generation cephalosporins and fluoroquinolones, increasing carbapenem resistance in Klebsiella pneumoniae and Acinetobacter baumannii, and ongoing methicillin resistance in Staphylococcus aureus.

Operations are centred on culture and sensitivity testing based on harmonised susceptibility standards, regular external quality assessments, and centralised data collection via a web-based reporting system. The annual AMR reports inform updates to treatment guidelines and hospital antibiotic stewardship programmes.

India has also broadened surveillance beyond tertiary centres by including state medical colleges and district hospitals, though coverage remains inconsistent. Efforts to integrate antimicrobial consumption data and private sector reporting are ongoing. One Health initiatives are progressing through collaboration with veterinary and food-sector surveillance under the national action plan on AMR. Overall, India's AMR surveillance has enhanced laboratory capacity and policy responsiveness, but challenges remain in geographic coverage, sustainability, and data integration.

India's second AMR surveillance network, operated by the National Centre for Disease Control (NCDC) under the Ministry of Health and Family Welfare, complements the ICMR network [27, 28]. It mainly focuses on public health surveillance by linking state public health labs and government medical colleges to monitor resistance in priority pathogens. This network emphasises standardised susceptibility testing, outbreak detection, and integration with the Integrated Disease Surveillance Programme (IDSP). It also supports capacity building, quality assurance, and data reporting to national authorities, strengthening epidemiological intelligence and early warning systems for AMR threats across states. Both networks analyse the extent and patterns of AMR across various regions.

Thailand's national AMR surveillance network [29] is coordinated by the Ministry of Public Health of Thailand and anchored by the Antimicrobial Resistance Surveillance Centre (ARSC). It links hospital laboratories nationwide to monitor resistance trends in key bacterial pathogens using standardised methods. Thailand has also integrated antimicrobial consumption monitoring and a strong One Health approach under its National Strategic Plan on AMR, producing regular national reports that guide stewardship policies and regulatory reforms.

It is now globally accepted that AMR surveillance is a vital tool for understanding, managing, and ultimately controlling the global threat of AMR.

11.7 Challenges in AMR Surveillance and Possible Solutions

AMR is one of the most pressing global public health threats of the twenty-first century. Surveillance of AMR is vital to track resistance trends, guide treatment, inform policies, and evaluate the effectiveness of interventions. Despite increased awareness and investment, AMR surveillance is still inconsistent and underdeveloped in many regions. Key global and regional challenges are outlined below, along with practical solutions.

11.7.1 Insufficient Political Commitment and Funding

Sustainable surveillance systems depend on long-term funding, which is often unavailable, especially in low- and middle-income countries (LMICs). Factors such as competing health priorities, limited awareness among policymakers, and the lack of legal frameworks lead to this neglect. To address this, advocacy and raising awareness among high-level leadership are essential to secure adequate and ongoing funding for comprehensive health system strengthening initiatives.

11.7.2 Inadequate Laboratory Infrastructure and Capacity

A major challenge is the shortage of sufficient and standardised microbiology laboratory infrastructure. Many LMICs do not have adequately equipped labs, dependable diagnostic tools, or trained staff. Even when infrastructure is present, there are differences in testing capabilities, quality control, and reporting standards.

Countries must invest adequately in developing and maintaining laboratory infrastructure using both domestic and international funds. Equally important is ensuring laboratories operate with a functional quality system to guarantee that the data produced is dependable and valuable. Building networks of sentinel, regional, and national reference laboratories to coordinate testing and data sharing enhances investment returns and allows for more exhaustive coverage with efficient processes.

11.7.3 Fragmented and Uncoordinated Surveillance Systems

Surveillance data is frequently fragmented across human health, animal health, and environmental sectors, which hampers the ability to produce comprehensive insights. While some networks generate significant data, it often remains unused because it is not translated into actionable insights. This issue may stem from a lack of awareness and limited analytical tools within the country. Implementing dashboards for consumers, such as clinicians and public health officials, along with developing and sharing policy briefs and providing feedback at all levels of data collection, should be prioritised.

National AMR programme managers should foster integrated surveillance across the human, veterinary, and environmental health sectors through a national AMR coordination body or task forces that connect ministries of health, agriculture, environment, and research. They should also efficiently use the analysed data to inform public health actions. To facilitate implementation, adopting standardised protocols from WHO, FAO, and WOAH—widely accepted worldwide—would help harmonise surveillance efforts.

11.7.4 Lack of Standardised Data and Reporting Mechanisms

AMR data often suffer from inconsistencies in definitions, methodology, and indicators, making cross-comparison difficult. Countries use different protocols, susceptibility breakpoints, and reporting templates. This can be overcome by encouraging enrolment in WHO GLASS, which promotes standardised methodologies and indicators. The use of currently available or newly created *digital platforms*, aligned with global databases, can be utilised for seamless data submission, access, and action. Many LMICs may not have an adequate number of skilled human resources. Continuous education for data managers and clinicians on standard terminology and practices is essential.

11.7.5 Poor Data Quality and Timeliness

Delayed reporting, missing data, manual entry errors, and limited real-time analytics reduce the utility of AMR surveillance data. This weakens timely response and early warning systems. The utilisation of Electronic Reporting Systems should be encouraged, and efforts should be made to *t*ransition to automated Laboratory Information Management Systems (LIMS). In addition, data validation protocols must be integrated into the entire data management to minimise errors.

11.7.6 Lack of Trained Human Resources

A worldwide shortage exists for skilled microbiologists, epidemiologists, and data analysts essential for AMR surveillance. Addressing this requires recruiting, training, and retaining enough qualified personnel across all levels of surveillance.

11.7.7 Surveillance Gaps in Community and Informal Settings

Most AMR surveillance happens primarily in hospitals, often missing community-acquired infections and informal healthcare settings where antibiotic misuse is common. To address this gap, developing community-based surveillance networks—such as at primary health centres or pharmacies—is crucial, along with conducting periodic point-prevalence surveys. Involving non-licenced drug sellers and traditional practitioners in surveillance activities and stewardship training is vital for comprehensive AMR management.

11.8 Global Inequities in Surveillance Coverage

High-income countries (HICs) often have robust surveillance systems (e.g. EARS-Net in Europe, CDC-NARMS in the U.S.), while many LMICs have minimal or no AMR surveillance. There is a global need to promote equitable support through WHO GLASS and other global alliances. HICs should share surveillance tools, software, and expertise with LMICs who should be encouraged and supported to use tools like the Tripartite AMR Country Self-assessment Survey (TrACSS) to track progress and identify gaps.

Effective AMR surveillance is fundamental to any strategy for combating AMR. Despite various systemic, infrastructural, and political hurdles, coordinated efforts at the global and national levels are starting to yield results. Key steps include implementing integrated One Health surveillance, enhancing laboratory and human resource capacities, standardising data collection and utilisation, and turning data into actionable insights. Continued political dedication and investment are crucial to ensure the sustainability of AMR surveillance and safeguard global health security.

References

1. FAO: antimicrobial resistance. Available at https://www.fao.org/antimicrobial-resistance/key-sectors/surveillance-and-monitoring/en/#:~. Accessed 14 Apr 2025.
2. Bengtsson-Palme J, Abramova A, Berendonk TU, Coelho LP, Forslund SK, Gschwind R, et al. Towards monitoring of antimicrobial resistance in the environment: for what reasons, how to implement it, and what are the data needs? Environ Int. 2023;178:108089. https://doi.org/10.1016/j.envint.2023.108089.
3. WHO. Global Antimicrobial Resistance and Use Surveillance System (GLASS). Available at https://www.who.int/initiatives/glass. Accessed 15 Apr 2025.
4. Jones RN. The emergent needs for basic research, education, and surveillance of antimicrobial resistance. Problems facing the report from the American Society for Microbiology task force on antibiotic resistance. Diagn Microbiol Infect Dis. 1996;25:153–61. https://doi.org/10.1016/s0732-8893(96)00099-5.
5. Núñez-Núñez M, Navarro MD, Palomo V, et al. The methodology of surveillance for antimicrobial resistance and healthcare-associated infections in Europe (SUSPIRE): a systematic review of publicly available information. Clin Microbiol Infect. 2018;24:105–9. https://doi.org/10.1016/j.cmi.2017.07.014.
6. Fuhrmeister AS, Jones RN. The importance of antimicrobial resistance monitoring worldwide and the origins of SENTRY antimicrobial surveillance program. Open Forum Infect Dis. 2019;6(Suppl 1):S1–4. https://doi.org/10.1093/ofid/ofy34.
7. de Kraker MEA, Lipsitch M. Burden of antimicrobial resistance: compared to what? Epidemiol Rev. 2022;43(1):53–64. https://doi.org/10.1093/epirev/mxab001.
8. WHO. Guidance on establishing national and local antimicrobial resistance surveillance systems in the Western Pacific region. Manila: World Health Organization Regional Office for the Western Pacific; 2024. Licence: CC BY-NC-SA 3.0 IGO.
9. Khadse SN, Ugemuge S, Singh C. Impact of antimicrobial stewardship on reducing antimicrobial resistance. Cureus. 2023;15(12):e49935. https://doi.org/10.7759/cureus.49935.

10. Alhassan MY, Ahmad AA. Antimicrobial resistance in a changing climate: a one health approach for adaptation and mitigation. Bull Natl Res Cent. 2025;49:26. https://doi.org/10.1186/s42269-025-01318-2.
11. Bengtsson-Palme J, Abramova A, Berendonk TU, Coelho LP, Forslund SK, Gschwind R, Heikinheimo A, et al. Towards monitoring of antimicrobial resistance in the environment: for what reasons, how to implement it, and what are the data needs? Environ Int. 2023;178:108089. https://doi.org/10.1016/j.envint.2023.108089.
12. WHO. GLASS. National antimicrobial resistance surveillance systems and participation in the Global Antimicrobial Resistance Surveillance System (GLASS) a guide to planning, implementation, and monitoring and evaluation. Available at https://iris.who.int/bitstream/handle/10665/251554/WHO-DGO-AMR-2016.4-eng.pdf?sequence=. Accessed 15 Apr 2025.
13. WHO. WHO implementation handbook for national action plans on antimicrobial resistance: guidance for the human health sector. Available at https://www.who.int/publications/i/item/9789240041981. Accessed 14 Apr 2025.
14. WHO. Global antimicrobial resistance & use surveillance system report 2022. Available at https://www.google.com/search?sa=X&cs=0&sca_esv=e8e3451742a7a0b0&q=Global+Antimicrobial+Resistance+and+Use+Surveillance+System+(GLASS)+Report+2022&si=. Accessed 3 Mar 2025.
15. WHO. WHO AMR surveillance and quality assessment collaborating centres network. Available at https://www.who.int/initiatives/glass/network#. Accessed 7 Mar 2025.
16. WHONET. The microbiology laboratory database software. Available at https://whonet.org/. Accessed 9 Mar 2025.
17. Manoj D, Vaghasiya J. Development and application of the WHONET software in hospital antibiogram. Clin Epidemiol Glob Health. 2023;24:101424. https://doi.org/10.1016/j.cegh.2023.101424.
18. European Centre for Disease Control and Prevention. EARS-Net (European Antimicrobial Resistance Surveillance Network). Available at https://www.ecdc.europa.eu/en/about-us/networks/disease-networks-and-laboratory-networks/ears-net-data. Accessed 29 Mar 2025.
19. WHO PAHO. Latin American and Caribbean Network for Antimicrobial Resistance Surveillance - ReLAVRA+. Available at https://www.paho.org/en/topics/antimicrobial-resistance/latin-american-and-caribbean-network-antimicrobial-resistance#. Accessed 3 Apr 2025.
20. WHO. Central Asian and European Surveillance of Antimicrobial Resistance (CAESAR). Available at https://www.who.int/europe/groups/central-asian-and-european-surveillance-of-antimicrobial-resistance-(caesar). Accessed 4 Apr 2025.
21. WHO. Western Pacific Regional Office. WPRACSS (Western Pacific Regional Antimicrobial Surveillance System). Available at https://www.who.int/westernpacific/health-topics/antimicrobial-resistance/wpracss. Accessed 5 Apr 2025.
22. Aboushady AT, Manigart O, Sow A, Fuller W, Ouedraogo A-S, Ebruke C, Babin F-X, Gahimbare L, Sombié I, Stelling J. Surveillance of antimicrobial resistance in the ECOWAS region: setting the scene for critical interventions needed. Antibiotics. 2024;13(7):627. https://doi.org/10.3390/antibiotics13070627.
23. Holm M, MacWright WR, Poudyal N, Shaw AG, Joh HS, Gallagher PF, Kim JH, Shaikh AT, Seo HJ, Kwon SY, Prifti K, Dolabella B, Taylor BEW, Yeats C, Aanensen DM, Stelling J, Marks F. Capturing data on antimicrobial resistance patterns and trends in use in regions of Asia (CAPTURA). Clin Infect Dis. 2023;77(Suppl 7):S500–6. https://doi.org/10.1093/cid/ciad567.
24. Cantón R, Gottlieb T, Coombs GW, Woo PCY, Korman TM, et al. Antimicrobial surveillance: a 20-year history of the SMART approach to addressing global antimicrobial resistance into the future. Int J Antimicrob Agents. 2023;62:107014. https://doi.org/10.1016/j.ijantimicag.2023.107014.

25. Frost I, Kapoor G, Craig J, Liu D, Laxminarayan R. Status, challenges and gaps in antimicrobial resistance surveillance around the world. J Glob Antimicrob Resist. 2021;25:222. https://doi.org/10.1016/j.jgar.2021.03.016.
26. US Centres for Disease Control and Prevention. National antimicrobial resistance monitoring system. Available at https://www.cdc.gov/narms/about/index.html. Accessed 16 Apr 2025.
27. National Centre for Disease Control. National AMR containment programme. Available at https://ncdc.mohfw.gov.in/national-programme-on-amr-containment/#:~. Accessed 16 Apr 2025.
28. Indian Council of Medical Research. India's antimicrobial resistance surveillance & research initiative. Available at https://iamrsn.icmr.org.in/. Accessed 1 May 2025.
29. Sumpradit N, Wongkongkathep S, Malathum K, Janejai N, Paveenkittiporn W, Yingyong T, Chuxnum T. Thailand's national strategic plan on antimicrobial resistance: progress and challenges. Bull World Health Organ. 2021;99(9):661–73. https://doi.org/10.2471/BLT.20.280644.

Chapter 12
AMR Surveillance in Veterinary Sector

Abstract Antimicrobial resistance (AMR) surveillance in the veterinary sector plays a crucial role in the One Health approach, enabling the early detection of resistance patterns and informing stewardship efforts. Unlike more developed human health surveillance systems, veterinary AMR monitoring is often fragmented, especially in low- and middle-income countries, due to limited lab capacity, inconsistent methods, and poor data integration across sectors. Effective surveillance depends on strong governance, reliable laboratory networks, trained personnel, and harmonised reporting standards. Global organisations such as WOAH, FAO, and WHO play a crucial role in delivering frameworks, technical assistance, and platforms like InFARM and GLASS for data collection and sharing. Regional efforts like EARS-Vet in Europe, NARMS in the USA, and CIPARS in Canada serve as models for integrated systems, while networks in Africa and Asia show emerging cooperation. Challenges like variable data quality, weak cross-sectoral links, and limited sustainability need to be tackled through capacity building, standardised protocols, digital tools, and stronger policy connections. Improving veterinary AMR surveillance is essential to protect animal and human health, maintain antibiotic effectiveness, and support sustainable food systems.

Keywords Antimicrobial resistance (AMR) · Veterinary surveillance · One Health · InFARM · EARS-Vet · CIPARS · NARMS

Surveillance involves the systematic, ongoing collection, organisation, and analysis of data, along with the quick dissemination of information to relevant parties, particularly those capable of taking action. Antimicrobial resistance (AMR) surveillance and monitoring track changes and trends in microbial populations, including bacteria resistant to antibiotics and their associated resistance traits, such as genes and mechanisms of resistance [1].

Monitoring AMR across health, agricultural, and environmental sectors is essential for understanding and fighting the spread of drug-resistant pathogens [2]. It provides vital data that support treatment choices, guide policy decisions, and evaluate the effectiveness of strategies designed to limit AMR.

R. Bhatia, *Drug-Resistant Infections*,
https://doi.org/10.1007/978-981-92-4190-3_12

12.1 AMR Surveillance in Veterinary Sector

AMR surveillance is vital for controlling the spread of drug-resistant microbes across humans, animals, plants, and the environment. These systems provide crucial data that deepen our understanding of AMR's complex epidemiology. The collected information is key to infection management, policymaking, and creating strategies to combat AMR.

AMR surveillance data is essential for countries to tackle AMR effectively, as it allows for proactive responses before crises escalate. This data plays an important role in designing, managing, and evaluating AMR control measures and interventions.

Surveillance frameworks in the food and agriculture sectors provide quick information regarding

(i) The prevalence of AMR in animals, plants, and environmental settings,
(ii) the application of antimicrobial drugs, and,
(iii) the concentration of antimicrobial residues in food products.

In contrast to human clinical surveillance, data on veterinary AMR is limited, inconsistent, and fragmented across various countries and regions.

Many countries, especially low- and middle-income (LMICs), need help to improve their capacity and resources for AMR surveillance and monitoring. This assistance would allow these nations to collect, generate, analyse, and interpret data on AMR, antimicrobial use patterns, antimicrobial residues in the food supply chain, and environmental AMR levels.

12.2 Key Elements of Veterinary AMR Surveillance

Several key components of veterinary AMR surveillance networks are essential for understanding the burden and trends of AMR. They also help demonstrate the success of interventions. High-quality surveillance data is vital for shaping AMR policies and creating effective programmes.

Efficient veterinary AMR surveillance systems generally consist of the following components:

Governance and Financing: National authorities need to lead, nurture and sustain the development, support, and oversight of a comprehensive national AMR surveillance network. This leadership is vital for mobilising resources, establishing standards, coordinating laboratories, data sharing and agreements, and ensuring alignment with national AMR action plans.

Quality Laboratory Support: As AMR surveillance depends entirely on laboratory analyses, it is essential to have laboratories capable of performing antimicrobial susceptibility testing following standardised international protocols such as European Committee on Antimicrobial Susceptibility Testing (EUCAST) [3] and Clinical and Laboratory Standards Institute (CLSI) [4]. Pathogens of public health importance should be identified and integrated into these protocols.

Creating a national laboratory network: It is essential for AMR surveillance, utilising statistically validated samples that accurately represent the ground realities. Members of this network should implement a laboratory quality management system that is regularly validated through external quality assessments.

Human Resources and Modern Technological Tools: Conducting surveillance activities, whether in the field or via data analysis, demands skilled personnel equipped with advanced technological tools and regular updates. This approach improves the responsiveness of surveillance to policy needs and public health initiatives.

Data Collection and Reporting Frameworks: Surveillance data are usually collected from infected (clinical isolates) or healthy animals via veterinary laboratories. Surveillance networks create essential datasets and metadata—including host species, sample type, antimicrobial tested, minimum inhibitory concentrations (MIC) values, and interpretative criteria—to maintain analytical consistency. The integration of AI, machine learning, and statistical modelling in AMR surveillance highlights a growing focus on predictive analytics, early warning systems, and decision support tools within One Health frameworks. However, their broad implementation by trained personnel remains limited.

Data Integration, Analysis, and Dissemination: Consolidated data should facilitate trend analysis, early recognition of emerging resistance, provide feedback for veterinary practitioners, and inform stewardship policies.

Linkages with One Health and Antimicrobial Stewardship (AMS) interventions: Surveillance systems contribute to AMS programmes, enabling veterinarians to tailor responsible antimicrobial prescriptions, monitor policy impacts, and coordinate with human sector surveillance within a One Health framework.

Unlike human health alone, animal-sector surveillance must address diverse production systems (including food-producing animals and aquaculture), various species, and the complexities of veterinary supply chains.

12.3 AMR Surveillance in Animals at the Global Level

The World Organisation for Animal Health (WOAH) plays a central role in global AMR surveillance within the animal sector [5]. It develops standards, publishes annual data reports, and promotes monitoring through its observatory process. WOAH's efforts include collecting data on antimicrobial agents used in animals and providing resources and guidance for national Veterinary and Aquatic Animal Health Services to report on drug use and resistance. Its position within the One Health framework enables WOAH to integrate veterinary surveillance with wider human and environmental health systems.

The UN's Food and Agriculture Organisation (FAO) highlights that surveillance and monitoring are key components of its approach to combating AMR [6]. FAO assists countries in developing and strengthening their AMR surveillance and laboratory infrastructures. This backing helps nations generate, collect, and analyse high-quality epidemiological data as part of their national AMR surveillance efforts in food and agriculture, facilitating cross-sector interpretation of the findings.

FAO's initiatives encompass:

- Developing and implementing tools to assess and enhance laboratory capacity, surveillance systems, and the utilisation of AMR data;
- Providing training on laboratory techniques for detecting and characterising AMR and on epidemiology for managing and analysing data;
- Establishing expert networks and broader partnerships with public and private-sector stakeholders;
- Publishing technical guidelines and scientific papers concerning FAO surveillance initiatives;
- Supporting the operationalisation of national surveillance programmes and implementing community-based surveillance approaches (both specific to the food and agriculture sectors and multi-sectoral One Health programmes).

12.3.1 InFARM

In 2022, FAO launched an IT platform for the International FAO Antimicrobial Resistance Monitoring (InFARM) [6]. The InFARM IT platform hosts AMR data for priority bacterial species relevant to public health, animal health, and indicator bacteria from animals and food, adhering to international standards (Table 12.1) and

Table 12.1 Priority bacteria to be reported to InFARM

Category	Bacterial species	Relevance
Public health	*Salmonella* spp.	Zoonotic; transmitted via food (meat, eggs, etc.)
	Campylobacter jejuni	Leading cause of foodborne illness; found in poultry
	Campylobacter coli	Significant in foodborne disease
	Escherichia coli (ESBL, AmpC, carbapenemase-producing)	Resistant strains pose serious risk to human health
Animal health	*Escherichia coli* (pathogenic strains)	Causes disease in animals (e.g. colibacillosis in poultry or calves)
	Staphylococcus aureus (including MRSA)	Causes infections in animals; MRSA is also zoonotic
Indicator bacteria	Commensal *Escherichia coli*	Used to track resistance trends in healthy animals and food chain
	Enterococcus faecalis	Commensal in the gut; indicator for resistance surveillance
	Enterococcus faecium	An indicator species; can carry resistance genes

the Codex Alimentarius recommendations [7] for integrated monitoring and surveillance of foodborne AMR and the animal health codes of the WOAH [8].

The InFARM platform supports national AMR surveillance efforts by:

- Formalising and establishing national surveillance networks;
- building capacity among national focal points and experts on data generation and sharing;
- adapting data management solutions and ensuring interoperability with Laboratory Information Management Systems.

The goals of the InFARM system and IT platform include:

- Helping countries collect, analyse, and use their AMR data related to animals and food to meet national goals. InFARM supports capacity building for the global standardisation of AMR data generated through laboratory-based surveillance. It will serve as a comprehensive resource with relevant contextual information on AMR and AMU monitoring programmes, including activities like national surveillance strategies and reports on FAO assessment tool usage.
- Encouraging countries to publicly share AMR data from food and agriculture sectors for global surveillance, supporting international efforts and advocacy.

InFARM accepts officially validated national data from both systematic and pilot surveillance efforts, following established data models and templates. To protect privacy, it provides two interfaces: a private one and a public one, with three confidentiality levels for data sharing. Participants can choose to keep data entirely private, accessible only to designated country users in the private interface (level 1), or share it publicly through regional or subregional aggregation, making it available to the global community.

InFARM promotes alignment with WOAH/FAO/WHO guidelines, facilitates data sharing, and encourages capacity building for national and regional reporting.

Contributions made by InFARM in the recent past InFARM has made significant progress in enhancing AMR surveillance within the food and agriculture sectors. Its recent reporting cycle featured the first annual open call for AMR data (2024), which attracted widespread global participation: 52 countries enrolled, 49 reported surveillance activities, and 28 submitted data on animal and food AMR, creating a strong foundation for international collaboration and evidence collection.

A major achievement has been capacity building. FAO organised regional training sessions for national focal points across Latin America, Sub-Saharan Africa, and Asia-Pacific, focused on improving skills in managing, analysing, and utilising AMR data. These trainings are essential for strengthening national surveillance systems and improving data quality.

Furthermore, InFARM is broadening its scope and usefulness. The platform now integrates AMR data collection with wider One Health goals, including plans to incorporate antimicrobial use (AMU) data in plant production—a critical step towards comprehensive surveillance in agrifood systems.

By combining an IT platform with capacity development, standardised data tools, and regional support, InFARM has transitioned from concept to practical application. This has helped build more robust national systems capable of producing reliable AMR evidence. This progress lays the groundwork for ongoing expansion and deeper integration with global surveillance initiatives.

World Health Organisation

The World Health Organisation (WHO) integrates animal-sector data into its One Health surveillance framework, aiming to link AMR data across human, animal, and environmental sectors [9]. The Global Antimicrobial Resistance and Use Surveillance System [10] (GLASS) is expanding to encompass this cross-sector approach, emphasising the critical need for interoperable data systems that include antimicrobial use in animals as a factor in resistance development.

Though GLASS continues to primarily focus on human health surveillance, it is increasingly incorporating One Health components that connect human, animal, and environmental AMR data. An example is the "Tricycle" model, which monitors resistant E. coli across different sectors. Although GLASS currently does not systematically collect veterinary AMR data, as specialised animal surveillance systems do, ongoing collaborations with the World Organisation for Animal Health and FAO indicate a shift towards a more integrated One Health surveillance approach.

12.4 Regional and Subregional Networks

Europe: EARS-Vet

The EU Joint Action on AMR and Healthcare-Associated Infections has started efforts to create the European AMR Surveillance network in veterinary medicine (EARS-Vet). The existing national systems for monitoring AMR in animal bacterial pathogens have been identified. EARS-Vet has defined its goals, scope, and standards. Pilot testing of the EARS-Vet surveillance system has been carried out to (i) assess the available data, (ii) perform cross-country analyses, and (iii) identify potential challenges and facilitate implementation [11].

North America

Initiatives such as the Canadian Integrated Programme for Antimicrobial Resistance Surveillance (CIPARS) [12] and the U.S. National Antimicrobial Resistance Monitoring System (NARMS) [13] include components that track antimicrobial use in food animals and resistance patterns in zoonotic and commensal bacteria. These national programmes contribute to global data synthesis, share methodologies, and often serve as benchmarks for middle- and low-income countries, improving their surveillance systems. In the USA, considerable efforts have been made to develop standardised national platforms [14].

12.5 Regional, Subregional, and Cross-Cutting Initiatives

Regional platforms and technical networks, such as those established through WOAH Collaborating Centres, support the exchange of best practices, external evaluations, and laboratory improvements. Reviews indicate that the advantages of surveillance—such as early detection and controlled usage—depend heavily on ongoing data sharing from regional hubs to inform national decisions [15].

12.6 MAAP (Mapping AMR & AMU Partnership)

Led by One Health Trust and supported by the Fleming Fund, this project analysed more than 819,000 AMR records from 205 labs across 14 African countries, establishing the first standardised overview of AMR prevalence in animal-sector isolates.

The Mekong Basin Disease Surveillance (MBDS) [16] consortium operates mainly on human zoonotic diseases. However, it demonstrates models of cross-border collaboration that could be adapted for animal AMR surveillance.

National Networks

In addition to developed nations such as Canada and the USA, only a few developing countries have established representative AMR surveillance networks in the animal health sector. One example is the Indian Network for Fishery and Animal AMR (INFAAR), which has established a baseline for the prevalence of resistant pathogens in India and is currently engaged in analysing AMR trends [17]. INFAAR is a national surveillance system for antimicrobial resistance in the veterinary and fisheries sectors, established by the Indian Council of Agricultural Research with support from the Food and Agriculture Organisation of the United Nations. Initiated in 2017, INFAAR unites laboratories from fisheries and livestock to systematically track antimicrobial resistance in food-producing animals and aquaculture, using standardised methods and quality-assured tools like WHONET. It produced India's first national AMR data report for 2019–22, highlighting notable resistance in pathogens such as *E. coli* and *Staphylococcus aureus*. FAO's support has enhanced training, data quality, and advisory oversight, with plans for ongoing expansion and capacity building.

Greece has implemented pilot projects and undertaken SWOT analyses to establish veterinary AMR surveillance systems, integrating them into EARS-Vet through national laboratories and veterinary authorities [18].

12.7 Challenges

Significant obstacles to AMR surveillance remain within the veterinary sector (Box 12.1).

Box 12.1 Key Challenges in AMR Surveillance in the Veterinary Sector

- Varying data quality, incomplete data coverage, and limited representativeness
- Inconsistent farm-level detail in low- and middle-income nations
- Disjointed systems and difficulties in data comparability
- Insufficient laboratory capacity and quality control systems
- Limited data management capabilities and infrastructure
- Absence of mechanisms to integrate data across sectors and along the value chain, diminishing the One Health potential of surveillance
- Lack of understanding in utilising AMR surveillance data for formulating policies and developing programmes at local, regional, and national levels
- Hesitance in data sharing among sectors, coupled with ownership and confidentiality concerns.

In many countries, surveillance initiatives are typically national, methodologically inconsistent, and employ differing antimicrobial susceptibility testing standards, thereby obstructing cross-border comparisons. A few years back, only around half of EU nations had functional national systems [19].

12.7.1 Challenges in AMR Surveillance in Developed World

Challenges in antimicrobial resistance (AMR) surveillance within the veterinary sector of developed countries involve both structural and operational issues despite robust regulatory frameworks. Harmonising data across nations remains difficult, with many countries adhering to standards from the World Organisation for Animal Health and regional bodies such as the European Food Safety Authority, yet differences in sampling methods, breakpoints, and reporting formats hinder direct comparison. Data integration of antimicrobial use (AMU) and resistance is often incomplete, especially at the farm level, where detailed prescription and treatment records may not be uniformly digitised. Surveillance of companion animals and aquaculture is less standardised compared to food-producing livestock. Additionally, private-sector data sharing is constrained by commercial sensitivities and data protection laws, thereby limiting transparency. Securing ongoing funding and political support remains challenging in developed nations, as AMR competes with other emerging animal health threats, similar to resource-limited settings.

12.8 Possible Solutions and Way Forward

Although establishing AMR surveillance can be challenging, it is feasible. As described earlier, several networks are already operating effectively. A strong commitment and determination from national authorities are urgently required. Here are some guiding operational principles:

Establish Governance and Operational Frameworks Quadripartite organisations have developed guidelines tailored to integrated surveillance for veterinary purposes that go beyond the human-oriented GLASS and align with One Health requirements.

Promote Engagement in Regional Networks Using a Harmonised and Standardised Strategy These networks should be developed via intercountry advocacy, collaborative planning, and joint implementation. Organisations such as FAO, WHO, WOAH, and UNEP, along with other international development partners, should provide resources and technical support to establish and manage these networks, recognising them as global public goods.

Standardise Testing and Reporting Protocols All surveillance entities need to operate following standardised protocols for testing and reporting. The global standards set by EUCAST and CLSI should be adopted.

Enhance Capacity Building By expanding initiatives such as FAO ATLASS [20], WOAH, and Fleming Fund's MAAP to support laboratory upgrades, training of personnel, and alignment with national action plans.

Establish Data-sharing Frameworks and Essential Digital Infrastructure Data sharing agreements should address privacy, stewardship, and laboratory accreditation and include feedback mechanisms. Digital platforms can support real-time monitoring, provide analytical dashboards, and enable open access to data.

Align Surveillance Efforts with Stewardship and Policy Initiatives The results from surveillance should directly inform AMS actions, guiding formulary choices, veterinary prescribing standards, regulatory policies on animal antibiotic use, and public awareness efforts.

Leverage Research and Technological Tools, such *as* geospatial modelling, genomic surveillance (including pathogen sequencing to identify resistance genes), AI-based analysis, and predictive modelling, to anticipate trends and optimise interventions.

12.8.1 Possible Support from International Development Partners

Monitoring AMR and antimicrobial use in the animal health sector is essential for managing resistance threats across the One Health continuum. Global organisations like WOAH, FAO (via InFARM), and WHO offer frameworks and platforms, while some regional networks demonstrate the advantages of standardised, policy-linked data. Despite progress, issues remain with data completeness, integration, and sustainability. Improving these systems through expanded coverage, better technical capacity, and cross-sector collaboration will be vital to prevent antimicrobial use in animals from undermining progress in both animal and human health.

AMR surveillance in the veterinary sector is still underdeveloped in many low- and middle-income countries, despite the crucial roles of livestock, aquaculture, and food systems in resistance transmission. This is mainly due to low prioritisation and weak infrastructure. International development partners can significantly contribute by advocating for policy change and providing sustainable financial and technical support to establish effective veterinary AMR surveillance systems. Key areas where international help can make a substantial impact include:

Long-term financing and infrastructure, which are vital given that many veterinary labs lack basic microbiology capabilities, cold chain systems, and biosafety infrastructure. Grants or concessional funding can be used to upgrade labs, equip regional diagnostic centres, and establish reference labs aligned with World Organisation for Animal Health standards, with an emphasis on decentralised networks to gather data from smallholder and commercial systems.

Technical assistance and standardisation efforts are essential, providing guidance on harmonised antimicrobial susceptibility testing, sampling protocols in livestock and aquaculture, and quality assurance, in collaboration with FAO and WHO to ensure alignment with global One Health frameworks.

Workforce development should be a priority, with support for training veterinary microbiologists, epidemiologists, and field officers, including specialised programmes and twinning arrangements with advanced labs to expedite capacity building.

Digital systems and data integration are also crucial; partners can help establish laboratory information management systems (LIMS), integrate antimicrobial use data, and develop national dashboards for real-time monitoring, linking veterinary AMR data with human and environmental systems for early warning.

Lastly, strengthening policies and regulations is urgent; technical support can assist countries in drafting legislation for antimicrobial use reporting, regulating veterinary drugs, and promoting stewardship programmes for responsible use. By combining funding, technical expertise, and policy development, international partners can help build sustainable veterinary AMR surveillance systems that safeguard both animal and human health.

Surveillance networks for AMR in veterinary medicine are evolving differently across the globe. Although human AMR monitoring is well-established with platforms like GLASS, veterinary AMR systems remain fragmented. An organised international effort is needed to strengthen veterinary AMR surveillance by standardising protocols, improving laboratory capabilities, integrating digital tools, and linking directly to stewardship and policy. Such an initiative is vital for safeguarding animal and human health, preserving antibiotic effectiveness, and protecting food systems and livelihoods worldwide.

References

1. FAO: antimicrobial resistance. Available at https://www.fao.org/antimicrobial-resistance/key-sectors/surveillance-and-monitoring/en/#:~. Accessed 15 Apr 2025.
2. Bengtsson-Palme J, Abramova A, Berendonk TU, Coelho LP, Forslund SK, Gschwind R, et al. Towards monitoring of antimicrobial resistance in the environment: for what reasons, how to implement it, and what are the data needs? Environ Int. 2023;178:108089. https://doi.org/10.1016/j.envint.2023.108089.
3. EUCAST. European Committee on Antimicrobial Susceptibility Testing. Available at https://www.eucast.org/. Accessed 19 Mar 2025.
4. CLSI. Clinical and Laboratory Standards Institute. Available at https://clsi.org/. Accessed 19 Mar 2025.
5. World Organization for Animal Health. Monitoring antimicrobial use and resistance. Available at https://www.woah.org/en/what-we-do/standards/observatory/implementation-of-standards-the-observatory-monitoring-report/monitoring-antimicrobial-use-and-resistance/#:~:text=. Accessed 23 Mar 2025.
6. FAO: The International FAO Antimicrobial Resistance Monitoring (InFARM) system and IT platform: InFarm. Available at https://openknowledge.fao.org/server/api/core/bitstreams/8fd532c0-b298-4de9-84f0-8a24eea71048/content. Accessed 19 Apr 2025.
7. Codex Alimentarius. Guidelines for integrated monitoring and surveillance of foodborne AMR. 2021. Available at https://www.fao.org/fao-who-codexalimentarius/sh-proxy/hu/?lnk=1. Accessed 9 Mar 2025.
8. WOAH. Standards. Available at https://www.woah.org/en/what-we-do/standards/#:~:text. Accessed 29 Mar 2025.
9. WHO. One health. Available at https://www.who.int/health-topics/one-health#tab=tab_1. Accessed 19 Apr 2025.
10. WHO. Global Antimicrobial Resistance and Use Surveillance System (GLASS). Available at https://www.who.int/initiatives/glass.
11. Lagrange J, Amat JP, Ballesteros C, Damborg P, Grönthal T, Haenni M, et al. Pilot testing the EARS-vet surveillance network for antibiotic resistance in bacterial pathogens from animals in the EU/EEA. Front Microbiol. 2023;14:1188423. https://doi.org/10.3389/fmicb.2023.1188423.
12. Avery BP, Parmley EJ, Reid-Smith RJ, Daignault D, Finley RL, Irwin RJ. Canadian integrated program for antimicrobial resistance surveillance: retail food highlights, 2003–2012. Can Commun Dis Rep. 2014;40(Suppl 2):29–35. https://doi.org/10.14745/ccdr.v40is2a05.
13. Karp BE, Tate H, Plumblee JR, Dessai U, Whichard JM, Thacker EL, Hale KR, et al. National antimicrobial resistance monitoring system: two decades of advancing public health through integrated surveillance of antimicrobial resistance. Foodborne Pathog Dis. 2017;14(10):545–57. https://doi.org/10.1089/fpd.2017.2283.

14. Ruzante JM, Harris B, Plummer P, Raineri RR, Loy JD, Jacob M, Sahin O, Kreuder AJ. Surveillance of antimicrobial resistance in veterinary medicine in the United States: current efforts, challenges, and opportunities. Front Vet Sci. 2022;9:1068406. https://doi.org/10.3389/fvets.2022.1068406.
15. Jacobsen AB, Jane O, Ekiri Abel B. Antimicrobial resistance interventions in the animal sector: scoping review. Front Antibiot. 2023;2:1–36. https://doi.org/10.3389/frabi.2023.1233698.
16. Mekong Basin Disease Surveillance. Available at https://www.cordsnetwork.org/networks/mbds/. Accessed 28 Mar 2025.
17. AMR Insights. Surveillance data from Indian Network for Fishery and Animal AMR. Available at https://www.amr-insights.eu/surveillance-data-of-the-indian-network-for-fishery-and-animal-antimicrobial-resistance-infaar-2/#:~:text. Accessed 1 Apr 2025.
18. Zafeiridis C, Valiakos G, Giakoupi P, Papadogiannakis E. Building the national antimicrobial resistance surveillance network in animals in Greece: a "one health" approach. Antibiotics. 2023;12(9):1442. https://doi.org/10.3390/antibiotics12091442.
19. Mader R, Bourély C, Amat JP, Broens EM, Busani L, Callens B, et al. Defining the scope of the European Antimicrobial Resistance Surveillance network in Veterinary medicine (EARS-Vet): a bottom-up and One Health approach. J Antimicrob Chemother. 2022;77:816–26. https://doi.org/10.1093/jac/dkab462.
20. FAO. FAO Assessment Tool for Laboratories and AMR Surveillance Systems (FAO-ATLASS). Available at https://www.fao.org/antimicrobial-resistance/resources/tools/fao-atlass/en/. Accessed 15 Apr 2025.

Chapter 13
Surveillance of Antimicrobial Consumption and Use

Abstract Surveillance of antimicrobial consumption (AMC) and antimicrobial use (AMU) is crucial to combating antimicrobial resistance (AMR), a global health threat driven by the inappropriate and excessive use of antibiotics in both humans and animals. AMC refers to aggregated data on antimicrobial volumes, while AMU involves patient- or farm-level usage details. Monitoring the AMC is vital for assessing prescribing patterns, stewardship efforts, and the impact of policies. Global frameworks, such as the WHO's GLASS, WOAH's ANIMUSE, and Europe's ESVAC, provide standardised methodologies for data collection, comparison, and reporting. Despite progress, especially in Europe, surveillance in many low- and middle-income countries remains limited, hindered by inadequate infrastructure, fragmented ownership, and inconsistent methodologies. Accurate AMC and AMU data link consumption with resistance trends, guiding stewardship, regulatory interventions, and global commitments to reduce the use of antibiotics in animals and humans. Innovative solutions—including standardised metrics, One Health integration, digital technologies, and advanced modelling—are essential to strengthen surveillance. Robust AMC and AMU estimation ensures accountability, informs global reduction targets, and safeguards the effectiveness of antibiotics for both human and animal health.

Keywords Antimicrobial consumption · Antimicrobial use · One Health surveillance · Stewardship programmes · Veterinary medicine · Global AMC monitoring frameworks

Antimicrobial use (AMU) refers to the data on the consumption of antibiotics by individual patients. This data is collected at the patient level and usually includes information about the treatment reason, the type of treatment, and patient characteristics. Although valuable for monitoring potential antimicrobial resistance (AMR) sources through prescribing patterns, gathering AMU data requires significant resources and is often challenging to implement nationwide, especially in the absence of electronic health records [1].

R. Bhatia, *Drug-Resistant Infections*,
https://doi.org/10.1007/978-981-92-4190-3_13

Antimicrobial consumption (AMC) involves aggregated data estimates, typically based on records from imports, manufacturers, or reimbursements [1]. Various private and government entities maintain these records and are often used as a proxy for antimicrobial use (AMU).

Need to Monitor AMC

Monitoring AMC is crucial because antibiotics are vital in treating infectious diseases, yet they are often misused or overprescribed. This excessive and improper use significantly contributes to the growth of AMR, which poses a major global health risk. Estimating AMC provides essential insights for assessing policy outcomes, including overall reductions and declines in key antibiotic categories [2]. Global data show that high antibiotic use in food-producing animals is a primary factor driving resistance, highlighting the importance of improved surveillance to track progress in reducing reliance and promoting better stewardship [3].

AMC Surveillance in Veterinary Sector

In AMC surveillance within the animal health sector, data on veterinary AMR are limited, inconsistent, and vary across countries and regions, especially when compared to human clinical surveillance. Effective surveillance involves two main strategies: measuring AMC (using methods like sales, prescriptions, or farm-level use) and assessing AMR phenotypes in animal pathogens or indicator organisms. These systems employ standardised metrics to enable comparison across different areas. Efforts to combine data strive to link consumption patterns with resistance trends, aiding targeted efforts to reduce high-risk antimicrobial use.

Several global and regional platforms have been established to oversee AMC within the veterinary sector. A brief overview of some of these platforms is provided below. Establishing similar mechanisms at the national, provincial, and local levels is vital for understanding local dynamics and implementing appropriate measures. AMC surveillance involves various methods and indicators. These systems typically monitor AMC through multiple approaches (Table 13.1). The effectiveness of the data points varies, and a range of metrics is employed, including standards such as the Defined Daily Dose (DDDvet) or Used Daily Dose, along with normalisation by population at risk (e.g. animal biomass) to facilitate comparisons.

Table 13.1 Possible methods and sources for estimating antimicrobial consumption

Mechanism	Feasibility	Related to AMC	Source/process
Production + import—Export—Waste/expiry	++	+	National authorities responsible for production, import/export and regulations of antibiotics
Distributors of veterinary pharma products	++	+	State drug controllers/regulators at local and national level
Point prevalence of sale from chemists/village shops	++	++	Planned studies by trained staff through a predefined protocol using smartphone
Inventory reviews of veterinary hospitals	++	++	Planned review by trained staff through a predefined protocol using smartphone
Time limited survey of prescribers	++	++	Survey by trained staff using a predefined protocol using smartphone
Time limited surveys of users for weekly consumption	+++	++++	Survey by trained staff using a predefined protocol using smartphone

13.1 Global Frameworks on AMC in Animal Health

13.1.1 WHO GLASS and Global Action Plans

The World Health Organisation (WHO) launched the Global Antimicrobial Resistance Surveillance System (GLASS) [4] under the Global Action Plan on Antimicrobial Resistance (2015) [5]. GLASS promotes harmonised surveillance of AMR across human, veterinary, and environmental sectors. Initially focused on human clinical data, GLASS aims to integrate veterinary and environmental antimicrobial use metrics under the One Health approach, endorsed by WHO, FAO, and the World Organisation for Animal Health (WOAH: earlier known as OIE).

13.1.2 WOAH's ANIMUSE Platform: A Global Digital Portal for AMC

WOAH has been monitoring antimicrobial use in food-producing animals since 2015 to limit the emergence of drug-resistant bacteria. The overuse of medically necessary antibiotics in these animals is a significant contributor to rising AMR rates.

In 2022–2023, WOAH launched the ANIMUSE platform to support country-level reporting of antimicrobial use in animals [6]. ANIMUSE allows comprehensive reporting, from national totals to detailed data on species, indications, dosage, and administration, promoting ongoing improvement. Recognising the significance of tracking antimicrobial use in animals, ANIMUSE [7] has been developed as an interactive, automated database that helps countries report, access, analyse, and share data on antimicrobials used in animals with various stakeholders. It offers simplified reporting, error detection, and data visualisation tools. Its goal is to enhance the practices of Veterinary and Aquatic Animal Health Services concerning antimicrobial use. Reporting to ANIMUSE is accessible to all countries, whether WOAH Members or non-members. National Veterinary Services can submit general data and, if quantitative details are available, select from various options based on the level of detail.

Each year, WOAH releases a report highlighting global and regional trends in antibiotic use in animals. This report is based on annual data collection conducted from September to May. The most recent report, published in May 2025, details antimicrobial use adjusted for animal biomass worldwide for 2022 and summarises the findings from the eighth year of data collection on animal antimicrobial use [8]. The report reveals that 34 of 157 responding countries (22%) still use antibiotics for growth promotion. These are mostly concentrated in the Americas and the Asia-Pacific regions. About 71% of responding countries (112 out of 157) confirmed that such non-veterinary medical use is no longer authorised, regardless of legislation. Notably, eight countries still report the use of colistin—a critically important antimicrobial for human health—despite a commitment made by all WOAH Members 10 years ago to phase out this practice [8].

WOAH estimates the global use of antimicrobial agents in food-producing animals for 2022 could be as high as 74,035 t, with tetracyclines and penicillin being the most prevalent, accounting for 28.29% and 17.75% of the total, respectively [8]. While both are classified as Veterinary Critically Important Antimicrobial (VCIA) agents in the WHO List of Antimicrobials of Veterinary Importance [9], they are not listed among the highest-priority critically important antimicrobial agents for human health by the WHO [10]. Among those that WHO lists in this category are fluoroquinolones (3.7%), polymyxins (1.8%), and third- and fourth-generation cephalosporins (0.9%).

ESVAC: Europe's Landmark Veterinary Consumption Surveillance

The European Surveillance of Veterinary Antimicrobial Consumption (ESVAC), managed by the European Medicines Agency from 2009 to 2023, gathered standardised data on veterinary antimicrobial sales and usage across EU/EEA countries. By using consistent units, such as population correction units, and enabling breakdowns by species like poultry, pigs, cattle, pets, and fish, ESVAC facilitated comparison between countries, trend analysis, and assessment of achievements of policy targets [11].

Low- and Middle-Income Countries

Developing countries, especially in Africa and Asia, have limited or nascent consumption reporting mechanisms; however, efforts are underway to encourage participation via ANIMUSE and AMU mapping initiatives [12].

13.2 Trends in Global Use of Antibiotics in Animals

The use of antibiotics in animal production has increased sharply in response to the global rise in demand for animal protein. Estimates suggest that approximately two-thirds of the growth in worldwide antimicrobial use is attributed to the expansion of food-animal production, particularly in low- and middle-income countries [3]. Conversely, some high-income regions have experienced a decline in veterinary antimicrobial use. Initiatives focusing on policies, stewardship, and regulations have contributed to significant reductions in usage levels in European countries, the UK, and the USA [13].

WOAH estimates that in 2022, antibiotic use ranged from 89 to 93 mg/kg of animal biomass. Globally, there was a 5% reduction in antibiotic usage across 81 countries in Europe, Africa, the Americas, and Asia. Conversely, Middle Eastern countries experienced a 43% increase during the same period [8].

Europe has seen notable progress in reducing antibiotic use in recent years. From 2011 to 2022, livestock antibiotic sales fell by 53%. In 2022, the EU implemented new regulations to eliminate routine antibiotic use on farms [14]. In the UK, antibiotic use in livestock has decreased by approximately 59% since 2014 [15].

New UK regulations—effective from 17 July 2024—are based on EU rules and prohibit routine antibiotic use, but do not ban prophylactic group treatments or require mandatory data collection on antibiotic use, unlike the EU.

13.3 Benefits of AMC Estimation

Excessive or inappropriate antimicrobial use is directly associated with rising levels of AMR. Surveillance systems gather essential data for analysing the links between consumption patterns and the development of resistance, supporting the creation of targeted stewardship and regulatory measures. This information helps inform effective policies and stewardship initiatives. Antimicrobial stewardship programmes (AMSP)—whether in hospitals, clinics, or farms—rely on consumption data to set goals, compare practices, and offer feedback. In veterinary medicine, AMSP promotes careful prescribing, optimised dosing, suitable treatment durations, and less environmental contamination from drug residues. Estimating AMC provides evidence for global efforts to reduce antibiotic use. At the Third Global High-Level Ministerial Conference on AMR in November 2022, nations committed to decreasing antimicrobial use in animals and agriculture by 30–50% by 2030 and to halting the use of medically necessary antimicrobials for growth promotion [16]. Monitoring consumption is vital for tracking progress towards these goals.

13.4 Challenges in AMC Surveillance

Inadequate Geographical Coverage While platforms like ANIMUSE and GLASS foster global participation, many countries—particularly low- and middle-income countries (LMICs)—report only basic or partial data on consumption. Capacity disparities create significant gaps in global visibility.

Insufficient Standardisation Even where data are available, they often lack breakdowns by animal species, disease indications, or administration routes, making comparative analysis and targeted stewardship difficult. Multiple metrics (e.g. DDDvet, usage per biomass) and inconsistent denominators further complicate cross-country harmonisation.

Poor Data Quality and Biases Sales-based surveillance may overestimate usage (as not all sold antibiotics are used) or underestimate black market or compounded usage. Farm-level data systems require regular updates and validation. Converting sales data into actual herd consumption demands sophisticated models and assumptions.

Inadequate Resources and Infrastructure LMICs often lack the necessary laboratory infrastructure, digital systems, and trained personnel to collect and analyse AMC data. Even willing countries may only provide high-level reports with minimal detail.

Fragmented Ownership and Non-integrated data Without integrated One Health frameworks, data remain siloed across ministries—health, agriculture, environment—hindering coordinated policy and intervention. Private veterinary practices or animal pharmaceutical archives may not consistently report usage.

13.5 Solutions to Improve AMC Data Management

International Development Partners (WOAH, FAO, and WHO) should

- Promote global engagement and capacity building by supporting countries in participating more fully in ANIMUSE and GLASS through technical support, guidance, and funding, especially for LMICs. This should include infrastructure, data systems, personnel training, and regulatory frameworks.
- Standardise metrics and reporting by harmonising methods for collecting and reporting antimicrobial consumption, including units (e.g. DDDvet), denominators (e.g. population-corrected units), species, and disease indications. This helps facilitate valid comparisons.
- Develop integrated One Health platforms by establishing templates and protocols that enable cross-sectoral data sharing for human, animal, and environmen-

tal resistance and consumption metrics. Digital systems must support interoperability across agencies within a One Health governance structure.
- Enhance data granularity by encouraging countries to transition from national totals to detailed datasets, including species, farm-level data, indications, dosages, and routes of administration. This will support targeted stewardship and policy decisions.
- Leverage technology and modelling, advocating for the adoption of AI, machine learning, and geospatial tools to estimate consumption in data gaps, identify misuse patterns, and fill reporting gaps, especially in resource-limited settings.

National Authorities should

- Develop national programmes to estimate AMC within the broader context of their national AMR action plans.
- Utilise consumption data to inform veterinary antimicrobial stewardship, establish reduction targets, monitor adherence to guidelines, and provide feedback to practitioners. This includes phasing out antibiotics used for growth promotion and used critically in human medicine.
- Promote transparency and accountability through public dashboards, national reports, and benchmarking across countries or regions. Engaging stakeholders, including farmers, veterinarians, and policymakers, is crucial.
- Incorporate technological advances such as geospatial modelling to estimate consumption or AMR prevalence in under-reported regions using environmental and epidemiological data. Similarly, machine learning and AI can help predict trends, detect anomalies, or estimate usage indirectly.

Monitoring AMU is essential in the worldwide fight against AMR. Without precise and prompt data—particularly in areas like livestock, aquaculture, companion animals, and the environment—efforts to curb misuse, shape policy, and maintain antibiotic effectiveness are significantly compromised. Enhancing surveillance by standardising methods, gathering detailed data, integrating across sectors, and connecting data directly to stewardship and policymaking allows governments and organisations to cut unnecessary consumption, track progress towards global reduction targets, and ultimately curb the spread of AMR [17].

13.6 Estimating Antimicrobial Use (AMU) in Humans

Understanding patterns of AMU is central to tackling AMR, as improper or excessive use in humans significantly contributes to resistance. By estimating AMU in human populations, policymakers, researchers, and healthcare professionals can track trends, evaluate stewardship efforts, and develop targeted strategies. However, accurate estimation faces challenges due to methodological, technical, and logistical issues. WHO highlights the importance of human AMU estimation, reviews various measurement methods, discusses difficulties encountered, and suggests solutions to enhance AMU surveillance and estimation globally. The WHO GLASS features AMU modules that promote standardised reporting by member states. ESAC-Net collects DDD data from pharmacies and hospitals for cross-country comparisons [18]. An Indian study estimated AMU through a point prevalence survey (PPS) in tertiary hospitals, and a private initiative (IQVIA data) evaluated retail antibiotic sales [19].

13.6.1 Importance of Estimating AMU in Humans

Understanding the Drivers of AMR The misuse and overuse of antibiotics accelerate the development of resistant pathogens. Estimating AMU helps identify sectors or settings, such as hospitals, communities, or informal healthcare providers, where antibiotics are overused, highlighting areas for potential intervention.

Evaluating Stewardship Programmes AMSP aim to optimise antibiotic use. Accurate data on usage enables the evaluation of AMSP outcomes, such as reductions in defined daily doses or changes in prescribing patterns.

Policy Development and Regulation Countries need AMU data to inform national strategies on AMR. Surveillance data are essential for drafting policies on antimicrobial prescribing, sales, and regulation, particularly in countries with high rates of self-medication.

Benchmarking and Global Comparisons Standardised AMU data facilitate comparisons between countries and regions, promoting accountability and knowledge sharing. This is central to initiatives like the WHO GLASS and the European Surveillance of Antimicrobial Consumption Network.

Research and Innovation AMU data are vital for operational research, including identifying knowledge gaps, understanding resistance patterns, and guiding innovation in diagnostics and treatment protocols.

13.6.2 Methods of Estimating AMU in Humans

Several methodologies are used to estimate AMU in human populations, each with its advantages and limitations.

Defined Daily Dose (DDD) Method
The DDD represents the estimated average daily dose of a drug used for its main indication in adults. The WHO employs it as a benchmark and for comparison, calculating DDD per 1000 inhabitants per day. This approach offers the benefit of a standardised method, enabling comparisons across multiple sites and countries. Nonetheless, it is not appropriate for use in paediatric populations.

Prescriptions and Sales Data
This data comes from various pharmacy dispensing records, insurance claim records, national prescription databases, and prescription audits. While readily accessible in high-income countries, it may not always accurately represent actual consumption and might miss over-the-counter use in low- and middle-income countries.

Point Prevalence Surveys (PPS)
Point prevalence surveys collect data at a specific moment in hospitals regarding patients on antibiotics. They offer detailed insights into prescribing habits and reasons for use. However, since they only capture a snapshot, they cannot determine trends unless they are conducted regularly.

Patient/Household Surveys
Community-based surveys gather data based on individuals' self-reports of antibiotic use. This approach documents informal and over-the-counter medication use but has limitations such as recall bias, misreporting, and a frequent lack of microbiological validation.

Electronic Health Records (EHRs) and Insurance Data
EHRs extract prescription data from digital systems. These datasets are timely and large-scale, but they require robust health information systems, which are often unavailable in LMICs.

Import and Production Data
This method is helpful in settings with weak regulatory oversight; however, the collected data does not accurately reflect actual use, as it includes wastage, exports, and veterinary use.

13.6.3 Challenges in Estimating AMU

Lack of Standardisation Differences in data sources, metrics (e.g. DDD vs. prescription count), and classification systems (ATC codes) hinder comparability.

Limited Data in LMICs Many LMICs lack robust prescription monitoring systems, EHRs, or regulatory frameworks to track antibiotic use, especially in the informal sector.

Inadequate Coverage of Informal Use In settings where antibiotics are available without prescriptions, traditional surveillance systems fail to capture a significant portion of AMU.

Fragmented Data Systems Countries with decentralised health systems often have data siloed across public and private providers, insurance systems, and retail pharmacies.

Paediatric and Special Populations DDD metrics are based on adult dosages and may not accurately reflect use in children or specific patient populations (e.g. patients with renal failure).

Resource and Capacity Constraints Human resource limitations, a lack of trained epidemiologists, and inadequate infrastructure for data collection and analysis hinder the accurate estimation of AMU.

Reluctance from the Private Sector Many private pharmacies and hospitals are hesitant to share sales or prescription data due to commercial confidentiality.

Timeliness and Data Lag Many estimates are retrospective and published years after data collection, limiting their usefulness for timely policy responses.

13.6.4 Strategies to Enhance AMU Estimation

Strengthening National Surveillance Countries should establish or expand their national AMU surveillance systems, following the GLASS methodology and national AMU guidelines, and integrate human and animal AMU reporting into a One Health framework.

Enforcing Regulations Rigorous enforcement of regulations governing prescription-only antibiotic sales is essential, particularly in LMICs where OTC access is common. Regulatory authorities need strengthening and empowerment.

Digital Technologies Use e-prescription platforms, health information exchanges, and mobile data collection tools to track antimicrobial prescribing.

Regular PPSs Standardised PPS should be conducted at least once a year in hospitals to analyse trends and inform stewardship. WHO offers toolkits and training to enhance capacity.

Private Sector Engagement Build trust and incentives for private providers and pharmacies to share anonymised sales data.

Standardisation Adopt internationally accepted metrics (e.g. DDD, ATC) and ensure compatibility with global databases, such as GLASS, through capacity-building workshops.

Transparency and Feedback Provide public dashboards, reports, and feedback to prescribers to foster data use and accountability.

Community Data Inclusion Expand surveys to collect data from pharmacies, general practitioners, and households to obtain a comprehensive picture.

Linking AMU and AMR Correlate antimicrobial use with resistance data at hospital or regional levels to understand resistance drivers and support targeted interventions.

13.7 Establishing National Antimicrobial Use and Antimicrobial Consumption Estimation Systems in Human and Veterinary Sectors

Without baseline AMR consumption and use data, countries cannot design evidence-based stewardship policies, regulate pharmaceutical markets effectively, or evaluate national AMR action plans. Countries need to develop and implement a phased, feasible, and cost-conscious roadmap to establish national AMU and AMC estimation systems across human and veterinary sectors under a One Health framework. It should align with global standards, including the GLASS and the ANIMUSE reporting platform, and be acceptable across the world. Given the political commitment and access to technical and financial resources, it should be possible to establish sustainable national reporting mechanisms that inform stewardship policies, guide regulatory reforms, and support international reporting obligations within 5 years.

In this endeavour, major challenges faced by developing countries include fragmented pharmaceutical sales data, weak veterinary drug monitoring systems, limited digital health information systems, inadequate integration between human and animal health sectors, and insufficient analytical capacity. As a result, national AMR action plans operate without reliable data on the drivers of antibiotic consumption and use.

For the national authorities to establish a sustainable national system for estimating, analysing, and reporting antimicrobial consumption (human sector) and antimicrobial use (animal sector) using standardised global methodologies within 5 years following strategic approaches can be considered:

Governance and Institutional Framework A National AMU/AMC Steering Committee should be established under the national AMR coordination mechanism, jointly led by the Ministry of Health, the Ministry of Agriculture/Livestock and the National Drug Regulatory Authority. This structure should set the standards, govern and manage data, undertake oversight and promote inter-sectoral coordination. If need be, this framework should be strengthened with a legal mandate in country-specific context.

Table 13.2 Possible phased roadmap for estimating AMC and AMU in developing countries

Phase	Duration	Salient objective	Major activities
Phase 1	Year 1	Establishing national baseline using sales and import data	Collect historical antimicrobial import and sales data Standardise units and classify active ingredients Estimate human per capita consumption Calculate animal biomass-adjusted use
Phase 2	Year 2–3	Develop sentinel surveillance systems to enable analysis of prescribing behaviour and misuse patterns	Human: Select representative hospitals (public/private) Implement electronic dispensing logs Conduct annual point prevalence surveys Veterinary: Select large poultry, dairy, and aquaculture farms Introduce standardised treatment logbooks Capture dosage and indication data
Phase 3a	Year 3–5	Digital integration	Routine reporting to integrate AMC reporting into national health information systems
Phase 3b	Year 3–5	Establish online veterinary drug sales reporting portals with mandate of annual pharmaceutical company reporting	Institutionalise annual national AMU/AMC reporting

Methodological Framework Global standards as set by WHO under its ATC/DDD methodology should be adopted as such. Core indicators that need to be integrated are Defined Daily Doses (DDD) per 1000 inhabitants per day (DID), proportion of Access, Watch, and Reserve (AWaRe) antibiotics and hospital DDD per 100 bed-days. To monitor progress through these indicators several data sources may be tapped including national procurement databases, import/export records, wholesale sales reports and sentinel hospital pharmacy data.

Veterinary Sector (AMU) This sector should adopt WOAH-recommended metrics with *c*ore indicators of mg of active ingredient per kg of animal biomass, *s*pecies-specific antimicrobial consumption and *p*roportion of critically important antimicrobials. The possible data sources for this information are veterinary pharmaceutical import records, feed premix sales, distributor declarations and *s*entinel commercial farms.

This roadmap can be implemented in a phased manner, as outlined in Table 13.2.

Analytical Framework Moving beyond data collection, countries must develop analytical capacity. The country should be able to conduct descriptive analyses of data to examine temporal trends, regional comparisons, AWaRe distribution, and species-specific consumption trends. To perform these tasks several tools are available, including Excel (initial phase), R/Python for advanced modelling, and GIS tools for hotspot mapping.

Policy Impact Evaluation These can be delineated through interrupted time series analysis to assess regulatory reforms, correlation analysis linking AMU and AMR laboratory data and facility benchmarking.

Risk Identification The AMR programme manager should identify risks by identifying high-consumption hospital departments, intensive livestock production zones and rapid increases in Watch or Reserve antibiotics. Their geospatial mapping supports targeted interventions.

Regulatory and Stewardship Linkage AMU/AMC data should guide, in the human sector, improvements in antibiotic stewardship programmes, essential medicines list revisions, prescription audits and insurance reimbursement controls. In the veterinary sector, this information should inform decisions on a ban on the use of antimicrobial growth promoters, *the* restriction of critically important antimicrobials, and the enforcement of prescription-only sales. These data, when placed in the public domain transparently, enhance accountability.

Capacity Development Requirements *Countries need to make* key investments in capacity enhancement through training in ATC/DDD and biomass calculations, data management and analytics training, veterinary dosage standardisation and establishment of national AMU analytical units. Partnerships with universities and other institutions of higher learning strengthen sustainability.

Financing Strategy All of the aforementioned activities require funding from domestic or international sources including domestic health and agriculture budgets, multilateral institutions and public-private partnerships. Estimates can be prepared for IT system development, for data analysts and epidemiologists, for training workshops, and for periodic surveys on outcomes and community engagement. Embedding costs into regulatory operations ensures long-term sustainability.

Expected Outcomes (5-Year Horizon) These include the following:

- Established national AMC baseline in humans.
- Species-adjusted AMU baseline in animals.
- Routine annual national reporting.
- Integration with global surveillance platforms.
- Evidence-based antibiotic stewardship policies.
- Reduction in inappropriate antimicrobial use.

In summary, developing countries can establish effective monitoring systems for antimicrobial use through a phased, pragmatic approach. Starting with data imports and gradually moving towards facility-level digital surveillance enables countries to build capacity step by step. When integrated with regulatory reforms and stewardship programmes, estimating antimicrobial use and consumption becomes a valuable policy tool to combat antimicrobial resistance within a One Health framework. They should begin by collecting national sales and import data to set a baseline, enforcing legally mandated pharmaceutical reporting within 2 years, establishing sentinel surveillance before expanding to nationwide digital systems, integrating AMU data with AMR laboratory surveillance, and ensuring ongoing domestic funding beyond donor support.

Estimating AMU in humans is vital for combating AMR. Despite numerous challenges, including data fragmentation, a lack of standardisation, and infrastructural and capacity constraints, practical strategies and tools exist to improve data quality and coverage. Moving forward, governments supported by global partners, such as the WHO, FAO, and WOAH, must prioritise integrating AMU surveillance into health systems, enforce regulations to prevent misuse, and leverage digital technology to bridge data gaps. Establishing a robust framework for AMU estimation is crucial for an effective response to AMR under the One Health approach.

References

1. WHO. GLASS. 3rd High-level technical consultation and meeting on surveillance of antimicrobial resistance and concerted actions, 2020. Available at https://cdn.who.int/media/docs/default-source/antimicrobial-resistance/amr-spc-sel-glass/glass-consultation-october-2020%2D%2D-march2021/theme-amc-amu-surveillance-model/glass-monitoring-hamc-q-a.pdf? Accessed 23 Mar 2025.
2. European Centre for Disease Control, EFSA, EMA. Fourth joint inter-agency report on integrated analysis of antimicrobial agent consumption and occurrence of antimicrobial resistance in bacteria from humans and food-producing animals in the EU/EEA JIACRA IV – 2019–2021. Antimicrobial consumption and resistance in bacteria from humans and food-producing animals. Available at https://efsaonlinelibrarywileycom/doi/full/102903/jefsa20248589#. Accessed 2 Mar 2025.
3. Mulchandani R, Wang Y, Gilbert M, Van Boeckel TP. Global trends in antimicrobial use in food-producing animals: 2020 to 2030. PLOS Glob Public Health. 2023;3(2):e0001305. https://doi.org/10.1371/journal.pgph.0001305.

4. WHO. Global action plan on antimicrobial resistance. 2015. Available at https://www.who.int/publications/i/item/9789241509763. Accessed 27 Mar 2025.
5. WHO. Global Antimicrobial Resistance and Use Surveillance System (GLASS). Available at https://www.who.int/initiatives/glass. Accessed 2 Mar 2025.
6. World Organization for Animal Health. ANIMUSE: use of antimicrobials in animals. Available at https://www.woah.org/en/article/animuse-monitoring-antimicrobial-use-in-animals/. Accessed 12 Mar 2025.
7. World Organization for Animal Health. ANIMUSE. Available at https://amu.woah.org/amu-system-portal/home. Accessed 27 Apr 2025.
8. World Organisation for Animal Health. 2025. Annual report on antimicrobial agents intended for use in animals. 9th report. Paris, 49 pp. https://doi.org/10.20506/woah.3584. Licence: CC BYSA 3.0 IGO.
9. World Organisation for Animal Health (WOAH). List of antimicrobial agents of veterinary importance. Paris: WOAH; 2024. Available at: https://www.woah.org/en/document/list-of-antimicrobial-agents-of-veterinary-importance. Accessed 27 Mar 2025.
10. World Health Organization (WHO). WHO medically important antimicrobial list. Geneva: WHO; 2024. Available at: https://www.who.int/news/item/08-02-2024-who-medically-important-antimicrobial-list-2024. Accessed 2 Mar 2025.
11. European Medicines Agency European Surveillance of Veterinary Antimicrobial Consumption (ESVAC): 2009–2023. Available at https://www.ema.europa.eu/en/veterinary-regulatory-overview/antimicrobial-resistance-veterinary-medicine/european-surveillance-veterinary-antimicrobial-consumption-esvac-2009-2023? m. Accessed 27 Apr 2025.
12. Schar D, Sommanustweechai A, Laxminarayan R, Tangcharoensathien V. Surveillance of antimicrobial consumption in animal production sectors of low- and middle-income countries: optimizing use and addressing antimicrobial resistance. PLoS Med. 2018;15(3):e1002521. https://doi.org/10.1371/journal.pmed.1002521.
13. Health for Animals. Global trends in animal antibiotic use. Available at https://healthforanimals.org/animal-health-in-data/antimicrobial-resistance/global-trends-in-animal-antibiotic-use/. Accessed 7 Apr 2025.
14. World Animal Protection. European Union bans the routine use of antibiotics in animal farms. Available at https://www.worldanimalprotection.org/latest/news/eu-bans-antibiotic-overuse-farmed-animals/. Accessed 1 Apr 2025.
15. CIDRAP. UK reports decade-low levels of antibiotic sales, resistance on farms. Available at https://www.cidrap.umn.edu/antimicrobial-stewardship/uk-reports-decade-low-levels-antibiotic-sales-resistance-farms#. Accessed 23 Aug 2025.
16. WHO. Quadripartite welcomes new political commitments in fight against antimicrobial resistance. Available at https://www.who.int/news/item/25-11-2022-quadripartite-welcomes-new-political-commitments-in-fight-against-antimicrobial-resistance#. Accessed 7 Apr 2025.
17. Zhao C, Wang Y, Mulchandani R, et al. Global surveillance of antimicrobial resistance in food animals using priority drugs maps. Nat Commun. 2024;15:763. https://doi.org/10.1038/s41467-024-45111-7.
18. Robertson J, Vlahović-Palčevski V, Iwamoto K, Högberg LD, Godman B, Monnet DL, Garner S, Weist K, ESAC-Net Study Group; WHO Europe AMC Network Study Group. Variations in the consumption of antimicrobial medicines in the European region, 2014-2018: findings and implications from ESAC-net and WHO Europe. Front Pharmacol. 2021;12:639207. https://doi.org/10.3389/fphar.2021.765748.
19. Bhattacharjee S, Mothsara C, Nusrat S, Panda PK, Rohilla R, Kaore S, et al. Antimicrobial prescription patterns in tertiary care centres in India: a multicentric point prevalence survey. EClinicalMedicine. 2025;82:103175. https://doi.org/10.1016/j.eclinm.2025.103175.

Chapter 14
Antimicrobial Stewardship to Control AMR

Abstract Antimicrobial stewardship (AMS) is a coordinated, evidence-based strategy designed to optimise antimicrobial use, improve patient outcomes, and reduce antimicrobial resistance (AMR). By ensuring the right drug, dose, route, and duration, AMS enhances clinical care while minimising unnecessary exposure to antibiotics. Hospitals implementing AMS benefit from improved treatment success, reduced mortality, shorter hospital stays, and significant cost savings. Beyond human health, AMS extends to veterinary systems, recognising the One Health link between human, animal, and environmental health. Effective programmes are built on strong leadership, multidisciplinary teams, local guidelines, robust monitoring, and feedback mechanisms. Interventions such as audit and feedback, formulary restrictions, IV-to-oral switches, and diagnostic stewardship have consistently demonstrated success globally. AMS effectiveness is evaluated through key metrics, including antibiotic consumption, clinical outcomes, and patterns of resistance. However, challenges such as resistance to change, resource limitations, knowledge gaps, and poor coordination hinder implementation. Addressing these requires advocacy, capacity building, interprofessional collaboration, and sustained investment. AMS remains essential for safeguarding antimicrobial efficacy across human and veterinary domains.

Keywords Antimicrobial stewardship (AMS) · Rational antibiotic use · Infection prevention and control (IPC) · Veterinary stewardship · Diagnostic stewardship

Antimicrobial stewardship (AMS) in hospitals is a coordinated effort designed to combat antimicrobial resistance (AMR). It involves actions that promote the correct use of antibiotics to enhance patient outcomes and prevent the rise of AMR. AMS takes a systematic approach, implementing various strategies and interventions to ensure patients receive the right medication, at the proper dose, for the correct duration, and through the appropriate route.

AMS is a holistic approach that emphasises collaboration, education, and ongoing monitoring to ensure the responsible use of antimicrobials and protect against the growing risks of AMR and related impacts.

R. Bhatia, *Drug-Resistant Infections*,
https://doi.org/10.1007/978-981-92-4190-3_14

14.1 Benefits of AMS

AMS offers various advantages to healthcare facilities and promotes the responsible use of antibiotics [1]. These include:

Effective Antimicrobial Use: AMS seeks to optimise therapy by choosing the most appropriate drug for each infection, taking into account factors like pathogen sensitivity, patient traits, and possible drug interactions.

Preventing AMR: By promoting responsible antimicrobial use, AMS helps slow down the emergence and spread of antibiotic-resistant bacteria, maintaining the effectiveness of current antimicrobials.

Proper Use of antibiotics can lead to improved patient outcomes, including quicker recovery, reduced mortality, and fewer antibiotic-related side effects.

Cost Savings: AMS can also lead to cost savings by reducing unnecessary antimicrobial prescriptions, hospital stays, and the need for expensive treatments for resistant infections.

Paediatrics and Special Populations: Paediatric stewardship adapts adult principles, emphasising weight-based dosing, reducing toxicity, encouraging vaccination synergy, and preventing unnecessary antibiotics for viral illnesses. In immunocompromised patients and critical care settings, stewardship collaborates with specialist teams to ensure effective, timely treatment while promoting early de-escalation.

Fosters Antibiotic Use according to WHO AWaRe Classification: The WHO's AWaRe classification categorises antibiotics into Access, Watch, and Reserve, supporting national targets (e.g. ≥60% of human use from Access) and procurement priorities [2].

14.2 Implementation of AMS

Figure 14.1 shows a detailed process for setting up an AMS programme [3, 4] in a healthcare facility. The key steps are as follows:

Engage Hospital Leadership: Strong support from the hospital administration is vital for successfully implementing AMS, including providing necessary resources and ensuring AMS is effectively integrated into overall quality improvement efforts.

Set up an Antimicrobial Stewardship Programme and Team: This team typically includes infectious disease physicians, pharmacists, infection control professionals, and other relevant healthcare professionals.

Create Policies and Guidelines: Developing evidence-based guidelines for antimicrobial use, based on local antibiograms and best practices, is essential.

Conduct Gap Assessment: Regularly review antibiotic prescriptions and provide feedback to prescribers to help identify areas for improvement.

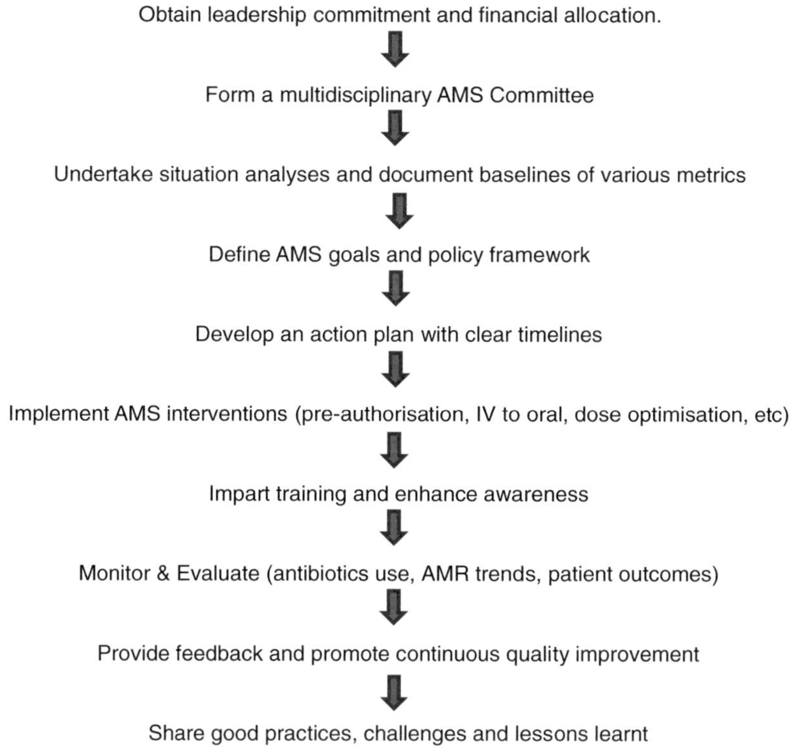

Fig. 14.1 Step-by-step for the Establishment of the AMS programme in hospital

Promote Education and Training: Educate healthcare staff on proper antimicrobial use, infection prevention, and the principles of AMS.

Utilise Technology: Use electronic health records, computerised prescriber order entry, and other technologies to support AMS efforts by offering alerts, reminders, and decision-support tools.

Strengthen Infection Prevention and Control: AMS is most effective when combined with strong infection prevention and control measures to reduce the risk of hospital-acquired infections.

14.3 Interventions That Work

AMS programmes in hospitals have demonstrated effectiveness in lowering antimicrobial use, reducing expenses, and enhancing patient outcomes. These initiatives focus on optimising antimicrobial use to combat AMR and boost patient safety through various evidence-based strategies. Some of these strategies include:

Prospective Audit and Feedback: Stewardship teams review ongoing treatments and offer case-specific recommendations, enhancing appropriateness and decreasing unnecessary broad-spectrum use without compromising outcomes [5].

Formulary restrictions and Preauthorization help limit access to broad-spectrum or last-line agents, reducing misuse. Adding this approach with PAF promotes sustainability and keeps clinicians involved.

Guideline and Pathway-based Prescribing involves local guidelines aligned with resistance patterns and clinical pathways for common syndromes such as pneumonia, UTI, and skin/soft tissue infections. This approach standardises best practices and minimises unnecessary treatment durations.

I*V-to-oral Switch Protocols*: Encourage earlier transition when equivalent oral options are available, which helps reduce the length of stay and complications.

Dose/interval Optimisation involves using pharmacokinetic/pharmacodynamic (PK/PD) methods, such as prolonged infusions for beta-lactams, and adjusting doses according to renal or hepatic function to improve both effectiveness and safety.

*Emphasis*e the importance of prompt and appropriate treatment for severe infections early on, then customise the strategy according to culture and molecular test results.

Surgical Prophylaxis Optimisation: By ensuring the correct agent is administered within 60 minutes of incision for most agents and limiting the duration to a single perioperative day, we can substantially reduce overuse.

Diagnostic Stewardship includes optimising testing timing and methods, avoiding reflex cultures when the pre-test probability is low, and preventing the misinterpretation of colonisation as infection, like asymptomatic bacteriuria. Working with laboratories to create reflex algorithms, set reporting thresholds, and provide interpretive comments can greatly reduce misuse.

Education and behaviour change strategies, such as audit-feedback, peer benchmarking, academic detailing, and clinical decision support, are more effective than simple didactic education alone [6].

Digital Decision Support and Analytics: Incorporating order sets, best-practice alerts, antibiogram integration, and default durations into electronic health records simplifies making the correct decision.

14.3.1 A Few Examples of Successful AMS Implementation

Examples of successful AMS implementation from different countries have been summarised by Huttner et al. [7]. In Australia, restrictions on fluoroquinolone use have correlated with lower resistance rates to these antibiotics [8]. A large private hospital network in South Africa has effectively implemented an AMS programme that reduced antibiotic use. The VINARES project [9] has enhanced AMS and infection control measures. Studies in the USA have demonstrated that AMS programmes can improve infection cure rates and reduce treatment failures [10].

14.4 AMS Complementarity with Other Interventions

Rapid testing methods like targeted PCRs, MALDI-TOF, and improved culture workflows can reduce turnaround times and allow hospitals to de-escalate treatments sooner. This results in more effective antimicrobial therapy. However, correct test ordering is crucial. Diagnostic stewardship ensures that the right test is performed for the right patient or animal at the right time, with proper support to avoid overtreatment of colonisation.

Besides diagnostic stewardship, crucial areas such as infection prevention and control (IPC), vaccination, sanitation, and water hygiene infrastructure are essential. Stewardship forms the foundation of any national strategy to combat AMR. The One Health approach, emphasising the link between human, animal, and environmental health, is central to contemporary stewardship policies and practices. [11–13].

14.5 Key Metrics to Measure Effectiveness

Several metrics are employed to evaluate the success of the AMS programme, focusing on antimicrobial use, clinical outcomes, and economic impact [14] (Table 14.1). These measures are essential in determining how effectively the programme enhances antimicrobial prescribing practices and boosts patient safety.

By linking consumption data with clinical and economic outcomes, hospitals can thoroughly evaluate their antimicrobial stewardship efforts and maximise their programme's impact on patient safety and care quality.

14.6 Veterinary Antimicrobial Stewardship

Animals derive significant benefits from antibiotics, but misuse in land and aquatic species promotes the spread of antibiotic resistance, posing risks to animal health, livelihoods, food security, and human health through direct contact, the food chain, and shared environments [6].

Effective animal health management aligns with human antibiotic stewardship goals, but also accounts for species-specific biology, production systems, and regulations. Various international agencies have set standards to promote the responsible use of antibiotics in animals (Table 14.2).

Table 14.1 Key metrics to measure the effectiveness of AMS

	Metric Group	Individual metric	Paramount measured	Indicative of
1	Antibiotics utilization	Days of Therapy/1000 patient days	Measures the total number of days a patient receives a specific antimicrobial divided by the total patient-days	Antimicrobial exposure over time
		Defined Daily Dose (DDD)	The amount of each antimicrobial used divided by the World Health Organisation's defined standard daily dose	Standardises drug consumption for comparison
		Antimicrobial cost in local currency	Tracks the expenditure related to antimicrobial agents but should not be the sole metric due to factors like drug shortages or patent expirations affecting costs	Cost of antimicrobial therapy
2	Clinical outcome metrics	All cause mortality	Overall death rate	Impact of AMS interventions on survival
		Length of stay	Hospital stay duration	Impact of AMS on recovery speed
		Readmission rate	Returning patients	Treatment failure or complications
3	Programme performance	Prescribing trends	Changes in prescribing patterns over time	Identifies areas for improvement
		Guidelines compliance	Adherence to guidelines	Conformity to hospital policies and protocols
		Resistance patterns	AMR patterns	Understanding trends in AMR

Table 14.2 Standards and guidelines for antimicrobial use in the veterinary sector

Organisation	Standard
World Organisation for Animal Health	Terrestrial Code, Ch. 6.10 [15]
European Union	Regulation 2019/6 [16]
European Medicines Agency	Categorises antibiotics for veterinary use into A–D (Avoid, Restrict, Caution, Prudence) to guide choice [17]
United States:	FDA Guidance for Industry (GFI) #213 [15]
European Medicines Agency	The European Surveillance of Veterinary Antimicrobial Consumption (ESVAC) [18]

14.6.1 Core Veterinary Stewardship Principles

Veterinary Oversight: Access to prescription-only medicines, where the veterinary-client-patient relationship plays a key role, is a fundamental aspect. Limiting medically essential antibiotics to veterinary oversight and therapeutic use helps prevent misuse. [17, 19].

Prioritise Prevention: Biosecurity, vaccination, husbandry, nutrition, and housing reduce disease pressure and antimicrobial need.

Judicious Therapeutic Use: Treat confirmed or strongly suspected bacterial infections, select narrow-spectrum agents whenever possible, optimise dose and duration based on PK/PD principles, and adhere to withdrawal periods to avoid residues in food.

Avoid Routine Prophylaxis and Metaphylaxis with Critically Important Agents: Reserve highest-priority critically essential antimicrobials (HPCIAs) for limited indications when no alternatives exist, with justification and, where applicable, susceptibility evidence [20].

Data Capture and Benchmarking: Monitor antimicrobial use (AMU) and results at the herd, flock, or clinic level using standardised metrics such as mg of active substance per population correction unit (mg/PCU), DDDvet, and DCDvet to identify opportunities for reduction and substitution [21, 22].

Many countries have observed notable declines in veterinary antimicrobial sales and usage after implementing reforms like enhanced oversight, tighter restrictions on growth promotion, stricter prophylaxis regulations, and increased use of vaccines and better husbandry practices. ESVAC data shows ongoing reductions in mg/PCU for essential classes across several EU countries. Farm and clinic programmes that focus on prevention strategies and diagnostics have achieved better clinical outcomes alongside reduced antimicrobial use.

14.7 Challenges in AMS implementation

Implementing AMS programmes faces multiple challenges, such as resistance to change, knowledge gaps, limited resources, and poor coordination. Overcoming these issues involves a comprehensive strategy that includes changing clinician behaviour, improving education and training, strengthening communication, and providing sufficient resources.

14.7.1 Resistance to Change and Lack of Awareness

Clinicians and healthcare professionals may resist changing prescribing practices, especially if they perceive AMS interventions as threatening to patient care or their independence. Furthermore, a lack of awareness about the importance of AMS and the risks of antimicrobial resistance can hinder its implementation.

14.7.2 Knowledge and Education Gaps

A lack of knowledge about appropriate antibiotic use, resistance patterns, and the principles of AMS among healthcare providers can lead to inappropriate prescribing practices.

14.7.3 Resource Limitations

Under-resourced healthcare systems may lack the necessary personnel, laboratory infrastructure, and financial resources to implement and sustain AMS programmes.

14.7.4 Communication and Coordination Issues

Ineffective communication between healthcare professionals, departments, and institutions can hinder the implementation and effectiveness of AMS efforts.

14.7.5 Lack of Administrative Support

Without strong administrative support, AMS programmes may struggle to gain traction and achieve sustainable change.

14.7.6 Interprofessional Relationships

In some cases, competing priorities or tensions between different healthcare professionals or departments can hinder collaboration on AMS initiatives.

14.7.7 Sustainability

Ensuring the long-term sustainability of AMS programmes requires ongoing commitment, funding, and evaluation.

14.8 Solutions and Way Forward

Solutions should stem from insights gained through in-house self-assessment. Various challenges, as shown in Box 14.1, can be tackled with different approaches, primarily emphasising advocacy, raising awareness, and enhancing stakeholders' capacity.

Box 14.1 Possible Solutions to Address AMS Implementation Challenges

- Advocate with all stakeholders, mainly clinicians, pharmacists, nurses, patients, and administrators.
- Promote a culture of stewardship through awareness, joint planning, and implementation.
- Providing comprehensive education and training on AMS principles, antimicrobial resistance, and appropriate prescribing practices is crucial.
- Encourage a culture of stewardship within healthcare facilities, where responsible antibiotic use is valued and prioritised.
- Strengthen communication and collaboration through clear communication channels.
- Leverage technology to improve data collection and facilitate informed decision-making.
- Develop guidelines that are aligned with national or WHO guidelines and policies.
- Secure adequate funding and resources.

By addressing these challenges and implementing effective strategies, healthcare facilities can enhance their AMS programmes and contribute to the global effort to combat antimicrobial resistance.

14.9 Establishing an Antimicrobial Stewardship Programme in a New Hospital

AMR threatens patient safety, increases mortality, prolongs hospital stays, and escalates healthcare costs. A new hospital has a unique opportunity to embed antimicrobial stewardship (AMS) into its governance and clinical culture from inception. An Antimicrobial Stewardship Programme (ASP or AMSP) ensures optimal antimicrobial use—right drug, dose, duration, and route—while minimising toxicity, resistance development, and unnecessary costs.

International guidance from the World Health Organisation, the Centres for Disease Control and Prevention, and the Infectious Diseases Society of America outlines core components of hospital-based stewardship programmes. The following framework translates those principles into a practical roadmap for a new hospital.

14.9.1 Governance and Leadership Commitment

The hospital board and chief executive must formally mandate the ASP as part of patient safety and quality assurance policy. A written antimicrobial stewardship policy should define goals and scope, assign authority to the ASP team, mandate compliance with prescribing guidelines and integrate AMS into accreditation and performance review. Leadership commitment should include dedicated budget allocation and sustainable staffing.

14.9.2 Composition of the ASP Team

A multidisciplinary team is essential to implementing this programme in the health facility. The core members must include the following:

- Infectious Disease (ID) Physician (Programme Lead).
- Clinical Microbiologist.
- Clinical Pharmacist (trained in infectious diseases).
- Infection Prevention and Control (IPC) Officer.
- Hospital Epidemiologist.
- Information Technology (IT) Representative.
- Nursing Representative.

In smaller hospitals where ID specialists are unavailable, trained general physicians can lead with remote mentorship support. The ASP team has important roles and responsibilities, including developing and updating antibiotic guidelines, reviewing antimicrobial prescriptions, monitoring consumption trends, conducting audits and feedback, and training healthcare staff on processes and guideline adherence.

14.9.3 Baseline Assessment

Before launching interventions, the hospital should conduct a situational assessment on current antibiotic formulary, the availability of microbiology laboratory, local resistance patterns, prescribing practices in different departments and infection prevention capacity. A new hospital shall lack resistance data. It should initially use national or regional antibiograms until facility-specific data are generated.

14.9.4 Core Stewardship Interventions

Two evidence-based strategies are considered foundational in any new hospital

Prospective Audit with Feedback that includes review of selected antibiotic prescriptions (e.g. carbapenems, colistin, vancomycin) within 48–72 hours, providing direct feedback to prescribers and recommending de-escalation, dose optimization, or discontinuation. This intervention promotes rational prescribing while preserving physician autonomy.

Formulary Restriction and Preauthorization to reserve certain broad-spectrum or high-cost antibiotics for approval by the ASP team, develop clear approval criteria and maintain documentation and periodic review.

14.9.5 Development of Clinical Guidelines

Standard Treatment Guidelines (STGs) should be developed based on local epidemiology, the WHO AWaRe classification, the National Essential Medicines List, and the available formulary. The guidelines should cover community-acquired pneumonia, urinary tract infections, sepsis, surgical prophylaxis and neonatal infections. Surgical prophylaxis protocols should clearly define single-dose or <24-hour duration policies.

14.9.6 Microbiology Laboratory Requirements

A functional microbiology laboratory is central to stewardship. It should be able to perform blood culture, pathogen isolation culture and sensitivity testing through standardised antimicrobial susceptibility testing methods and regular quality control. Turnaround time for culture and susceptibility results should ideally be ≤72 hours. The laboratory should develop annual antibiograms, share monthly resistance reports with clinicians, and participate in external quality assurance programmes, with demonstrated strong performance.

14.9.7 Surveillance and Monitoring Systems

The hospital must use standardised metrics, viz. Defined Daily Doses (DDD) per 100 bed-days and Days of Therapy (DOT) per 1,000 patient-days. The monitoring should include department-wise consumption, ICU vs non-ICU comparison and

AWaRe category distribution. Beyond these broad categories, the AMS Team should track resistance trends for priority pathogens, identify multidrug-resistant organisms (MDROs), and monitor hospital-acquired infection rates. A data integration system should be in place between the pharmacy and microbiology systems to enhance impact.

14.9.8 Education and Training

Continuous education ensures operational sustainability. Target groups to be prioritised are physicians, nurses, pharmacists and laboratory staff. Must-trained topics include principles of AMR, rational prescribing, interpretation of antibiograms, and infection prevention practices. New employee orientation should include AMS training.

14.9.9 Information Technology and Data Systems

Electronic systems significantly improve stewardship efficiency. Various tools can assist in electronic prescribing systems with decision support, alerts for duplicate therapy, automatic stop orders for surgical prophylaxis and integration with laboratory reporting. If digital systems are unavailable, structured manual data-collection tools must be implemented.

14.9.10 Infection Prevention and Control (IPC) Integration

Stewardship and IPC are complementary. ASP must coordinate with IPC on hand hygiene compliance, isolation precautions, environmental cleaning, and device-associated infection prevention bundles. Reducing hospital-acquired infections directly reduces antimicrobial use.

14.9.11 Key Performance Indicators (KPIs).

For a programmatic and systematic approach several key performance indicators should be developed. Quarterly reporting to hospital leadership strengthens accountability. These KPIs may include the following:

- Reduction in broad-spectrum antibiotic use.
- Increase in Access antibiotic proportion.

- Compliance with surgical prophylaxis duration.
- Reduction in carbapenem consumption.
- Reduction in MDRO rates.
- 30-day mortality for key infections.

14.9.12 Regulatory and Accreditation Linkages

AMS should be embedded in hospital accreditation standards, clinical audit systems, physician performance appraisal, and pharmacy procurement policies. This ensures institutionalisation beyond individual champions.

14.9.13 Implementation Timeline

Figure 14.2 shows the AMSP implementation timeline in a new hospital

14.9.14 Sustainability Strategy for New Hospital Management

- Institutionalise ASP in hospital bylaws.
- Continuous training cycles.
- Annual review of guidelines.
- Participation in national AMR networks.
- Benchmarking against peer hospitals.

A new hospital can embed antimicrobial stewardship into its operational DNA by integrating governance, clinical guidelines, laboratory capacity, surveillance

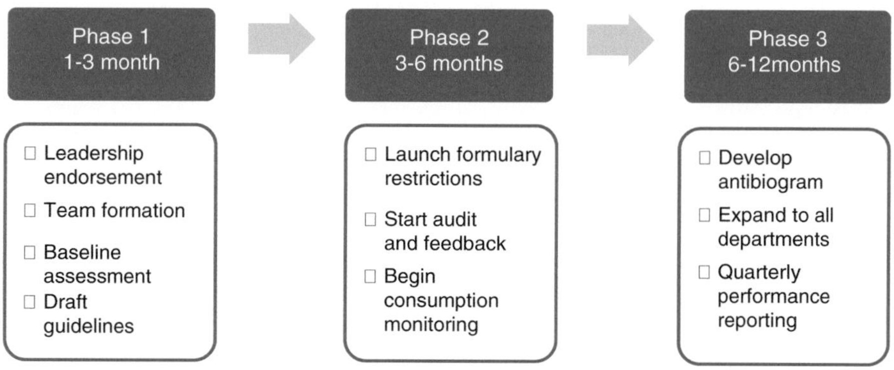

Fig 14.2 Suggested AMSP phased implementation timeline in a new hospital

systems, education, and digital support from the outset. When leadership commitment, microbiological diagnostics, and continuous audit mechanisms function together, stewardship programmes reduce inappropriate antibiotic use, lower resistance rates, improve patient outcomes, and decrease costs.

Embedding stewardship early avoids the difficult corrective reforms required in older institutions and positions the hospital as a model centre for quality and patient safety in the fight against antimicrobial resistance.

Antimicrobial stewardship is essential for preserving the effectiveness of important drugs in both human and veterinary medicine. Evidence-based strategies—emphasising leadership, team collaboration across disciplines, and data-driven feedback—enhance results, reduce side effects, and cut costs. In veterinary care, prevention methods such as proper husbandry, veterinary oversight, and careful therapeutic use greatly reduce antimicrobial pressure without compromising animal health or productivity.

References

1. Eyre DW, Pill G, Ng BY, Herin C, O'Riordan B, Izzard D, et al. The impact of antimicrobial stewardship ward rounds on antimicrobial use and predictors of advice, uptake, and outcomes. J Infect. 2025;90:106419. https://doi.org/10.1016/j.jinf.2025.106419.
2. WHO. WHO AWaRe system for antimicrobial stewardship. Available at https://www.who.int/teams/surveillance-prevention-control-AMR/control-and-response-strategies/AWaRe. Accessed 23 Apr 2025.
3. WHO. Antimicrobial stewardship programmes in health-care facilities in low- and middle-income countries. A practical toolkit. Geneva: World Health Organization; 2019. Licence: CC BY-NC-SA 3.0 IGO
4. Centres for Disease Control and Prevention. Core elements of hospital antibiotic stewardship programs. Atlanta: CDC; 2019. Available from: https://www.cdc.gov/antibiotic-use/core-elements/hospital.html. Accessed 13 Apr 2025.
5. Davey P, Marwick CA, Scott CL, Charani E, McNeil K, Brown E, et al. Interventions to AImprove antibiotic Prescribing for Hospital Inpatients. Cochrane Database Syst Rev. 2017;2:CD003543. https://doi.org/10.1002/14651858.CD003543.pub4.
6. Huttner B, Harbarth S, Carlet J, Cosgrove S, Goossens H, Holmes A, et al. Antimicrobial resistance and the practice of antimicrobial stewardship. Lancet Infect Dis. 2013;13(12):1009–11. https://doi.org/10.1016/S1473-3099(13)70312-9.
7. Huttner B, Harbarth S, Nathwani D. Success stories of implementation of antimicrobial stewardship: a narrative review. Clin Microbiol Infect. 2014;20:954–62. https://doi.org/10.1111/1469-0691.12803.
8. Cheng AC, Turnidge J, Collignon P, Looke D, Barton M, Gottlieb T. Control of fluoroquinolone resistance through successful regulation, Australia. Emerg Infect Dis. 2012;18(9):1453–60. https://doi.org/10.3201/eid1809.111515.
9. Vu TVD, Do TTN, Rydell U, Nilsson LE, Olson L, Larsson M, Hanberger H, et al. VINARES consortium. Antimicrobial susceptibility testing and antibiotic consumption results from 16 hospitals in Viet Nam: the VINARES project 2012-2013. J Glob Antimicrob Resist. 2019:269–78. https://doi.org/10.1016/j.jgar.2029.06.002.
10. Khadse SN, Ugemuge S, Singh C. Impact of Antimicrobial Stewardship on Reducing Antimicrobial Resistance. Cureus. 2023;15(12):e49935. https://doi.org/10.7759/cureus.49935.

11. Tripartite and UNEP. One Health Joint Plan of Action (2022–2026). FAO, UNEP, WHO, WOAH; 2022. Available from: https://www.who.int/publications/i/item/9789240059139. Accessed 23 Apr 2025.
12. Food and Agriculture Organization, World Organisation for Animal Health, World Health Organization. Antimicrobial resistance: a manual for developing national action plans. FAO/WOAH/WHO; 2016. Available from: https://www.fao.org/antimicrobial-resistance/resources/publications. Accessed 3 Apr 2025.
13. World Health Organization. Antimicrobial resistance and the One Health approach. WHO; 2017. Available from: https://www.who.int/health-topics/antimicrobial-resistance. Accessed 23 Apr 2025.
14. Public Health Ontario. Antimicrobial Stewardship Programs (ASPs) Metrics Examples. Available at https://www.publichealthontario.ca/-/media/documents/A/2017/asp-metrics-examples.pdf. Accessed 2 Apr 2025.
15. US FDA. CVM GFI #213 New Animal Drugs and New Animal Drug Combination Products Administered in or on Medicated Feed or Drinking Water of Food-Producing Animals. Available at https://www.fda.gov/regulatory-information/search-fda-guidance-documents/cvm-gfi-213-new-animal-drugs-and-new-animal-drug-combination-products-administered-or-medicated-feed. Accessed 23 Apr 2025.
16. European Union. Regulation (EU) 2019/6 of the European Parliament and of the Council on veterinary medicinal products. Official Journal of the European Union; 2019. Available from: https://eur-lex.europa.eu/eli/reg/2019/6/oj. Accessed 23 Apr 2025.
17. World Organisation for Animal Health (WOAH). Responsible and prudent use of antimicrobial agents in veterinary medicine (Terrestrial Code, Ch. 6.10). Paris: WOAH; 2019 (and updates). Available from: https://www.woah.org. Accessed 23 Apr 2025.
18. EMA: https://www.ema.europa.eu/en/veterinary-regulatory-overview/antimicrobial-resistance-veterinary-medicine/european-surveillance-veterinary-antimicrobial-consumption-esvac-2009-2023. Accessed 1 Apr 2025.
19. U.S. Food and Drug Administration. Veterinary Feed Directive (VFD) final rule. FDA; 2015. Available from: https://www.fda.gov/animal-veterinary/development-approval-process/veterinary-feed-directive-vfd Accessed 23 Mar 2025.
20. World Organisation for Animal Health (WOAH). List of antimicrobial agents of veterinary importance and guidance on use. Paris: WOAH; 2021. Available from: https://www.woah.org. Accessed 3 Apr 2025.
21. European Medicines Agency. European Surveillance of Veterinary Antimicrobial Consumption (ESVAC) report: sales of veterinary antimicrobial agents in 31 European countries, 2011–2021. Amsterdam: EMA; 2023. Available from: https://www.ema.europa.eu. Accessed 2 Apr 2025.
22. National Antimicrobial Resistance Monitoring System (NARMS). Integrated report. U.S. FDA/CDC/USDA; 2021. Available from: https://www.fda.gov/animal-veterinary/national-antimicrobial-resistance-monitoring-system. Accessed 3 Apr 2025.

Chapter 15
Infection Prevention and Control, Biosecurity and AMR

Abstract Antimicrobial resistance (AMR) is one of the most pressing global health challenges, threatening to undermine decades of medical progress. Infection Prevention and Control (IPC) and biosecurity serve as the first line of defence by reducing the incidence and spread of diseases, thereby minimising the need for antibiotics. IPC primarily focuses on healthcare facilities, encompassing practices such as hand hygiene, sterilisation, use of personal protective equipment, and safe waste management to prevent healthcare-associated infections (HAIs). Biosecurity extends beyond healthcare, addressing risks in livestock, veterinary settings, laboratories, and the environment, to prevent the introduction and dissemination of resistant pathogens. Weak IPC and biosecurity practices result in increased infections, higher antibiotic consumption, economic losses, and ethical concerns about patient and worker safety. Strengthened IPC and farm-level biosecurity, combined with surveillance, training, and a robust One Health approach, are essential to tackling AMR. Integrating these strategies across human, animal, and environmental domains is critical to reduce reliance on antibiotics, preserve their effectiveness, and safeguard global health.

Keywords Antimicrobial resistance · Infection prevention and control
Biosecurity · One Health · Healthcare-associated infections · Veterinary biosecurity · Multisectoral collaboration

Antimicrobial resistance (AMR) has become one of the top global health threats of the twenty-first century. If not addressed, it could result in 10 million deaths annually by 2050, along with significant economic consequences [1]. AMR undermines progress in modern medicine, threatening the effective treatment of common infections, surgeries, and those who are on immunosuppressive therapies. Combatting AMR requires a broad approach that extends beyond just developing and managing drugs. Key components include Infection Prevention and Control (IPC) in healthcare settings and biosecurity efforts across human, animal, and environmental sectors.

R. Bhatia, *Drug-Resistant Infections*,
https://doi.org/10.1007/978-981-92-4190-3_15

While antimicrobial stewardship (AMS) targets the appropriate use of drugs, IPC and biosecurity address the root causes by preventing infections early on and decreasing the demand for antibiotics. Consequently, IPC and biosecurity serve as the initial barrier against AMR, supporting the One Health approach that emphasises the links between human, animal, and environmental health.

15.1 Definitions and Concepts

- IPC refers to a set of practices and policies designed to prevent infections in healthcare and community settings. Effective IPC reduces healthcare-associated infections (HAIs), lowering the need for antibiotics. It prevents the spread of multidrug-resistant organisms (MDROs) within hospitals and communities [2]. The World Health Organisation (WHO) defines IPC as "scientific approaches and practical solutions designed to prevent harm caused by infection to patients and health workers" [2]. IPC encompasses a range of interventions in hospitals, clinics, and community settings aimed at interrupting the transmission of infectious agents.
- *Biosecurity* in the context of AMR is a broad term. It encompasses measures designed to protect people, animals, plants, and the environment from harmful biological agents.
- In *animal husbandry*, biosecurity helps prevent infections in livestock, thereby reducing the need for non-therapeutic antibiotic use. World Organisation for Animal Health (WOAH) defines biosecurity in the Terrestrial Animal Health code as "a set of management and physical measures designed to reduce the risk of introduction, establishment and spread of animal diseases, infections or infestations to, from and within an animal population" [3]. *Farm biosecurity* controls diseases like avian influenza or salmonella outbreaks without the need for mass antibiotic use.
- In *laboratories and research centres*, biosecurity ensures containment of resistant pathogens to avoid accidental release. Laboratories handling resistant organisms require strict containment to prevent accidental release. Breaches can lead to the environmental spread of resistant strains. Similarly, in hospitals, biosecurity includes access control, waste management, and sterilisation of reusable medical devices.
- *Environmental biosecurity* prevents contamination of water, soil, and food chains with resistant microorganisms [4]. It prevents untreated pharmaceutical waste discharge that drives AMR.
- *Biosecurity has a strong One Health perspective* and is crucial across human, animal, and environmental sectors to contain resistant organisms and genes.
- Both IPC and biosecurity aim to reduce the risk of infection, thereby reducing antimicrobial use and the emergence/spread of AMR.

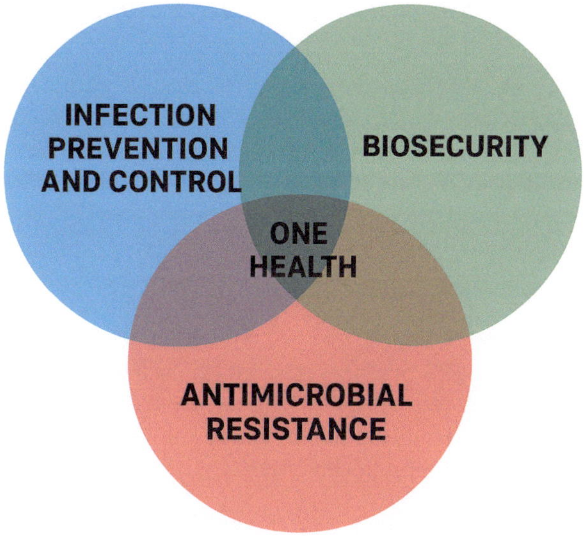

Fig. 15.1 Convergence of AMR, IPC, and biosecurity in One Health

- IPC is more *healthcare-focused*, while biosecurity spans *human, animal, and environmental systems.*
- Together, they form a *preventive shield* against AMR within the *One Health framework* (Fig. 15.1).

15.2 Consequences of Poor IPC in Health Facilities

Poor IPC practices in healthcare settings can cause serious issues such as higher rates of HAIs, AMR, increased mortality, strain on healthcare resources, and rising costs.

15.2.1 Increased HAIs, AMR, and Associated Mortality

Inadequate IPC practices directly facilitate the spread of HAIs, affecting both patients and healthcare workers [5]. These infections can lead to longer hospital stays, more severe illnesses, and even death. The overuse and misuse of antibiotics for HAIs, often caused by poor IPC, contribute to the rise of AMR. This makes infections more difficult to treat and increases the likelihood of treatment failure. HAIs significantly impact mortality rates, particularly among vulnerable groups and in low- and middle-income countries (LMICs). Poor IPC procedures worsen this issue by increasing the risk of infections and related complications.

15.2.2 Strain on Healthcare Resources

HAIs and AMR result in longer hospital stays, greater use of antibiotics and medications, and escalate healthcare costs for both facilities and patients. The costs associated with treating HAIs, combating AMR, and dealing with the consequences of insufficient IPC are substantial for healthcare providers and individuals.

15.2.3 Ethical Concerns

Inadequate IPC practices raise ethical issues related to patient safety and healthcare facilities' duty to ensure a safe environment. Poor IPC increases healthcare workers' risk of acquiring HAIs, which can result in illness, absences from work, and possible long-term health effects [6].

15.2.4 Reduced Quality of Care

Overall, poor IPC compromises the quality of healthcare services [7], erodes public trust in healthcare facilities, and undermines efforts to improve healthcare outcomes.

15.3 Implementation of IPC in Health Facilities

Implementing IPC in health facilities demands a multifaceted strategy [8] (Table 15.1), emphasising standard precautions, specific isolation measures, and fostering a robust organisational culture.

Table 15.1 Key elements of implementation of IPC in health facilities

	Major area	Key elements
1	Leadership and policy with resource commitment	Prioritise IPC and allocate necessary resources. Develop and implement facility-level IPC policies, SOPs, and guidelines.
2	IPC team	Establish multispecialty dedicated IPC team. Define their roles and responsibilities.
3	Training and education	Provide comprehensive training to all healthcare staff on IPC principles, practices, and procedures. Regularly update training materials and conduct refresher courses.

(Continued)

Table 15.1 (Continued)

	Major area	Key elements
4	Core components of IPC programme	*Hand hygiene* Emphasise the importance of hand hygiene as a primary measure to prevent infection transmission. Provide accessible hand hygiene stations and promote regular handwashing. *Personal protective equipment* (PPE) Ensure appropriate and readily available PPE for all healthcare workers, and train them on proper usage. *Sterilisation and disinfection* Implement robust procedures for cleaning, disinfecting, and sterilising medical equipment and devices, following established protocols. *Patient placement and isolation* Implement appropriate patient placement strategies, including isolation precautions when necessary, particularly for patients with infectious diseases. *Safe injection practices* Follow safe injection practices and proper handling of sharps to prevent needle stick injuries and infections. *Waste management* Implement proper waste management protocols, including segregation and disposal of infectious waste. *Environmental cleaning* Establish routine and targeted cleaning and disinfection protocols for environmental surfaces, paying attention to high-touch areas. *Laundry management* Ensure safe handling of textiles and laundry, including proper washing and disinfection procedures. *Water, sanitation, and hygiene (WASH)* Integrate IPC with WASH programmes to improve overall hygiene and sanitation in the facility.
5	Priority actions/ areas	Respiratory hygiene Injection safety Catheter-associated infections Surgical site infections
6	Monitoring and evaluation	Implement a robust monitoring and evaluation system to assess the effectiveness of IPC practices. Conduct regular audits, collect data on infections, and provide feedback to staff. Establish clear feedback mechanisms to address identified issues and improve IPC practices.

Key areas encompass hand hygiene, PPE use, correct handling of medical equipment and waste, vaccinating all healthcare workers, and ensuring effective communication. A multimodal approach that combines system modifications, education, monitoring, and feedback is essential for successful adoption.

15.4 Impact of IPC on AMR and HAI

15.4.1 IPC and Reduction of Antimicrobial Use

Effective IPC helps prevent infections like ventilator-associated pneumonia, surgical site infections, and bloodstream infections. Preventing these infections reduces the need for antibiotics, which in turn decreases the selective pressure that fosters resistance [9]. For example, hand hygiene alone can decrease HAIs by up to 40% [10].

15.4.2 IPC and Containment of Resistant Pathogens

Hospitals are common sites for resistant organisms such as methicillin-resistant *Staphylococcus aureus* (MRSA*), carbapenem-resistant Enterobacteriaceae* (CRE)*,* and *vancomycin-resistant Enterococci* (VRE)**.** IPC measures are essential to stop these pathogens from transferring between patients. Outbreak studies consistently reveal that failures in hand hygiene and sterilisation are key factors in the spread of AMR [11].

15.4.3 Implementing Biosecurity Measures in the Health Sector

Implementing biosecurity measures in the health sector is crucial for preventing HAIs and AMR and for protecting patients and staff. Global guidelines from organisations such as WHO, WOAH, FAO, and CDC provide comprehensive frameworks for establishing robust biosecurity systems aligned with a One Health approach.

Governance and Regulations Effective biosecurity starts with solid governance and regulation, requiring national policies that mandate IPC programmes across all healthcare facilities, supported by laws, accreditation, and accountability. Health ministries should align national IPC guidelines with the WHO core components, defining clear procedures for isolation, outbreak response, laboratory safety, and waste management. Assigning a biosecurity or IPC focal point at each facility ensures leadership and compliance.

Essential Infrastructure Infrastructure prerequisites include reliable water, sanitation, hygiene (WASH), power, ventilation, and designated isolation areas. Hand hygiene facilities, including alcohol-based dispensers, are essential. Labs handling infectious agents should meet biosafety level standards, featuring controlled access, safety cabinets, sterilisation, and secure specimen transport. Engineering controls like negative-pressure rooms help reduce airborne infection spread.

Capacity Building of Health Workforce Workforce training is equally important, covering standard and transmission-based precautions, PPE use, sterilisation, and spill response. Regular drills and professional development promote ongoing compliance.

Institute Surveillance System Surveillance systems enable early detection of HAIs and resistant organisms, guiding responses and stewardship efforts. Risk assessments identify infrastructure or process vulnerabilities for corrective action.

Establish Efficient Supply Chain Sound supply chain management ensures availability of PPE and disinfectants, with procurement adhering to quality standards. Antimicrobial stewardship reduces antibiotic misuse, limiting resistance development.

Manage Waste as per Local Regulations Waste management protocols, including waste segregation, transportation, and treatment, are vital for containment. Routine cleaning with approved disinfectants minimises pathogen persistence. Water system monitoring prevents outbreaks of waterborne pathogens like Legionella.

Monitoring and Evaluation Monitoring and evaluation, including audits and accreditation, track compliance, with indicators such as hand hygiene rates, HAI incidence, and PPE stocks. Transparent reporting fosters trust.

Engage Communities Engaging communities through clear communication during outbreaks builds public trust and compliance. Integrating biosecurity into broader health system efforts, including universal coverage, supports sustainability.

Overall, effective biosecurity demands coordinated governance, infrastructure, training, surveillance, and continuous improvement, aligned with global standards and a One Health approach, to enhance resilience against emerging infectious threats and ensure long-term health security.

15.5 Biosecurity in Livestock and AMR

Across the globe, animals are given more antibiotics than humans, mainly for growth promotion and disease prevention. Factors such as poor farm hygiene and overcrowding contribute to high antibiotic usage. Enhancing biosecurity—by improving ventilation, restricting personnel access, disinfecting equipment, and vaccinating herds—reduces infection risks and lowers antibiotic dependence [12]. Denmark reduced antibiotic use in pigs by 50% through improved biosecurity and herd management, while maintaining productivity [13]. Similarly, in a broiler farm, there was no direct link between biosecurity measures and antibiotic use; however, farms with better biosecurity showed a tendency towards reduced antibiotic use. Misusing antibiotics can promote the development of AMR [14].

15.6 Why Is AMR Increasing in Livestock and Poultry?

15.6.1 Weak Farm Biosecurity

Poorly maintained facilities, inadequate hygiene practices, and a lack of visitor protocols can facilitate the occurrence of disease outbreaks, necessitating the use of antimicrobials.

15.6.2 Inadequate IPC in Veterinary Clinics

Lack of proper disinfection procedures, inadequate hand hygiene, and improper use of protective equipment can contribute to the spread of resistant bacteria among animals and staff.

15.6.3 Lack of Awareness and Training

Insufficient knowledge among farmers and veterinarians about the importance of IPC and biosecurity, as well as the risks of AMR, can lead to poor practices and increased antimicrobial use.

15.7 Consequences of Weak Biosecurity in Animal Husbandry

Weak IPC and biosecurity practices in veterinary services play a major role in the emergence and spread of AMR. Insufficient measures increase disease rates, prompting higher antimicrobial use (AMU). This overuse and misuse apply selective pressure, encouraging resistant bacteria to survive and spread [15]. The key outcomes are outlined in Box 15.1.

Box 15.1 Consequences of Inadequate Biosecurity in Animal Husbandry
Reduced disease prevention
Greater reliance on antibiotics
Widespread inappropriate dosing further contributes to resistance development
Enhanced pathogen transmission within the farm, between farms and increased zoonoses
Environmental contamination
Establishing environmental reservoirs
Overburdened veterinary services that have limited resources
Erosion of trust of farmers in veterinary advice and practices

15.7.1 Increased Disease Prevalence and Antimicrobial Use

Inadequate IPC and biosecurity practices facilitate the easy transmission of infectious agents both within and across animal populations. This results in higher infection rates, leading to increased dependence on antibiotics for treatment and prevention. The absence of effective biosecurity measures, like proper hygiene and isolation protocols, worsens the situation by enabling diseases to spread quickly and extensively [16].

15.7.2 Selective Pressure and AMR Development

Frequent use of antibiotics exerts selective pressure on bacteria, promoting the survival and reproduction of resistant strains. This process, known as AMR development, can render treatments ineffective, leading to longer illness duration, higher mortality, and increased healthcare costs. Misuse of antibiotics, such as their use for growth promotion or for other inappropriate purposes, accelerates the spread of AMR.

15.8 Impact on One Health

The dissemination of AMR among animal populations directly impacts human health. Resistant bacteria originating from animals can spread to humans via direct contact, contaminated food, or environmental sources, leading to treatment failures in human infections and potentially severe illness or mortality.

Biosecurity in human and animal health sectors is fundamentally connected through the One Health approach, which recognises that human, animal, and ecosystem health are intertwined. Emerging infectious diseases, AMR, and foodborne pathogens often cross species and environmental boundaries. As a result, isolating biosecurity efforts within either the human or animal sector is ineffective; coordinated action across sectors is crucial.

The global champion of the One Health framework is the Quadripartite collaboration between FAO, WHO, WOAH, and UNEP, which stresses that biosecurity measures—whether in hospitals, laboratories, farms, or markets—are part of a shared defence against biological threats.

In human health, biosecurity emphasises IPC, safe laboratory practices, surveillance, and containment of high-risk pathogens. Hospitals adopt standard precautions, isolation, sterilisation, and antimicrobial stewardship to prevent healthcare-associated infections and combat AMR. Laboratories follow biosafety level standards to handle infectious agents safely.

In animal health, biosecurity encompasses farm-level actions such as controlled access, vaccination, sanitation, quarantining new animals, safe feed and water, and disease surveillance. Preventing zoonoses such as avian influenza, brucellosis, and rabies at their source reduces the risk of spillover to humans.

The connection becomes clearest in zoonotic disease control. About 60–75% of emerging human infectious diseases originate from animals. Poor farm biosecurity can lead to pathogen spread among livestock, increasing exposure for farmers, vets, and consumers. Similarly, weak hospital IPC during outbreaks can enable human-to-human transmission. Thus, coordinated biosecurity fortifies the entire prevention chain.

AMR further exemplifies this interdependence. Antibiotic use in animals for treatment, prevention, or growth promotion can lead to antibiotic-resistant bacteria that can reach humans through food, contact, or the environment. Strong animal biosecurity reduces disease, lowers antibiotic use, and supports antimicrobial stewardship. Shared surveillance of AMR patterns across sectors helps detect resistance trends early and guides policies.

Environmental biosecurity is the third pillar of One Health. Waste from hospitals, pharma, and farms can pollute water and soil with resistant organisms or drug residues. Proper waste management, water sanitation, and environmental monitoring are vital to prevent cross-sector transmission.

Implementing One Health involves joint risk assessments, data-sharing platforms, coordinated outbreak response, and cross-sector training. Exercises, joint surveillance, and harmonised rules boost readiness. Political commitment and sustainable funding are essential to sustain these efforts.

It is well-established now that human and animal biosecurity are interconnected. Failures in one can jeopardise the other. The One Health approach bridges these gaps, ensuring that prevention is coherent, collaborative, and comprehensive. Strengthening biosecurity through One Health improves global health security, protects livelihoods, and enhances resilience against future pandemics.

15.9 Implementation of Biosecurity in Livestock Farms

Implementing biosecurity measures on livestock farms requires a comprehensive approach to prevent disease introduction and spread, including AMR. Essential strategies involve controlling the introduction of new animals, reducing contact with external

Table 15.2 Key elements of biosecurity implementation in animal husbandry

	Major area	Key elements
1	Control animal introduction	Reduce number of animals purchased Procure from reputed sources with known low disease risk Implement quarantine for new animals in dedicated facility Isolate sick animals in dedicated isolation facility Maintain detailed records for traceability
2	Limit external threats	Control visitors access Ensure all vehicles and equipment entering the farm are thoroughly cleaned and disinfected Implement fencing to prevent contact with wild animals and manage pest and rodent populations
3	Maintain hygiene and waste management	Regularly clean and disinfect facilities, including feeding and watering equipment, bedding, and handling areas Implement effective manure management practices to minimise disease transmission and prevent contamination of water sources Ensure feed and water are clean and free from contamination
4	Vaccination and health monitoring	Implement recommended vaccination programme to protect animals against common diseases. Conduct regular health checks on animals Promptly investigate any signs of illness and take appropriate action, including diagnostic testing and treatment
5	Staff hygiene	Ensure staff follow strict hygiene protocols, including handwashing and changing clothes when moving between healthy and sick animals
6	Responsible antimicrobial use	Use antibiotics only under the guidance of a veterinarian, following recommended dosages and treatment durations Maintain detailed records of all antimicrobial use, including dates, dosages, and treated animals Properly dispose of any unused or expired antibiotics and antifungals

threats, maintaining good hygiene and waste management practices, and establishing quarantine and isolation protocols. Additionally, vaccination, consistent health monitoring, and responsible antimicrobial use are vital components [17] (Table 15.2).

15.10 Possible Solution to Enhance Biosecurity in Animal Sector

Enhancing IPC and biosecurity in veterinary services is vital for decreasing antimicrobial use and stopping the spread of AMR. A One Health approach, which fosters collaboration between human and animal health sectors, is key to tackling the complex issue of AMR effectively. The solutions involve:

- Robust Implementation of biosecurity protocols on farms.
- Improved hygiene practices in veterinary clinics.

- Enhanced awareness, knowledge, and skills of farm workers in implementing biosecurity.
- Strengthened veterinary services, including diagnostic capabilities.

15.10.1 Implementation of Biosecurity in Poultry Farms in Developing Countries

- Effective poultry farm biosecurity is crucial for preventing transboundary animal diseases such as highly pathogenic avian influenza (HPAI) and Newcastle disease, reducing antimicrobial use, and safeguarding farmers' livelihoods. Global standards by the World Organisation for Animal Health (WOAH) and guidance from the Food and Agriculture Organisation (FAO) offer practical frameworks adaptable to developing countries. Successful implementation requires phased, risk-based, and cost-effective strategies tailored to local systems.
- *Governance and Regulation.* National veterinary bodies should develop clear biosecurity regulations aligned with the WOAH Terrestrial Animal Health Code. Licencing farms, hatcheries, and live bird markets should require minimum safety standards, such as perimeter fencing, visitor logs, and disease reporting. Public–private partnerships can aid in disseminating guidelines and encouraging compliance via certification and market benefits.
- Farm Zoning and Access Control. Defining clean and dirty zones on farms is key. Using perimeter fencing, single entry points, and locked gates limits unauthorised access. Disinfectant footbaths, vehicle dips, and designated parking areas help prevent pathogen entry. Restrict visitor access, maintain logs, and ensure that only essential personnel enter poultry houses, with strict adherence to hygiene protocols.
- *Infrastructure Improvements.* Incremental upgrades significantly boost biosecurity, even with limited resources. Poultry houses should prevent contact with wild birds through netting and sealed openings. Feed must be stored rodent-proof and dry, water sources treated or chlorinated, and drainage improved to reduce standing water. All-in–all-out systems help break disease cycles when feasible.
- *Cleaning and Waste Managem*ent. Routine cleaning and disinfecting are vital. Houses should be cleaned after each cycle, including washing, application of disinfectant, and a downtime period before restocking. Proper litter disposal and prompt removal of dead birds—via burial, incineration, or composting—are necessary. Manure should be handled to prevent runoff contamination.
- *Health Monitoring and Surveillance.* Regular veterinary oversight and disease monitoring are fundamental. Vaccination should follow national programmes for diseases like Newcastle and infectious bursal disease. Rapid reporting through surveillance systems and regional laboratories helps manage outbreaks. Keeping records of mortality, feed, and production aids early detection of issues.

- *Worker Training and Behaviour.* Human practices are often weak links. Continuous training on hygiene, clothing, and symptom recognition is essential. Workers should avoid backyard poultry and live markets without proper precautions. Using local languages and visual aids for education improves compliance.
- *Supply Chain Biosecurity.* Extending biosecurity to hatcheries, transport crates, feed mills, and vehicles is critical. Disinfecting equipment and ensuring feed quality prevent contamination. Contract farming models can help standardise practices.
- *Monitoring and Incentives.* Regular inspections and audits promote ongoing compliance. Certification programmes offering market or export advantages motivate farmers. Digital reporting tools and insurance schemes further incentivise adherence.
- *Linking Biosecurity to AMR Control.* Improved farm biosecurity reduces disease incidence and antibiotic use, thereby supporting antimicrobial stewardship aligned with WHO and WOAH guidance. Improved husbandry, vaccination, and hygiene help lower reliance on antibiotics.
- Implementation in developing countries must consider affordability and scale. Governments and development partners should support training, subsidise infrastructure like fencing and disinfectants, and strengthen veterinary services. A gradual, risk-focused approach—especially in dense poultry areas—can lead to meaningful reductions in outbreaks and economic losses.

15.10.2 Implementation of Biosecurity at the Backyard Poultry Level

- Backyard poultry is common in developing countries, crucial for household nutrition and income, but often faces high disease risks due to low biosecurity and contact with wild birds. Simple, low-cost measures can greatly improve safety.
- First, housing birds in basic enclosures or night shelters minimises scavenging and contact with wild birds. Separating ducks from chickens and avoiding mixing new birds with existing flocks without isolation reduces disease transmission.
- Second, hygiene promotion through community groups led by veterinary workers is vital. Handwashing, dedicated footwear, and keeping children away from sick birds are key. Local materials can make footbaths.
- Third, early reporting of unusual deaths supports disease detection; community surveillance systems under FAO and WOAH have been shown to be effective.
- Finally, vaccination campaigns for diseases such as Newcastle disease can be scaled up through outreach. Thermostable vaccines suitable for rural settings are especially useful.
- By combining affordable housing, education, and integration with veterinary services, backyard poultry biosecurity can significantly lower disease risks while supporting livelihoods and food security.

15.11 Challenges in Implementation of IPC and Biosecurity

Despite global recognition, IPC and biosecurity face significant barriers:

Resource Limitations: Many LMICs lack infrastructure for IPC (hand hygiene stations, isolation wards) and farm biosecurity (vaccination, veterinary oversight).

Behavioural Barriers: Compliance with hand hygiene and protective measures is often poor due to cultural and behavioural factors.

Surveillance Gaps: The limited surveillance of AMR across hospitals, farms, and the environment weakens evidence-based policy.

Weak Enforcement of Regulations: The over-the-counter sale of antibiotics, inadequate enforcement of waste management, and insufficient monitoring of animal antibiotic use exacerbate risks.

Cross-sectoral Silos: A lack of coordination between the human health, veterinary, and environmental sectors undermines One Health action.

15.12 Way Forward

Implementing the processes outlined earlier across health facilities at all levels and in animal farms will significantly reduce the irrational use of antibiotics. The only evidence-based way to address this challenge is through a sustained, multisectoral, and multidisciplinary One Health approach. Key actions are summarised in Table 15.3.

Table 15.3 Critical actions to improve IPC and biosecurity

	Broad Group	Critical actions
1	*Integrated One Health Surveillance*	Strengthen data sharing between health, veterinary, and environmental sectors. Monitor resistant organisms and antimicrobial consumption across domains.
2	*Strengthen Healthcare IPC:*	Establish IPC committees in all hospitals. Ensure availability of hand hygiene facilities and PPE. Conduct regular training and audits of healthcare staff.
3	*Invest in Farm-Level Biosecurity*	Improve housing, ventilation, and vaccination of livestock. Restrict access to farms, enforce disinfection of vehicles/equipment. Phase out non-therapeutic antibiotic use.
4	*Environmental Biosecurity*	Regulate effluent discharge from hospitals and pharmaceutical industries. Promote safe disposal of unused medicines. Invest in wastewater treatment technology.
5	*Workforce Training and Behavioural Change*	Incorporate IPC and biosecurity training into medical, nursing, and veterinary curricula. Use behavioural science to improve compliance with IPC guidelines.
6	*Adopting One Health approach*	Ensure active cooperation of human, animal, and environmental health partners [18].

AMR threatens to reverse decades of medical progress. While stewardship and innovation are essential, preventing infections is the most effective strategy against AMR. Establishing infection prevention and control (IPC) in healthcare, biosecurity on farms and in the environment, and connecting these efforts via the One Health approach form a robust prevention framework. Promoting these actions will save lives, reduce healthcare costs, and preserve the efficacy of antimicrobials for future generations.

Implementing these biosecurity measures allows livestock farms to greatly lower the risk of disease outbreaks, reduce reliance on antimicrobial treatments, and support overall animal health and welfare.

References

1. O'Neill J. Tackling drug-resistant infections globally: final report and recommendations. Review on Antimicrobial Resistance. 2016. Available at https://amr-review.org/sites/default/files/160518_Final%20paper_with%20cover.pdf. Accessed 2 May 2025.
2. WHO. WHO. Infection prevention and control. World Health Organisation. 2020. Available at https://www.who.int/teams/integrated-health-services/infection-prevention-control/about. Accessed 12 May 2025.
3. World Organisation for Animal Health (OIE) Terrestrial Code Online Access, OIE 2021. https://www.oie.int/en/what-we-do/standards/codes-and-manuals/terrestrial-code-online-access/. Accessed 5 May 2025.
4. Alawneh JI, Hassan MM, Camac J, et al. Plant biosecurity and one health: government and industry roles as risk creators and mitigators. One Health Outlook. 2025;7:27. https://doi.org/10.1186/s42522-025-00150-y.
5. Magadze TA, Nkhwashu TE, Moloko SM, Chetty D. The impediments of implementing infection prevention control in public hospitals: nurses' perspectives. Health SA. 2022;27:2033. https://doi.org/10.4102/hsag.v27i0.2033.
6. Edward MJ, Witness M, Elton I, Jennifer N, Odilia B, Daniel K et al. Challenges of compliance with Infection Prevention and Control (IPC) Standard Procedures among Healthcare Workers: a hospital-based cross-sectional study. J BioMed Res Rep 5(2);2024;3:1–07. https://doi.org/10.59657/2837-4681.brs.24.067
7. Markus RJ, Japhet S, Gabriel A, M. Infection prevention and control: implication on quality health care delivery. Int J Creative Res Thoughts. 2024;2024(12):2320–882. https://www.researchgate.net/publication/383155323
8. Sonpar A, Hundal CO, Totté JEE, Wang J, Klein SD, Twyman A, Allegranzi B, Zingg W. Multimodal strategies for the implementation of infection prevention and control interventions—update of a systematic review for the WHO guidelines on core components of infection prevention and control programmes at the facility level. Clin Microbiol Infect. 2025;31:948–57. https://doi.org/10.1016/j.cmi.2025.01.011.
9. WHO. IPC and antimicrobial resistance. Available at https://www.who.int/teams/integrated-health-services/infection-prevention-control/ipc-and-antimicrobial-resistance#
10. Alshagrawi S, Alhodaithy N. Determinants of hand hygiene compliance among healthcare workers in intensive care units: a qualitative study. BMC Public Health. 2024;24:2333. https://doi.org/10.1186/s12889-024-19461-2.
11. Russotto A, Rolfini E, Paladini G, Gastaldo C, Vicentini C, Zotti CM. Hand hygiene and antimicrobial resistance in the COVID-19 era: an observational study. Antibiotics (Basel). 2023;12(3):583. https://doi.org/10.3390/antibiotics12030583.

12. Butucel E, Balta I, McCleery D, Morariu F, Pet I, Popescu CA, Stef L, Corcionivoschi N. Farm biosecurity measures and interventions with an impact on bacterial biofilms. Agriculture. 2022;12(8):1251. https://doi.org/10.3390/agriculture12081251.
13. Levy S. Reduced antibiotic use in livestock: how Denmark tackled resistance. Environ Health Perspect. 2014;122(6):A160–5. https://doi.org/10.1289/ehp.122-A160.
14. Ziebe SD, Vougat Ngom R, Akoussa AMM, Bogning HP, Zangue HA. Impact of biosecurity on production performance and antimicrobial usage in broiler farms in Cameroon. Animals (Basel). 2025;15(12):1771. https://doi.org/10.3390/ani15121771.
15. Hasan M, Ali T, Khan AKMD, et al. Determinants of indiscriminate antimicrobial use in commercial chicken farms in Bangladesh and their impact on food safety and public health. Sci Rep. 2025;15:30103. https://doi.org/10.1038/s41598-025-14108-7.
16. World Organization of Animal Health. Implementing stronger biosecurity to avoid disease spread to new areas Available https://www.woah.org/en/implementing-stronger-biosecurity-to-avoid-disease-spread-to-new-areas. Accessed 1 May 2025.
17. Wierup M, Allard Bengtsson U, Vågsholm I. Biosafety considerations and risk reduction strategy for a new veterinary faculty building and teaching hospital in Sweden. Infect Ecol Epidemiol. 2020;10(1):1761588. https://doi.org/10.1080/20008686.2020.1761588.
18. US CDC. About One Health. https://www.cdc.gov/one-health/about/index.html#:~. Accessed 27 Apr 2025.

Part IV
Prevention and Therapeutic Innovations

Chapter 16
Role of Vaccines in Reducing AMR

Abstract Antimicrobial resistance (AMR) is a significant global threat, weakening the effectiveness of antibiotics and increasing morbidity, mortality, and healthcare costs due to various infections. Vaccines are a powerful, yet underused, tool to combat AMR by preventing infections, reducing antibiotic use, and limiting the spread of resistant bacteria. The vaccines achieve this through various mechanisms, including lowering infection rates, promoting herd immunity, decreasing bystander selection, preventing secondary bacterial infections, and slowing resistance development. Evidence from vaccines against pneumococcus, Hib, typhoid, rotavirus, and influenza shows notable declines in antibiotic prescriptions, treatment failures, and resistant infections. Global data suggest that expanding vaccine coverage, especially in low- and middle-income countries, could avert millions of antibiotic courses, hospitalisations, and deaths. Challenges such as serotype replacement, unequal coverage, and data gaps for certain pathogens remain. Future vaccines targeting high-burden resistant bacteria like *Klebsiella*, Group B *Streptococcus*, and extraintestinal pathogenic *Escherichia coli* (ExPEC) are promising. Incorporating vaccination into national AMR action plans, aligning it with antimicrobial stewardship, WASH, and infection prevention efforts, and prioritising AMR impact in investments are vital. Vaccination is a cost-effective, sustainable strategy that should be fully utilised within global efforts to combat AMR.

Keywords Antimicrobial resistance · Vaccines · Antibiotic stewardship · Herd immunity · Pneumococcal conjugate vaccine · Typhoid conjugate vaccine, Hib vaccine · Gavi

Antimicrobial resistance (AMR) is a major global public health issue that impairs the effectiveness of antibiotics and other antimicrobials, leading to higher rates of illness, death, and healthcare costs. Vaccines offer a practical and often underused strategy for preventing infections and lowering both drug-sensitive and resistant disease cases. By preventing infections, vaccines help slow resistance development, reduce co-infections that necessitate antibiotic use, boost herd immunity, and lessen the need for antimicrobial treatments [1]. Successful vaccination initiatives include

R. Bhatia, *Drug-Resistant Infections*,
https://doi.org/10.1007/978-981-92-4190-3_16

pneumococcal conjugate vaccines, rotavirus vaccines, and flu vaccines. Integrating vaccination strategies into national and international AMR policies is both cost-effective and essential for sustainable AMR management [1].

16.1 Role of Vaccines in Containing AMR

Antibiotic use exerts selection pressure that promotes AMR, but the main factor is infection incidence. Vaccines help reduce infections, thereby decreasing opportunities for antibiotic use and the pressure for resistance. Studies by the World Health Organisation (WHO) [2] and Gavi [3] emphasise that vaccinations are both crucial and cost-effective in tackling AMR comprehensively. Vaccines can prevent bacterial infections, such as *Streptococcus pneumoniae*, *Haemophilus influenzae* type b, and typhoid, all of which pose concerns about resistance. The vaccines can also prevent viral infections such as influenza and respiratory syncytial virus, which often lead to unnecessary antibiotic use, and diarrhoeal diseases that may require antibiotics.

Although vaccinations can strengthen the immune system against different pathogens before an infection begins or intensifies, their impact on reducing AMR has not been sufficiently recognised. Vaccinated individuals typically suffer fewer illnesses, which helps prevent secondary infections that might lead to hospitalisation or the need for antibiotics.

Three broad categories of vaccines that influence the reduction in AMR are:

1. These vaccines defend against "community-acquired infections," which are bacterial illnesses commonly contracted in everyday life. By decreasing carriage—the silent spread of infection—these vaccines protect community members from bacterial diseases. They help reduce antibiotic use, lowering the risk of bacteria developing resistance and transmitting to others.
2. Vaccines also protect against "hospital-acquired infections," or bacterial illnesses often contracted in healthcare settings, like hospitals. Given the risk of bacterial transmission and related health issues, multidrug-resistant infections in healthcare environments are particularly concerning.
3. The vaccines guard against viruses, which are crucial, as many unnecessary prescriptions are written for viral infections.

16.2 Mechanisms by Which Vaccines Reduce AMR

Vaccines reduce AMR through several complementary mechanisms (Box 16.1):

Box 16.1 Possible Mechanisms by Which Vaccines Reduce AMR
Reducing the burden of infections through their prevention
Inducing herd immunity
Reducing bystander selection
Preventing secondary bacterial infections
Slowing the evolution of resistance and reducing the transmission of resistant clones

16.2.1 Reducing the Burden of Infections Through Their Prevention

When vaccination prevents a bacterial infection that would otherwise require antibiotics, it reduces antibiotic use and decreases the selection pressure for resistant bacteria. This is the simplest mechanism. For instance, pneumococcal conjugate vaccines (PCVs) help prevent pneumococcal disease, thereby reducing the need for antibiotics such as beta-lactams and macrolides, which are often used to treat ear infections, septicaemia, and pneumonia [4].

16.2.2 Inducing Herd Immunity

Vaccines provide indirect protection to unvaccinated individuals by limiting disease transmission among vaccinated populations. When vaccine-targeted serotypes become resistant, their decline reduces the overall prevalence of resistance in the community. Herd immunity also decreases the circulation of both susceptible and resistant strains. PCVs exemplify how vaccination can diminish drug-resistant pneumococci in the community by significantly reducing vaccine-targeted serotypes linked to resistance.

16.2.3 Reducing Bystander Selection

Antibiotics used to treat one infection exert selection pressure on the entire microbiota, promoting resistance not only in the target pathogen but also in other bacteria, such as commensals that could later cause infection [5]. Vaccines help reduce this pressure across multiple species by preventing infections that would otherwise necessitate antibiotic use.

16.2.4 Preventing Secondary Bacterial Infections

Viral infections frequently raise the risk of secondary bacterial infections, such as bacterial pneumonia, that can occur after influenza. Vaccinating against viral pathogens thus helps lower the chances of these secondary infections and reduces the need for antibiotics. Studies have shown that flu vaccination results in fewer antibiotic prescriptions for respiratory illnesses [6].

16.2.5 Slowing Evolution of AMR and Reducing Transmission of Resistant Clones

Vaccines alter the selective environment that fosters resistant mutations and clones by reducing antibiotic use and infection rates. This may eventually influence the AMR evolution, reducing the speed at which resistance appears and spreads [5]. Furthermore, targeted bacterial vaccines can directly interrupt transmission chains of resistant clones by decreasing the carriage of strains with resistance genes.

16.3 Evidence from Specific Vaccines' Impact on AMR

Empirical evidence from observational studies, surveillance data, and modelling supports the role of vaccines in reducing AMR. Below are several well-documented examples.

16.3.1 Pneumococcal Conjugate Vaccines (PCVs)

Conjugate vaccines for pneumococcal disease (PCVs), including PCV7, PCV10, PCV13, and now PCV20, have significantly decreased the rates of pneumonia, otitis media, and invasive pneumococcal disease in vaccinated children and, through herd immunity, in older populations. These vaccines often target serotypes with antibiotic-resistance determinants, highlighting their importance for combating resistant microbes. Many settings observed notable reductions in *S. pneumoniae* resistance to penicillin and macrolides, along with a decrease in antibiotic prescriptions for respiratory illnesses, following the widespread use of PCV. A multicountry study after PCV implementation confirmed significant drops in antibiotic consumption and resistant pneumococcal infections [3]. Overall, the impact on resistance and antibiotic use has been positive, since reducing the carriage of resistance genes can interrupt transmission of resistant clones. However, some gains were offset by shifts to non-vaccine serotypes, known as serotype replacement.

Enhanced PCV coverage has averted approximately 718,100 treatment failures, resulting in a 27% decline in deaths related to AMR between 2011 and 2017 [7]. With 70% coverage, administering PCV to children under two in 18 low- and middle-income countries (LMICs) could prevent approximately 23.8 million antibiotic-treated acute respiratory infections each year [3]. Ethiopia avoided over 100,000 antibiotic treatment failures from 2011 to 2017 through PCV use [8]. In Indonesia, achieving 85% PCV coverage over two years, followed by 99% coverage over three years, may reduce antibiotic treatment failures by up to 13% [3].

In Northern California, the introduction of PCV resulted in a decrease of 35 antibiotic prescriptions per 100 vaccinated children, suggesting that about 1.4 million antibiotic prescriptions each year could be avoided with PCV in the USA [9]. Similarly, after including PCV in routine childhood immunisations in the USA, the incidence of penicillin-non-susceptible invasive pneumococcal disease fell by 81% among children under 2 years old [10].

16.3.2 Haemophilus influenzae *Type b (Hib) Vaccine*

Children vaccinated against *Haemophilus influenzae* type b (Hib) experienced a significant decline in Hib meningitis and other invasive diseases [11]. Vaccination prevents Hib-related illnesses, leading to fewer hospitalisations and reducing the use of antibiotics, including broad-spectrum ones in children, even though Hib resistance is not the primary concern in AMR. The public health advantages of the Hib vaccine also demonstrate how preventing invasive bacterial diseases indirectly contributes to AMR reduction by decreasing antibiotic demand. Research in China indicates that the Hib vaccine is cost-effective and may help lower AMR [12].

16.3.3 Typhoid Conjugate Vaccine

Typhoid fever is becoming more associated with multidrug-resistant and extensively drug-resistant Salmonella enterica serovar Typhi worldwide. Typhoid conjugate vaccines (TCVs) help lower the incidence of clinical typhoid, decreasing the need for extended antibiotic use and helping to prevent the spread of resistant strains. In countries affected by extensively drug-resistant (XDR) typhoid outbreaks, deploying TCV has been a crucial step to address AMR. The Gavi and WHO [13] have highlighted the importance of TCV as an effective tool against drug-resistant typhoid.

A Gavi-supported modelling study across 73 countries indicated that introducing TCV combined with a catch-up campaign for children aged 15 and under could avert 21.2 million cases of multidrug-resistant typhoid, prevent 826,000 deaths, and save 44.4 million disability-adjusted life years (DALYs) over ten years [3].

In Pakistan, where XDR typhoid cases are rising [14], a cohort study utilising census data indicates that TCV provides over 90% protection for young children against XDR Salmonella Typhi (S. Typhi) [15].

16.3.4 Rotavirus Vaccination

Many LMICs frequently administer antibiotics to children with diarrhoeal illnesses because of limited diagnostics and concerns about bacterial coinfection. Nevertheless, rotavirus is a viral pathogen, and antibiotics are ineffective against viral diarrhoea. Following the introduction of rotavirus vaccination, antibiotic use has decreased, as have hospitalisations and clinic visits for severe diarrhoea. Recent research and systematic reviews indicate a reduction in antibiotic usage following the vaccine's roll-out. This decline may also help minimise the development of antibiotic-resistant enteric bacteria within the gut microbiome [16]. Gavi estimates that Rotavirus vaccines, with 77% coverage in children under two years old in 18 LMICs, could avert 13.6 million (31%) episodes of antibiotic-treated diarrhoea annually [3].

16.3.5 Influenza Vaccination

Respiratory tract infections are the primary reason for antibiotic prescriptions in outpatients. However, many of these prescriptions are unnecessary because the illnesses are viral. Vaccination reduces the incidence of influenza, and multiple studies indicate a modest yet significant decrease in antibiotic prescriptions for respiratory diseases in outpatient clinics [6]. Improving influenza vaccination coverage could further cut antibiotic use and help reduce the development of antibiotic-resistant bacteria [17].

16.4 Promising Vaccines of Future

Researchers are working on candidate vaccines for illnesses that frequently need antibiotics, such as urinary tract infections (UTI) caused by extraintestinal pathogenic *E. coli* (ExPEC) and neonatal sepsis due to Group B *Streptococcus*. These vaccines have the potential to decrease future antibiotic dependence. Early clinical trials and proof-of-concept studies have shown that developing these vaccines is feasible. If they effectively reduce disease occurrence and antibiotic use, they could also play a role in preventing antibiotic resistance [6].

Table 16.1 Global impact of vaccines on AMR and related parameters

Vaccine category	Deaths averted	DALY's reduced in millions	Productivity loss prevented in billion USD	Hospital cost saved in million USD	Reduced antibiotics use in million DDD
Existing	106,000	9.1	5.9	861	142
Late stage development	135,000	5	2.2	1200	1900
Early clinical development	408,000	23	17.7	3000	548

16.5 Global Impact of Vaccines on AMR

Recent studies have evaluated the global influence of vaccines on antibiotic resistance. WHO and partners have modelled how greater use of existing vaccines—such as pneumococcal, Hib, rotavirus, and typhoid—and new vaccine introductions could notably decrease antibiotic consumption and related deaths (Table 16.1) [18], especially in LMICs.

Gavi's analysis indicates that fully expanding key childhood vaccines could save hundreds of thousands of lives from antibiotic-resistant infections and eliminate the use of tens of millions of antibiotic doses annually in Gavi-eligible countries alone. While various models have different assumptions and results, they all concur that vaccines are among the most cost-effective strategies to combat AMR, more so than solely developing new antibiotics or stewardship efforts. WHO estimates that vaccines targeting 23 identified pathogens could decrease antibiotic consumption by 22%, which equates to about 2.5 billion defined daily doses each year [19].

16.6 Gavi's Contribution to Preventing AMR

Gavi is a leading global organisation involved in all stages of vaccine development, manufacturing, distribution, and investment. It supports vaccines for 20 infectious diseases, including some highly effective against AMR, such as pneumococcal, typhoid, and *Haemophilus influenzae* type b (Hib). Six Gavi-backed vaccines help prevent AMR by reducing the transmission of both sensitive and resistant strains, thereby preventing severe infections that are difficult to treat. Many vaccines in Gavi's portfolio, such as those for measles and COVID-19, contribute to combating AMR by reducing unnecessary antibiotic use and lowering the risk of secondary bacterial infections, which often necessitate antibiotics. Recognising vaccines' role in combating AMR, Gavi's Vaccine Investment Strategy 2024 [20] highlights "impact on AMR" as a key indicator of a vaccine's contribution to global health security. Increasing investments in vaccines could save lives from AMR, reduce antibiotic consumption, and lower costs associated with resistant infections.

16.7 Challenges in Vaccination as an AMR Containment Strategy

Vaccines are effective, but they cannot be the sole solution to AMR. Although mentioned in the Global Action Plan on AMR and the 2024 UNGA Political Declaration on AMR, their full potential in AMR prevention has yet to be recognised. For instance, an analysis of 108 national AMR plans found that only 13%, or 14 plans, included immunisation efforts and highlighted strengthening immunisation programmes as a key strategy to prevent and combat AMR [21].

The Immunisation Agenda 2030 (IA2030)[1] clearly highlights the critical role of vaccines in preventing AMR. It notes that vaccines are widely regarded as essential in combating emerging infectious diseases by preventing the spread of resistant bacteria [22]. A WHO Resolution on AMR at the 77th World Health Assembly in 2024 underscored the need for advancing research and development in vaccines, diagnostics, and treatments. It also emphasised the importance of integrating IA2030 into the WHO's global infection prevention and control strategies [23].

Despite several initiatives, vaccines remain undervalued as a tool against AMR and face numerous obstacles. Some of these include:

16.7.1 Serotype Replacement and Evolving Pathogen Populations

Some vaccines target only specific strains or serotypes, which can lead to an increase in non-vaccine types that may also carry resistance genes. This phenomenon is known as serotype replacement. Consequently, the overall effect on AMR depends on the resistance characteristics of the emerging strains and antibiotic usage patterns [7]. The experience with PCVs demonstrates notable net benefits but also highlights the importance of surveillance to identify and address the replacement phenomenon [4].

[1] The Immunisation Agenda 2030 (IA2030) is a global strategy for 2021–2030, endorsed by the World Health Assembly, with the vision that everyone, at every age, fully benefits from vaccines for improved health and well-being.

16.7.2 Vaccine Coverage Gaps and Inequities

The benefits of vaccines in reducing AMR depend on sufficient uptake [3]. Gaps in coverage—both within and across countries—restrict herd immunity and allow disease reservoirs and antibiotic use to persist. Historically, many national AMR strategies have overlooked immunisation; therefore, integrating immunisation efforts with AMR strategies is crucial for achieving optimal results.

16.7.3 Vaccines Against Non-bacterial Pathogens Have Only Indirect Effects

Vaccines targeting viruses like influenza and rotavirus mainly cut down on antibiotic use by preventing unnecessary prescriptions or secondary bacterial infections. However, they do not directly influence the selection of bacterial pathogens, except through decreased bystander selection [14]. Nonetheless, these indirect effects can be significant, especially in environments with high rates of inappropriate antibiotic prescribing.

16.7.4 Evidence Gaps for Some Pathogens and Settings

For a few pathogens, vaccine candidates show promise, yet data on phase III efficacy and real-world effectiveness remain limited. Additional research is essential to assess the impacts of AMR in various health systems and to understand the long-term evolutionary influence of vaccines on resistance [24].

16.8 Pathogens in Urgent Need of Vaccines

WHO has published a list of 17 high-priority pathogens for vaccine research and development, aiming to combat endemic diseases worldwide and promote equitable access to vaccines. These pathogens are chosen based on their significant public health burdens, antibiotic resistance, and socioeconomic effects, especially in low- and middle-income countries. They are ranked according to factors such as mortality rates, resistance levels, and regional disease impact [25]. The 17 prioritised pathogens are divided into three groups based on the current stage of vaccine development (Table 16.2) [26].

Table 16.2 WHO List of pathogens requiring vaccines urgently

Category of vaccines	Examples
Pathogens requiring new vaccine research: New vaccines for these pathogens are urgently needed to address unmet health challenges worldwide.	Group A *Streptococcus*, hepatitis C virus, HIV-1, and *Klebsiella pneumoniae*.
Pathogens needing further vaccine development: These pathogens present significant health and economic burdens, particularly in regions where AMR rates are rising	Cytomegalovirus, *Leishmania* species, influenza virus, *Plasmodium falciparum,* non-typhoidal *Salmonella*, norovirus, *Shigella* species, and *Staphylococcus aureus*.
Pathogens approaching regulatory approval: Vaccines in this category are nearing policy recommendations and potential public use.	Dengue virus, Group B *Streptococcus*, extra-intestinal pathogenic *E. coli*, *Mycobacterium tuberculosis*, and respiratory syncytial virus.

16.9 Importance of Animal Vaccines in Control of AMR

It is well known that a key factor driving AMR is the frequent and often excessive use of antibiotics in livestock and poultry to treat diseases, prevent infections, and, in some regions, promote growth. This practice has led to the rise and spread of resistant bacteria across animals, the environment, and, more recently, in humans through food and direct contact. Resistant bacteria *can transfer between animals and humans* directly or via food, water, and environmental pathways.

Vaccines break this cycle by stopping infections in animals, which decreases the need for antibiotics, reduces bacterial disease cases, and lessens the selection pressure for resistance. This concept is key to worldwide "One Health" strategies that connect human, animal, and environmental health efforts to fight AMR.

16.9.1 How Vaccines Reduce AMR in Livestock and Poultry

Vaccines contribute to AMR control through several mechanisms:

Preventing disease and reducing the need for antibiotics involves protecting animals from certain infectious agents, which results in fewer infections and thus fewer antibiotic treatments. This decline in antibiotic use lessens the selective pressure that leads to resistant strains developing and spreading. For instance, in aquaculture, the use of vaccines against bacterial pathogens has significantly lowered antibiotic reliance. In Norway, vaccines targeting furunculosis and other diseases in salmon have nearly eliminated routine antibiotic treatments, making antimicrobial resistance in fish pathogens rare. According to efeedlink (2020), 99% of Norwegian salmon were produced without antibiotics [27].

Reducing Secondary Infections. Many viral infections predispose animals to bacterial superinfections, which are often treated with antibiotics. Vaccines against these viruses (e.g. porcine circovirus in pigs) reduce secondary bacterial disease and thus antibiotic use.

Reducing the spread of resistant bacteria: Vaccines help control disease outbreaks, lowering pathogen circulation in animal populations. This decreases the chances for resistant strains to spread among animals and potentially reach humans involved in handling or consuming animal products.

Enhancing overall herd or flock health leads to animals that grow more efficiently, experience fewer illnesses, and need fewer antibiotics throughout their lives. This comprehensive advantage is especially crucial in intensive production systems where antibiotic use has historically been substantial.

16.9.2 Veterinary Vaccines with Demonstrated Efficacy in Preventing AMR

Many vaccines have already demonstrated tangible benefits in lowering antibiotic usage and the risk of antimicrobial resistance in livestock and poultry, including in developing regions.

Newcastle Disease Vaccines (Poultry) The Newcastle disease virus significantly impacts poultry mortality, especially among smallholder and backyard flocks in Asia and Africa. Vaccination efforts, including thermostable vaccines designed for hot climates, have greatly lowered disease rates and reduced the need for antibiotics to treat secondary bacterial infections [28]. Initiatives in Nepal and India with community vaccinators have enhanced survival and productivity.

Vaccines for Salmonella and pathogenic E. coli help lower antibiotic use by preventing enteric infections. Live attenuated or recombinant vaccines trigger targeted immune responses, decreasing the need for broad-spectrum antibiotics [29]

Pig Vaccines The Porcine Circovirus Type 2 (PCV-2) virus leads to immune suppression and makes pigs more vulnerable to bacterial infections. Vaccinating herds in Europe and North America has greatly decreased antibiotic use and enhanced performance metrics [30].

Fish Vaccines Vaccines against bacterial fish pathogens have almost eliminated intensive antibiotic use in Norwegian salmon aquaculture, providing a model for sustainable practises.

Other Livestock Vaccines Although less frequently quantified, several clostridial vaccines, leptospirosis vaccines (cattle and pigs), and respiratory disease vaccines are widely used to control diseases that would otherwise require antibiotic treatment.

Vaccination interventions in many low- and middle-income countries (LMICs) have shown positive results, though data specific to AMR outcomes is still growing:

16.9.3 Global Vaccine Coverage Gaps

Although vaccines offer advantages, coverage for key livestock diseases like foot-and-mouth disease and brucellosis is still limited in developing countries, especially where veterinary infrastructure is weak. Improving access to and affordability of effective animal vaccines could significantly lower the risk of antimicrobial resistance (AMR) in these regions.

In many developing countries, veterinary services and vaccine supply chains lack sufficient resources. The costs associated with vaccines and their delivery can be prohibitive for smallholders unless supported by subsidies or community programmes.

Effective protection depends on matching vaccine strains with circulating pathogens. Diverse bacterial strains in different regions can reduce effectiveness if vaccines are not locally tailored.

Farmers and producers often overlook the long-term advantages of vaccination compared to immediate antibiotic use, particularly when antibiotics are inexpensive and easily accessible. Education and extension services are crucial to encourage the adoption of vaccines.

Vaccination should be part of a broader AMR mitigation strategy that includes improved hygiene, biosecurity, sound husbandry, and prudent antibiotic use, guided by veterinary oversight.

Vaccines have the potential to be crucial in preventing antimicrobial resistance stemming from livestock and poultry. They directly lower infection rates and reduce antibiotic use, which helps decrease the selection pressure for resistant bacteria. This not only safeguards animal health and boosts productivity but also indirectly protects human health by supporting safer food systems. Evidence from both high- and low-resource environments—such as successful poultry vaccination initiatives and fish vaccine programmes—demonstrates the real impact of immunisation in cutting down antibiotic dependency.

However, to expand these benefits worldwide, it is necessary to enhance veterinary services, increase vaccine access and affordability, incorporate vaccine strategies into national AMR plans, and maintain research on vaccines for key animal pathogens. When integrated into One Health approaches, vaccines go beyond disease prevention—they become vital tools in the ongoing effort to combat AMR sustainably.

16.10 Way Forward

Given the evidence, the following solutions should be considered by the national authorities, international agencies, civil society, and the communities in general:

16.10.1 Treat Vaccination as an Explicit Pillar of National AMR Plans

National action plans for AMR should include specific targets for immunisation, strategies for procurement, and financing mechanisms. Current evidence shows that many national AMR plans do not adequately focus on vaccination, which is an urgent gap that can be addressed. Stakeholders involved in AMR and immunisation need to recognise the crucial role of vaccines in reducing AMR. Vaccines should be integrated into global, regional, and national AMR and immunisation strategies and implementation plans to encourage their widespread adoption and incorporation.

16.10.2 Prioritise Impactful Vaccines and Accelerate the Introduction of New Vaccines

Policymakers should prioritise broad vaccination campaigns that have demonstrated benefits in combating AMR. Key vaccines include PCVs, Hib, rotavirus, TCV, and seasonal influenza, especially in LMICs, where antibiotic misuse is widespread and AMR poses a major threat. Gavi and supporting donors can be approached for providing the funding necessary to expand these initiatives.

The pace of introducing existing vaccines should be hastened, and their coverage should be expanded. All currently available paediatric vaccines should meet the immunisation targets of IA2030, and consideration should be given to the use of these vaccines among older age groups. The effects of existing vaccines on AMR should be analysed to guide policy-making decisions.

16.10.3 Use AMR Impact as a Criterion in Vaccine Investment Decisions

Donors and decision-making bodies should account for the potential to reduce AMR when making vaccine introduction and funding choices. Gavi has started integrating the impact of AMR into its investment decisions, and other funders, as well as national immunisation technical advisory groups, are encouraged to follow this example.

16.10.4 Enhance Monitoring That Connects Vaccination, Antibiotic Usage, and AMR

Effective, integrated monitoring systems that link vaccination rates, antibiotic usage (in both community and hospital settings), and microbial resistance trends are essential for evaluating the impact of vaccines on AMR and identifying shifts in serotypes or strains. Molecular surveillance can help elucidate the evolving genetic landscape of resistance.

16.10.5 Integrate Vaccination with Stewardship, WASH, and IPC

To effectively combat AMR, vaccination efforts should be integrated into a broader strategy that also emphasises prudent antibiotic use, improvements in water, sanitation, and hygiene (WASH), infection prevention and control in healthcare environments, and measures to promote animal health. Evidence suggests that combining these approaches can achieve substantially greater reductions in illness and mortality associated with AMR compared to implementing any single intervention. Investing in research and development for new vaccines that can significantly mitigate AMR is crucial.

Supporting the development and clinical testing of vaccines for high-AMR pathogens—such as ExPEC, *Klebsiella*, *E. coli* UTI vaccines, as well as improved typhoid and non-typhoidal *Salmonella* vaccines—is essential. Collaborations between public and private sectors, combined with innovative financing strategies, can address the challenges faced in researching and developing new vaccines.

16.10.6 Continuous Assessment of the Impact of Vaccines on AMR

Evaluate the health and economic impacts of AMR and use this data to support including vaccination in AMR mitigation efforts. It is essential to gather information on how vaccines affect AMR rates and antibiotic use, as well as to develop comprehensive value assessments for new vaccines in development.

Immunisation stands out as a highly effective, economical, yet underused strategy to fight AMR. By preventing infections, lowering antibiotic consumption, curbing the spread of resistant bacteria, and reducing bystander selection, vaccines target both immediate and long-term causes of AMR. Evidence from randomised clinical trials, observational research, surveillance, and modelling consistently supports integrating vaccination into national and global efforts against AMR. To maximise its benefits, countries and funding bodies should focus on expanding access to key vaccines (notably pneumococcal conjugate vaccines, Hib, rotavirus, tetanus, diphtheria, and influenza), enhancing integrated surveillance systems that combine immunisation and AMR data, and continuing investment in vaccine research and development for high-AMR pathogens [31]. Although vaccination alone cannot eradicate AMR, it remains a vital and sustainable element of a comprehensive strategy.

References

1. WHO. Antimicrobial resistance. Available at https://www.who.int/news-room/fact-sheets/detail/antimicrobial-resistance#:~. Accessed 7 May 2025.
2. WHO. Vaccines and antimicrobial resistance. Available at https://www.who.int/teams/immunization-vaccines-and-biologicals/product-and-delivery-research/anti-microbial-resistance. Accessed 17 May 2025.
3. Gavi. Vaccines: a key tool to combat antimicrobial resistance. Available at https://www.gavi.org/news-resources/knowledge-products/vaccines-key-tool-tackle-antimicrobial-resistance-amr. Accessed 7 May 2025.
4. Dagan R, Klugman KP. Impact of conjugate pneumococcal vaccines on antibiotic resistance. Lancet Infect Dis. 2008;8:785–95. https://doi.org/10.1016/S1473-3099(08)70281-0.
5. Micoli F, Bagnoli F, Rappuoli R, et al. The role of vaccines in combating antimicrobial resistance. Nat Rev Microbiol. 2021;19:287–302. https://doi.org/10.1038/s41579-020-00506-3.
6. Smith ER, Fry AM, Hicks LA, Fleming-Dutra KE, Flannery B, Ferdinands J, et al. Reducing antibiotic use in ambulatory care through influenza vaccination. Clin Infect Dis. 2020;71(11):e726–34. https://doi.org/10.1093/cid/ciaa464.
7. Ben-Shimol S, Givon-Lavi N, Greenberg D, Stein M, Megged O, Bar-Yochai A, Negari S, Dagan R, Israel Bacteremia and Meningitis Active Surveillance Group. Impact of pneumococcal conjugate vaccine introduction on antibiotic resistance of Streptococcus pneumoniae meningitis in children aged 5 years or younger, Israel, 2004–2016. Euro Surveill. 2018;23(47):1800081. https://doi.org/10.2807/1560-7917.ES.2018.23.47.1800081.
8. Ozawa S, Chen H-H, Rao GG, Eguale T, Stringer A. Value of pneumococcal vaccination in controlling the development of antimicrobial resistance (AMR): case study using DREAMR in Ethiopia. Vaccine. 2021;39:6700–11. https://doi.org/10.1016/j.vaccine.2021.04.024.
9. Fireman B, Black SB, Shinefield HR, Lee J, Lewis E, Ray P, et al. Impact of the pneumococcal conjugate vaccine on otitis media. Pediatr Infect Dis J. 2003;22:10–6. https://doi.org/10.1097/00006454-200301000-00006.
10. Kyaw MH, Lynfield R, Schaffner W, Craig AS, Hadler J, Reingold A, et al. Effect of introduction of the pneumococcal conjugate vaccine on drug-resistant Streptococcus pneumoniae. N Engl J Med. 2006;354:1455–63. https://doi.org/10.1056/NEJMoa051642.
11. Gilsdorf JR. Hib vaccines: their impact on *Haemophilus influenzae* Type b disease. J Infect Dis. 2021;224(12 Suppl 2):S321–30. https://doi.org/10.1093/infdis/jiaa537.
12. Zhang H, Garcia C, Yu W, Knoll MD, Lai X, Xu T, et al. National and provincial impact and cost-effectiveness of Haemophilus influenzae type b conjugate vaccine in China: a modelling analysis. BMC Med. 2021;19(1):181. https://doi.org/10.1186/s12916-021-02049-7.
13. WHO. Typhoid vaccines. Position Paper. Available at https://www.who.int/publications/i/item/whio-wer9313. Accessed 7 Apr 2025.
14. Yousafzai MT, Karim S, Qureshi S, Kazi M, Memon H, Junejo A, et al. Effectiveness of typhoid conjugate vaccine against culture-confirmed Salmonella enterica serotype Typhi in an extensively drug-resistant outbreak setting of Hyderabad, Pakistan: a cohort study. Lancet Glob Health. 2021;9(8):e1154–62. https://doi.org/10.1016/S2214-109X(21)00255-2.

15. Abdullah MA, Shaikh BT, Ashraf M, Khan SA. XDR typhoid in Pakistan: a threat to global health security and a wake-up call for antimicrobial stewardship. PLoS Negl Trop Dis. 2025;19(5):e0013067. https://doi.org/10.1371/journal.pntd.0013067.
16. Simhachalam Kutikuppala LV, Cozma MA, Maddineni G, Chorya HP, Tummala N, et al. Exploring the impact of rotavirus vaccination on antibiotic prescription and resistance: a comprehensive systematic review. World J Virol. 2024;13(2):92586. https://doi.org/10.5501/wjv.v13.i2.92586.
17. He WQ, Gianacas C, Muscatello DJ, Newall AT, McIntyre P, Cheng AC, Liu B. Effectiveness of influenza vaccination in reducing influenza-like illness and related antibiotic prescriptions in adults from a primary care-based case-control study. J Infect. 2022;85(6):660–5. https://doi.org/10.1016/j.jinf.2022.10.028.
18. WHO. Estimating the impact of vaccines in reducing antimicrobial resistance and antibiotic use: technical report. Geneva: World Health Organization; 2024. Licence: CC BY-NC-SA 3.0 IGO
19. WHO. Better use of vaccines could reduce antibiotic use by 2.5 billion doses annually. Available at https://www.who.int/news/item/10-10-2024-better-use-of-vaccines-could-reduce-antibiotic-use-by-2.5-billion-doses-annually%2D%2Dsays-who. Accessed 7 May 2025.
20. Gavi. Vaccine Investment Strategy 2024. Available at https://www.gavi.org/our-alliance/strategy/vaccine-investment-strategy-2024. Accessed 27 May 2025.
21. Charani E, Mendelson M, Pallet SJC, et al. An analysis of existing national action plans for antimicrobial resistance—gaps and opportunities in strategies optimising antibiotic use in human populations. Lancet Global Health. 2023;11:e466–74. https://doi.org/10.1016/S2214-109X(23)00019-0.
22. WHO. Immunization Agenda 2030, A global strategy to leave no one behind: https://www.who.int/teams/immunization-vaccines-and-biologicals/strategies/ia2030. Accessed 7 Apr 2025.
23. WHO. EB154/CONF//7, 23 January 2024. Antimicrobial resistance: accelerating national and global responses. Available at https://apps.who.int/gb/ebwha/pdf_files/EB154/B154_CONF7-en.pdf. Accessed 7 Apr 2025.
24. Tadesse BT, Keddy KH, Rickett NY, Zhusupbekova A, Poudyal N, Lawley T, et al. Vaccination to reduce antimicrobial resistance burden-data gaps and future research. Clin Infect Dis. 2023;77(Suppl 7):S597–607. https://doi.org/10.1093/cid/ciad562.
25. WHO. WHO study lists top endemic pathogens for which new vaccines are urgently needed. Available at https://www.who.int/news/item/05-11-2024-who-study-lists-top-endemic-pathogens-for-which-new-vaccines-are-urgently-needed. Accessed 27 Mar 2025.
26. Hasso-Agopsowicz M, Hwangb A, Hollm-Delgadoa M-G, Umbelino-Walkerb I, Karrond RA, Raoe R, et al. Identifying WHO global priority endemic pathogens for vaccine research and development (R&D) using multi-criteria decision analysis (MCDA): an objective of the Immunization Agenda 2030. eBioMedicine. 2024;110:105424. https://doi.org/10.1016/j.ebiom.2024.105424.
27. efeedlink. 99% of Norwegian salmon produced antibiotics free, 2020. Available at https://www.efeedlink.com/contents/11-06-2020/6da0616e-7993-447b-9dcd-a6b635a8d822-1752.html#:~:text. Accessed 6 Feb 2026.
28. Habibi H, Firuzi S, Nili H, Asasi K, Mosleh N. Efficacy of thermostable newcastle disease virus Strain I-2 in broiler chickens challenged with highly virulent newcastle virus. Arch Razi Inst. 2020;75(1):31–7. https://doi.org/10.22092/ari.2019.122830.1228
29. Hasso-Agopsowicz M, Sparrow E, Cameron AM, Sati H, Srikantiah P, Gottlieb S. The role of vaccines in reducing antimicrobial resistance: a review of potential impact of vaccines on AMR and insights across 16 vaccines and pathogens. Vaccine. 2024;42:S1–8. https://doi.org/10.1016/j.vaccine.2024.06.017.
30. Rose N, Andraud M, Bigault L, Jestin A, Grasland B. A commercial PCV2a-based vaccine notably reduces PCV2b transmission in experimental settings. Vaccine. 2016;34:3738–45. https://doi.org/10.1016/j.vaccine.2016.06.005.
31. Bhatia R. Vaccines as a tool to contain antimicrobial resistance. Indian J Med Microbiol. 2019;37(1):1–4. https://doi.org/10.4103/ijmm.IJMM_19_223.

Chapter 17
Research Priorities for AMR

Abstract Antimicrobial resistance (AMR) research is essential to prevent a global health and development crisis. AMR necessitates several key research priorities, including new drug discovery, understanding resistance mechanisms, optimising antimicrobial use, and guiding policy through evidence-based strategies. It is important to emphasise the leadership of the World Health Organisation in shaping global AMR research agendas, especially the 2023 framework that focuses on prevention, diagnostics, treatment, and cross-cutting issues within a One Health approach. Major public, private, multilateral, and philanthropic organisations play a role in advancing research, although funding and coordination remain fragmented and inadequate, especially in low- and middle-income countries.

National research agendas, such as that of Australia, provide guiding principles for tailoring priorities to local contexts, supporting innovation, and promoting cross-sectoral collaboration. Veterinary research must focus on surveillance, stewardship, alternatives to antibiotics, and addressing transmission pathways between animals, humans, and the environment. Environmental research is equally critical in understanding pollution, farming practices, and AMR gene transfer. Despite progress, challenges of inadequate prioritisation, limited funding, and a shrinking research workforce persist. Overcoming these requires global coordination, equitable financing, and strong interdisciplinary collaboration to develop sustainable AMR solutions.

Keywords Antimicrobial resistance · Research priorities · One Health approach
Antimicrobial stewardship · Veterinary sector · Environmental transmission
Global health policy

Research on antimicrobial resistance (AMR) is essential for addressing the global health threat it presents. Research enables the development of new antibiotics, enhances understanding of resistance mechanisms and their behaviour across different environments, optimises current treatments, and guides policy decisions to fight AMR. Without ongoing research, the world faces a future where common infections may become impossible to treat, leading to higher death rates, increased healthcare expenses, and significant economic impacts.

R. Bhatia, *Drug-Resistant Infections*,
https://doi.org/10.1007/978-981-92-4190-3_17

17.1 Importance of Research in AMR

Some of the key benefits from research in any AMR programme are outlined in Table 17.1.

Table 17.1 Importance of research in AMR

Research priority area	Key focus areas
Developing Novel Antimicrobials	Discovering and developing new drugs, vaccines, and alternative therapies to combat resistant pathogens Exploring novel classes of antibiotics and repurposing existing ones Understanding how resistance develops and spreads
Understanding Resistance Mechanisms	Studying molecular and cellular mechanisms of resistance Developing strategies to overcome resistance and predict new resistant strains Designing diagnostics for rapid identification of resistant infections
Optimising Antimicrobial Use	Identifying effective and appropriate use of existing antimicrobials Optimising dosing, treatment duration, and usage across patient populations Developing diagnostics for accurate infection identification and treatment
Informing Policy and Public Health Strategies	Supporting policy development and implementation with research evidence Addressing antimicrobial use in human and animal health, infection control, and AMR surveillance Raising public awareness and promoting responsible use
Addressing Socioeconomic Impacts of AMR	Quantifying economic burden (healthcare, productivity, agriculture). Justifying investments in AMR research Studying social and behavioural contributors to AMR and informing corrective interventions

17.2 Major Organisations Supporting AMR Research

Since 2014, the World Health Organisation (WHO) has played a prominent role among various organisations supporting and promoting AMR research.

17.2.1 WHO Leadership in Setting Global Research Agenda for AMR

The WHO promoted increased research on AMR with its 2014 report, "Antimicrobial Resistance: Global Report on Surveillance."[1]. This has been the WHO's first comprehensive effort to assess the scope of AMR worldwide. The report highlighted significant gaps in surveillance, poor coordination, and the urgent need to enhance laboratory and monitoring systems globally by conducting focused research on various aspects of AMR containment. It recommended five key areas, including research and development, for international attention (Table 17.2) and identified 40 priorities out of which seven are related to tuberculosis.

This report was followed by discussions at the 67th World Health Assembly (May 19–24, 2014), which resulted in empowering the WHO to create a Global Action Plan on AMR [2] and urged Member States to increase support for research activities related to AMR.

Recognising the importance of R&D and innovation for executing national action plan components, the WHO released an AMR research agenda in 2023 [3]. It outlines 40 essential research priorities to be tackled by 2030, stressing the urgent necessity of ongoing investment and collaboration in this vital field.

Figure 17.1 highlights the key areas outlined in the WHO's Agenda. These encompass policy, governance, epidemiology, the burden of AMR, and its drivers, as well as prevention, diagnosis, and treatment, plus multiple cross-cutting topics.

A simplified version of overview of the key elements in the WHO AMR Research Agenda has been shown in Table 17.3.

Table 17.2 AMR focus areas recommended in WHO 2014 report

Area	2014 WHO focus/priority
Surveillance	Establish baseline, coordinate global AMR data collection and reporting
Stewardship & Regulation	Strengthen drug management systems and rational antibiotic use policies
One Health Approach	Incorporate human, animal, environmental health sectors in AMR strategy
R&D & Capacity Building	Improve diagnostics, laboratories, stewardship; explore new funding models
Attention to LMIC Needs	Emphasize affordability, accessibility, and capacity support for low-and-medium-income countries (LMICs)

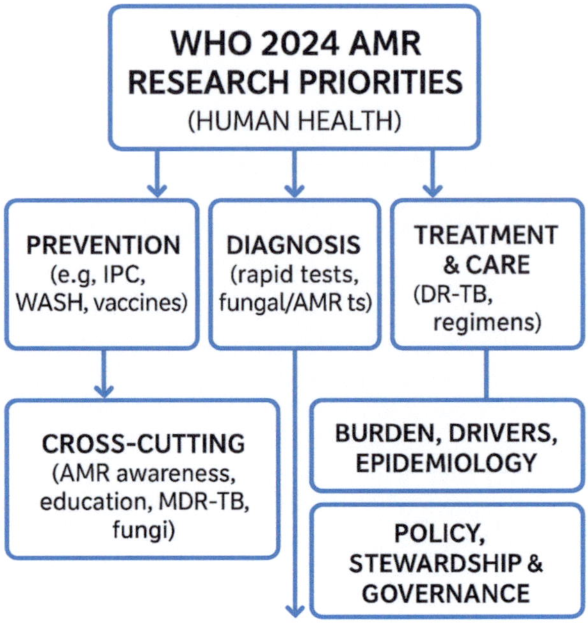

Fig. 17.1 Salient areas that require research and innovation (WHO AMR Research Agenda [3])

Table 17.3 Key elements of WHO AMR research agenda (2023)

	Broad area	Key elements
1	Main Pillars	Prevention: IPC, WASH, vaccination Diagnosis: Rapid tests, fungal/AMR diagnostics Treatment and Care: Drug-resistant TB, AMR treatment regimens
2	Cross-cutting Areas	Burden, Drivers, Epidemiology Stewardship and Policy Public awareness, education Fungal pathogens and MDR-TB
3	One Health Additions	WASH in healthcare and community Transmission pathways Integrated surveillance Behavioural insights and economics

Antimicrobial researchers form the foundation of the antibiotic development necessary to protect everyone from the rising threat of AMR. They constantly develop new treatments, tackle resistance challenges, and support public health. However, the AMR sector has been gradually losing essential scientific and research talent for the past twenty years [4]. Nonetheless, various organisations—including public, multilateral, philanthropic, and private sectors—are funding R&D efforts related to AMR, as shown in Table 17.4.

Worldwide, progress has been slow in raising awareness of AMR, monitoring and optimising antimicrobial use, and implementing infection prevention and control (IPC) programmes. Funding for AMR research has been insufficient. From

Table 17.4 Major organisations financing research on AMR

Funding source	Type	Focus areas	Geographic focus
National Institutes for Allergy and Infectious Diseases (NIIAD), USA [5]	Public (National)	Basic research, drug development, surveillance	Global, mainly USA
UK Research and Innovation (UKRI) [6]	Public (National)	AMR in One Health, diagnostics, policy	Global, mainly UK and LMICs
European Union (Horizon Europe, IMI) [7]	Public (Regional)	R&D, public–private partnerships, surveillance	EU and partner countries
Global AMR R&D Hub	Multilateral Platform	Coordination, transparency, funding analysis	Global
CARB-X (Combating Antibiotic-Resistant Bacteria Biopharmaceutical Accelerator) [13]	Public–Private Partnership	Early-stage therapeutics, diagnostics, vaccines	Global, focus on LMIC-applicable tools
GARDP (Global Antibiotic Research and Development Partnership) [12]	Public–Private Partnership	Antibiotic development for public health needs	LMICs
Wellcome [8]	Philanthropic	One Health, behavioural research, policy, diagnostics	Global, emphasis on LMICs
Gates Foundation [9]	Philanthropic	AMR in agriculture, vaccines, health systems	Global, strong LMIC focus
World Health Organization (WHO) [2]	Multilateral Agency	Policy, surveillance (GLASS), capacity building	Global
World Bank [10]	Multilateral Agency	Health systems strengthening, AMR investment frameworks	LMICs
Innovative Medicines Initiative (IMI) Accelerator Programme [11]	Public–Private Partnership	Collaborative R&D for antibiotics and alternatives	Europe
Pharmaceutical Companies (e.g. Pfizer, GSK)	Private Sector	Antibiotic R&D, stewardship, education programmes	Global
AMR Industry Alliance	Private Sector	Discovery of new antibiotics and diagnostics	Global

2017 to 2021, the Global AMR R&D Hub estimated that global investments in AMR research amounted to just US$8.9 billion [14].

The Global AMR R&D Hub is a collaboration among countries, non-governmental donors, and intergovernmental organisations aimed at tackling challenges and enhancing coordination and cooperation in global AMR R&D through a One Health approach. Launched in May 2018, it is guided by a Board of Members. The Secretariat functions under DZIF, the German Centre for Infection Research.

Private sector investment in AMR research remains limited because of the low returns on antibiotic development. Initiatives such as CARB-X and GARDP have been established to address this issue, but their effectiveness is constrained without continuous and predictable public funding [12].

GARDP is dedicated to creating new antibiotics to combat drug-resistant infections, aligning with the WHO bacterial priority list. Additionally, CARB-X (Combating Antibiotic Resistant Bacteria Biopharmaceutical Accelerator) [13] supports the development of novel antibacterial therapies.

CARB-X aims to speed up the development of new antibiotics and other strategies to combat drug-resistant bacterial infections. Public funding for research and reducing risks for private sector investments are also beneficial. Organisations like CARB-X are supporting dozens of small companies, providing crucial support for their researchers to keep their important work going. In 2021, the $1 billion AMR Action Fund was launched to offer short-term funding for innovative antibiotic companies, with seven investments made so far.

17.3 National AMR Research Guiding Principles

A national research agenda is essential for any country's AMR action plan. Australia's agenda can serve as a model for other nations in creating their own [15]. It should highlight sector-specific priorities, like gathering baseline data on AMR in the environment, and also focus on cross-sector issues such as transmission risks among humans, animals, and the environment.

The national AMR research agenda can direct resource allocation and focus efforts on areas needing discoveries, technological advances, or best-practice initiatives. It will also identify opportunities for international research collaboration and promote efficiency within Australian R&D by reducing duplication. Establishing a mechanism for national coordination, with sector representation aligned with a One Health approach, will further enhance coordination of Australia's research and development activities.

17.3.1 Guiding Principles for National AMR Research Agenda

The following are a few guiding principles for developing a comprehensive and action-oriented national AMR research agenda.

- Establish a flexible national AMR research and development agenda and maintain dedicated funding for it, including partnerships between private and public sectors.
- Support the translation of research findings into new approaches, applications, and policies to combat the AMR agenda that strives for innovation

- Coordinate and share research and development activities
- Develop research priorities in the veterinary sector.

17.4 Research Priorities in the Veterinary Sector

Research priorities in the veterinary sector for AMR should emphasise prevention, surveillance, and responsible antimicrobial use. This involves exploring infection prevention strategies, enhancing diagnostic tools, understanding AMR transmission and drivers, and promoting stewardship programmes to optimise antimicrobial use—particularly by phasing out antibiotics as growth promoters. Key areas in veterinary research that require actionable insights include:

Prevention efforts should prioritise identifying effective, multimodal strategies to prevent infections and minimise the use of antimicrobials. This involves studying the effects of vaccination programmes and enhancing biosecurity measures on AMR. Further research is essential to understand how WASH (Water, Sanitation, and Hygiene) contributes to reducing AMR, especially in community and healthcare environments. Understanding the effectiveness of various hygiene practices in limiting the spread of resistant bacteria between animals and through the food chain to humans is crucial.

Research should begin to gather evidence on integrated surveillance systems by developing and deploying robust methods to monitor AMR in animals and their environment, as well as tracking antimicrobial use and resistance patterns.

Research should identify which pathogens of veterinary importance and antibiotics of human use should be prioritised for surveillance, focusing on critical and high-priority pathogens in the veterinary sector. Additionally, affordable, practical, and efficient data sharing tools should be evaluated for generating and sharing surveillance data, as well as for facilitating collaboration across different sectors to gain a comprehensive understanding of AMR trends.

Responsible antimicrobial use is a crucial area requiring targeted research. This includes developing and assessing the effectiveness of antimicrobial stewardship programmes across different animal production systems. Research is needed to understand antimicrobial consumption (AMC) and analyse patterns of antimicrobial use (AMU) in various animal populations, focusing on the reasons behind their use and the resulting impact on AMR.

Development of alternatives to antibiotics and strategies for disease prevention and treatment, such as probiotics, prebiotics, and immunomodulators, to reduce reliance on antibiotics. Researching and developing rapid and accurate diagnostic tools to identify resistant bacteria and inform appropriate treatment decisions is another key research priority.

There's growing interest in alternative antimicrobial strategies like bacteriophage therapy [16], antimicrobial peptides (AMPs) [17], and CRISPR-Cas antimicrobials [18]—which promise specificity, evolvability, and minimal immunogenicity. AI-powered discovery of AMPs is an area of active research (Chap. 19).

The One Health approach underscores research priorities for AMR in the veterinary sector. Key areas include understanding how AMR is transmitted among animals, humans, and the environment, creating rapid diagnostic tools, and encouraging responsible use of antimicrobials. This also involves exploring how the environment, such as water and waste management systems, contributes to AMR spread. Additionally, studying the economic factors driving AMR and crafting effective policies to ensure responsible antibiotic use in animals are critical research priorities.

Addressing Knowledge Gaps: There are a few areas that have knowledge gaps and require research in the local context to understand:

- *Impact of AMR on Animal Health and Welfare*: Researching the impact of AMR on animal health, productivity, and welfare.
- *Emergence and Spread of AMR*: Investigating the mechanisms of AMR emergence and spread in different animal populations and environments.
- *Behavioural Insights*: Understanding the factors that influence antimicrobial use practices in different settings and developing interventions to promote behavioural changes.
- Phasing out growth-promotion use where overlap exists with human-use antibiotics
- Monitoring usage and resistance, and safety evaluations of new products before regulatory approval.

17.5 Research Priorities for AMR in the Environment

Aligning human health, animal health, environmental science, and social disciplines enables the development of comprehensive and effective strategies against AMR. It is urgent to identify barriers to collaboration and bring together diverse stakeholders [19]. This will help develop a strong One Health surveillance system, crucial for tracking AMR trends across humans, animals, and the environment. However, these systems often face difficulties in data sharing and coordination between sectors, which requires further operational research to resolve.

Research may explore the environmental pathways of AMR transmission and the connections between ecological pollution and AMR. It is crucial to examine how AMR genes and bacteria move among animals (such as livestock, pets, and wildlife), humans, and the environment.

Understanding how environmental variables—such as wastewater, soil, or agricultural runoff—drive the evolution of AMR. These outcomes can inform Water, Sanitation, and Hygiene (WASH) interventions across all sectors and waste management policies.

Agricultural practices and crops are now believed to have a significant influence on AMR epidemiology. More detailed research is needed to understand how different farming practices—such as antibiotic use in livestock and manure management—affect the emergence and dissemination of AMR.

17.6 Consolidation of Academic AMR Research Outputs to Benefit NAP Implementation

Consolidating research outputs from academic institutions to effectively implement a national action plan (NAP) on antimicrobial resistance (AMR) is both a strategic necessity and a governance challenge. Universities and research institutes generate valuable data on antimicrobial use (AMU), resistance patterns, diagnostics, behavioural drivers, infection prevention, and policy interventions. However, much of this evidence remains fragmented, unpublished in actionable formats, or disconnected from policy decision-making. Systematic consolidation can bridge this gap and accelerate NAP implementation.

Mapping and Cataloguing Existing Research Is Essential Governments, through national AMR secretariats or coordinating bodies, should establish a centralised repository of research outputs. This should include peer-reviewed publications, theses, surveillance datasets, operational research findings, and implementation studies across the human health, veterinary, agricultural, and environmental sectors. A digital, searchable knowledge platform hosted by a national public health institute or ministry can ensure access for policymakers and implementers.

Standardisation and Harmonisation of Research Protocols and Data Academic research often uses diverse methodologies, definitions, and indicators. Aligning research outputs with national and global frameworks—such as standardised AMR surveillance indicators, antimicrobial consumption metrics, and One Health reporting standards—enhances comparability and policy relevance. National technical working groups can review research findings and synthesise them into policy briefs aligned with NAP objectives.

Institutionalisation of Structured Policy–Academia Interfaces Regular forums, technical advisory committees, and thematic working groups enable researchers to present findings directly to policymakers. Embedding academic experts on NAP steering committees ensures that emerging evidence informs regulatory reforms, stewardship guidelines, vaccination strategies, and infection prevention measures. Conversely, policymakers can communicate priority research gaps to academia, promoting demand-driven research rather than purely academic pursuits.

Translation of Research into Policy Formulation and Programme Development Is Vital Translating research into implementation tools is essential. Evidence must be converted into actionable guidance—clinical protocols, standard treatment guidelines, veterinary advisories, training curricula, and community awareness materials. Universities can collaborate with ministries to develop operational manuals and training modules based on locally generated data. This approach improves contextual relevance and ownership compared with adopting generic international guidance.

Applied Research Consolidation should include economic and behavioural research outputs. Cost-effectiveness studies of stewardship programmes, vaccination campaigns, diagnostic tools, and infection control interventions inform resource allocation within NAP budgets. Behavioural and social science research can inform risk communication strategies targeting prescribers, farmers, pharmacists, and communities.

Open Access and Ease of Data Access Strengthening open-access and data sharing mechanisms is crucial. Memoranda of understanding between academic institutions and government agencies can facilitate ethical data sharing while protecting intellectual property. National funding agencies can mandate that publicly funded AMR research be shared in national repositories and summarised in policy-relevant formats.

Capacity Building Capacity-building initiatives can enhance utilisation. Policymakers may need support to interpret complex epidemiological or genomic data. Short courses, policy dialogues, and joint analysis workshops foster mutual understanding between researchers and implementers.

Monitoring and Evaluation Monitoring and evaluation systems should integrate academic evidence into NAP performance reviews. Annual NAP progress reports can include synthesised research findings, highlighting how evidence has informed interventions and identifying emerging threats. This creates a feedback loop in which research continuously refines implementation strategies.

Consolidating academic research outputs for NAP implementation requires institutional mechanisms, standardised data systems, structured policy engagement, knowledge translation processes, and robust governance. When effectively integrated, academic evidence becomes a dynamic engine for evidence-based AMR control rather than a passive repository of publications.

17.7 Operational Research for AMR

Operational research (OR)[1] on AMR is vital for aligning policy goals with actual implementation. Although NAPs offer strategic guidance, their success relies on how interventions operate within intricate health systems, veterinary services, food production processes, and community environments. Operational research supplies tailored evidence to enhance these interventions, boost efficiency, and promote sustainability.

[1] Operational research (OR) is a scientific approach to problem-solving and decision-making that uses advanced analytical methods—such as mathematical modeling, statistics, and optimization—to improve organizational performance.

17.7.1 Need for Operational Research on AMR

AMR results from multiple factors such as clinical practices, pharmaceutical supply chains, agricultural use, gaps in infection prevention, behavioural factors, and regulatory weaknesses. While traditional epidemiological surveillance detects resistance patterns, it doesn't clarify why certain interventions succeed or fail. OR addresses this gap by analysing processes, bottlenecks, and system performance in real-world settings.

Implementation gaps are frequent. For instance, antimicrobial stewardship guidelines might be in place but poorly followed because of workload pressures, limited diagnostics, or financial incentives. Likewise, regulations that restrict over-the-counter antibiotic sales can be bypassed by informal markets. Operational research plays a key role in uncovering these obstacles and suggesting practical solutions.

AMR interventions frequently demand substantial investments, including diagnostic labs, surveillance systems, vaccination efforts, biosecurity protocols, and awareness initiatives. Policymakers rely on evidence of cost-effectiveness and scalability. OR assesses whether interventions achieve their expected results in routine programme settings, not just in controlled pilot studies environments.

AMR presents a One Health challenge spanning human, animal, and environmental sectors. Coordinating these sectors is operationally demanding. OR aids in testing integrated strategies like joint surveillance, shared labs, and cross-sector stewardship, confirming their feasibility and sustainability.

AMR patterns change quickly. Operational research offers adaptive learning, helping programmes to respond flexibly to new resistance trends, technological advances, and changing behaviours.

17.7.2 Mechanisms for Undertaking Operational Research

Embedding OR Within NAP Structures National AMR coordinating bodies should formally incorporate operational research into their implementation framework. Establishing dedicated research components, allocating budgets, and forming technical working groups can help ensure that OR is prioritised as a core function rather than an afterthought.

Defining Priority Questions Research should focus on specific programmatic gaps, such as: Why is hospital antibiotic guideline compliance low? What factors drive antibiotic use in poultry farms? How successful are community awareness campaigns? Conducting priority-setting workshops with policymakers, implementers, and researchers helps ensure the research aligns with national priorities.

Multidisciplinary Collaboration OR on AMR necessitates cooperation among clinicians, veterinarians, microbiologists, epidemiologists, social scientists, economists, and policymakers. Universities and public health institutes can oversee technical design, while health facilities and veterinary services handle implementation platforms.

Incorporate Mixed Methods Quantitative techniques, such as prescription audits, AMU data analysis, and surveillance trends, should be combined with qualitative methods like interviews, focus groups, and workflow observations to explore behavioural and systemic factors.

Capacity Building Training frontline healthcare workers and veterinary officers in fundamental OR methods enhances local ownership. This includes short courses, mentorship programmes, and fellowships in operational research can build sustainable capacity.

Ethical and Governance Frameworks It is crucial to have clear protocols for ethical approval, data protection, and dissemination. To prevent delays, governments should streamline ethical review procedures, especially for public health–focused OR.

Knowledge Translation and Feedback Loops Findings should be converted into policy briefs, implementation guidelines, and corrective actions. Regular review meetings between researchers and programme managers facilitate quick adoption of results.

Monitoring Impact OR It should include measurable indicators like decreased antibiotic use, better adherence to guidelines, reduced infection rates, or cost savings. Monitoring these results shows the value of the initiative and supports ongoing investment.

Operational research is frequently overlooked, yet it consistently turns AMR control from a static policy into a flexible, adaptive process. Through systematically pinpointing barriers, testing potential solutions, and fine-tuning implementation tactics, OR guarantees that NAPs lead to tangible decreases in antimicrobial use and resistance. Especially in resource-limited environments, operational research offers the critical evidence needed for effective, context-specific, and sustainable AMR strategies.

17.8 Challenges in AMR Research and Possible Solutions

AMR is a complex challenge that demands collaboration across human health, animal health, and environmental sectors. However, these sectors frequently face coordination issues and capacity gaps. One Health research on AMR is constrained by limited funding, especially flexible funds needed for cross-sectoral efforts, and by inadequate infrastructure in some regions. There is a shortage of researchers with expertise in human health, animal health, and environmental science, which are essential for a true One Health approach.

In summary, three major challenges are being faced globally in executing meaningful research on AMR. These are

- Inadequate prioritisation
- Limited funding
- Inadequate number of researchers

17.8.1 Inadequate Prioritisation of AMR Research

The inadequate prioritisation of AMR research results from several factors, such as limited funding, competing priorities, and a lack of awareness about its long-term consequences. The perception of AMR as a "slowly emerging disaster"—in contrast to rapidly spreading infectious diseases—also leads to delays or insufficient action. Additionally, there is a general lack of awareness regarding the importance of prioritising research within the health sector [20]. Global engagement of the private sector in the national AMR research agenda remains suboptimal. Addressing this requires recognising the roles of national authorities and international organisations—both public and private—in elevating AMR research on their agendas. Strong advocacy from influential bodies like the UNGA, the WHO, and the FAO is essential to prioritise AMR research and raise awareness about its potential impact on human development.

17.8.2 Limited Funding

AMR research funding is fragmented, poorly coordinated, and heavily skewed towards high-income nations. A comprehensive global funding analysis reveals significant disparities. Data from the Global AMR R&D Hub indicates that from 2017 to 2023, nearly 80% of AMR R&D funding was contributed by just five countries, primarily the U.S. and the U.K. Meanwhile, LMICs, which bear the highest burden of AMR, receive minimal support, hindering research on local pathogens, resistance mechanisms, and health systems.

Furthermore, most funding concentrates on basic science and pharmaceutical R&D, particularly in developing new antibiotics. While vital, this narrow focus often overlooks other critical areas, such as diagnostics, infection prevention and control, environmental surveillance, and behavioural sciences. The lack of interdisciplinary research funding impedes the development of comprehensive, One Health-based strategies to combat AMR.

Effectively tackling AMR involves shifting funding priorities both in focus and geography. Increasing investments in LMICs, fostering innovation within the One Health approach, and enhancing global cooperation are essential steps. Implementing transparent monitoring systems for AMR R&D funding and including AMR in broader health and development budgets can help maintain progress. Without prompt, equitable, and strategic investments, AMR could reverse decades of medical advancements and threaten global health security. For example, seven of the last ten antibiotics were launched by companies that are now defunct, either bankrupt or acquired cheaply [21].

According to the global AMR R&D Hub's dynamic dashboard [14], a total of US$16.68 billion has been invested in AMR research from 2017 to 2024. One hundred one countries use this funding through 3529 organisations. Nearly 90% of the investment targets research and development on bacterial pathogens, with about a third—roughly $4.3 billion in the US—focused on priority bacterial pathogens for new therapeutic development [14].

Securing substantial funding is crucial for advancing a multidisciplinary research agenda on AMR with clear priorities. In addition to increasing funding, the global community should promote investment by governments and funders, while also drawing the attention of policymakers, researchers, and the private sector to critical knowledge gaps that need evidence. Addressing these gaps will support the effective development and implementation of AMR policies and interventions.

17.8.3 Inadequate Number of Researchers

Research from the AMR Industry Alliance [22] shows approximately 3,000 researchers dedicated to AMR, compared to 46,000 for cancer and 5,000 for HIV/AIDS. The number of authors publishing on AMR, often seen as a sign of laboratory expertise, halved from 1995 to 2020. Similarly, the group of researchers with three or more publications decreased proportionally. This decline is especially pronounced in antibiotics research. In 2022, academic journals published about 5.5 times more articles on HIV/AIDS than on priority bacteria, even though estimates suggest that AMR causes more deaths annually than AIDS [23].

Unfortunately, this problem extends beyond researchers. Clinicians are also crucial members of the antimicrobial and antifungal R&D teams. However, in countries where AMR research is concentrated, there are few infectious disease specialists, and the field is losing new entrants. In 2022, the US saw 44% of infectious disease fellowships remain vacant—more than double the vacancy rate across all specialities.

Research on AMR encounters numerous challenges, such as poor coordination, insufficient funding, and reliance on traditional research methods that may not suit complex, multisectoral issues. Addressing these requires a comprehensive strategy that includes improved surveillance, responsible antibiotic use, the development of new diagnostics and treatments, and the fostering of interdisciplinary cooperation.

Since AMR is a multifaceted problem involving human health, animal health, agriculture, and the environment, better integration across these sectors is essential. Currently, research efforts often lack the necessary collaboration and coordination. Research and development (R&D) for new antibiotics and alternative therapies, especially novel antimicrobials, is frequently underfunded. Many interventions are evaluated with inadequate study designs, producing unreliable results that impede effective policy-making.

A strong need exists to greatly increase investment in R&D for new diagnostic methods, alternative treatments such as phage therapy and immunotherapy, and innovative antimicrobial drugs [23]. Finally, it is crucial to promote collaboration among researchers across different fields, including microbiology, pharmacology, epidemiology, and social sciences.

References

1. WHO. Antimicrobial resistance: Global Report on Surveillance, 2014. Available at https://apo.who.int/publications/i/item/9789241564748? Accessed 5 June 2025.
2. WHO. Global action plan on antimicrobial resistance. Geneva: World Health Organization; 2015. Available at https://iris.who.int/handle/10665/193736. Accessed 15 June 2025.
3. WHO. Global research agenda for antimicrobial resistance in human health- Policy brief, 2023. Available at https://www.who.int/publications/i/item/9789240102309#. Accessed 5 June 2025.
4. Fabbro E, Lamichhane U, Sudbrak R, Ogilvie L, Vitiello A, Zovi A, Sabbatucci M. Investment gaps in antimicrobial resistance research & development: trends in Europe, 2017-2021. Eur J Health Econ. 2025; https://doi.org/10.1007/s10198-025-01796-1.
5. National Institutes for Allergy and Infectious Diseases. Research initiatives of antimicrobial resistance. Available at https://www.niaid.nih.gov/research/recent-initiatives-antimicrobial-resistance. Accessed 15 June 2025.
6. UK Research and Innovation. Antimicrobial Resistance. Available at https://www.ukri.org/what-we-do/browse-our-areas-of-investment-and-support/antimicrobial-resistance/. Accessed 5 May 2025.
7. European Commission. Public Health. Research, projects and studies. Available at https://health.ec.europa.eu/antimicrobial-resistance/research-projects-studies_en#:~:text. Accessed 15 June 2025.
8. Wellcome. Antimicrobial Resistance: it is time for global action. Available at https://wellcome.org/our-priorities/infectious-disease/antimicrobial-resistance?gad_source. Accessed 3 June 2025.
9. Gates Foundation. Philanthropic partnership launches new initiative tackling antimicrobial resistance. Available at https://www.gatesfoundation.org/ideas/media-center/press-releases/2025/02/amr-bacteria-treatment-discovery. Accessed 5 April 2025.
10. World Bank. Antimicrobial Resistance. Available at https://www.worldbank.org/en/topic/health/brief/antimicrobial-resistance-amr. Accessed 5 June 2025.
11. Innovative Medicines Initiative (IMI) Accelerator Programme. Available at https://amr-accelerator.eu/. Accessed 25 June 2025.
12. Global Antibiotic Research & Development Partnership GARDP: Available at https://gardp.org. Accessed 5 June 2025.
13. CARB X. Combating antibiotic-resistant bacteria. Available at https://carb-x.org/.0. Accessed 25 June 2025.

14. Global AMR R&D Hub. Dynamic dashboard. Available at https://dashboard.globalamrhub.org/reports/investments/overview. Accessed 11 Apr 2025.
15. Australian Government. Antimicrobial Resistance. Australia's National Antimicrobial Resistance Strategy 2020 and beyond. Available at https://www.amr.gov.au/resources/australias-national-antimicrobial-resistance-strategy-2020-and-beyond. Accessed 5 June 2025.
16. Brives C, Pourraz J. Phage therapy as a potential solution in the fight against AMR: obstacles and possible futures. Palgrave Commun. 2020;6:100. https://doi.org/10.1057/s41599-020-0478-4.
17. Yuchen H, Qing K, Haijin M, Huaxi Y. Antimicrobial peptides: classification, design, application and research progress in multiple fields. Front Microbiol. 2020:11. https://www.frontiersin.org/journals/microbiology/articles/10.3389/fmicb.2020.582779/full. Accessed 17 Apr 2025
18. Harris CT, Cohen S. Reducing immunogenicity by design: approaches to minimize immunogenicity of monoclonal antibodies. BioDrugs. 2024;38(2):205–26. https://doi.org/10.1007/s40259-023-00641-2.
19. Cameron A, Esiovwa R, Connolly J, Hursthouse A, Henriquez F. Antimicrobial resistance as a global health threat: the need to learn lessons from the COVID-19 pandemic. Glob Policy. 2022;13(2):179–92. https://doi.org/10.1111/1758-5899.13049.
20. Jeleff M, Haddad C, Kutalek R. Between superimposition and local initiatives: Making sense of 'implementation gaps' as a governance problem of antimicrobial resistance. SSM Qual Res Health. 2023;4:100332. https://doi.org/10.1016/j.ssmqr.2023.100332.
21. KFF Health News. As big pharma loses interest in new antibiotics, infections are only growing stronger. Available at https://kffhealthnews.org/news/article/big-pharma-new-antibiotics-infections-growing-stronger/. Accessed 23 Aug 2025.
22. AMR Industry Alliance. Vanishing workforce: an antimicrobial resistance threat. Available at https://www.amrindustryalliance.org/mediaroom/vanishing-workforce-an-antimicrobial-resistance-threat/. Accessed 30 Apr 2025.
23. Ahmed SK, Hussein S, Qurbani K, Ibrahim RH, Fareeq A, Mahmood KA, Mohamed MG. Antimicrobial resistance: impacts, challenges, and future prospects. J Med Surg Public Health. 2024;2:100081. https://doi.org/10.1016/j.glmedi.2024.100081.

Chapter 18
New Antibiotics: Needs, Challenges, and Status

Abstract The accelerating rise of antimicrobial resistance (AMR) poses a profound threat to global health, demanding urgent development of new antibiotics. Existing drugs are losing effectiveness against critical pathogens, including carbapenem-resistant *Enterobacterales*, multidrug-resistant *Acinetobacter baumannii*, and rifampicin-resistant *Mycobacterium tuberculosis*. The World Health Organisation's 2024 Bacterial Priority Pathogens List highlights urgent gaps, particularly for Gram-negative bacteria, which remain resistant to last-resort treatments. Despite incremental progress, the current antibiotic pipeline remains fragile, characterised by limited innovation and an over-reliance on modifications of existing molecules. Between 2017 and 2024, only a few novel agents were approved, with even fewer representing entirely new classes. Barriers include high research and development costs, scientific complexity, limited market incentives, and stringent regulatory requirements. Innovative solutions—such as AI-enabled discovery, novel β-lactamase inhibitors, pathogen-specific agents, and non-traditional approaches—show promise but require sustained investment to fully realise their potential. Strengthened public–private partnerships, global collaboration, economic pull incentives, and improved diagnostics are essential to revitalise antibiotic development. Without urgent reforms, the world risks entering a post-antibiotic era where common infections and medical procedures become life-threatening.

Keywords Antimicrobial resistance · Antibiotic pipeline · Priority pathogens · Drug development challenges · Public–private partnerships · Novel antibiotics · Global health

Addressing the needs, challenges, and current status of new antibiotics to fight antimicrobial resistance (AMR) is vital because the threat of drug-resistant infections is increasing, leading to higher death rates, rising healthcare costs, and longer hospital stays. Major obstacles include a stagnant pipeline for antibiotics, limited research and development, and the overuse and misuse of existing antibiotics. A

R. Bhatia, *Drug-Resistant Infections*,
https://doi.org/10.1007/978-981-92-4190-3_18

comprehensive approach is required, which includes developing new antibiotics, improving diagnostics, supporting stewardship programs, and strengthening infection control measures [1].

18.1 Need for New Antibiotics

To keep pace with the increasing AMR, it is imperative to develop new and affordable antibiotics to overcome several challenges (Box 18.1).

Box 18.1 Major Challenges that Warrant New Antibiotics

Many infections are becoming increasingly resistant to existing antibiotics, rendering them ineffective.

Medical procedures, such as surgeries and organ transplants, are becoming riskier as infections become increasingly challenging to treat.

Healthcare costs are increasing, hospital stays are getting prolonged, and there are potential economic losses due to reduced productivity.

Common infections and minor injuries are becoming life-threatening.

Several important pathogens are becoming resistant to multiple drugs.

18.2 Major Pathogens Urgently Requiring New Antibiotics

The World Health Organisation (WHO) published its updated Bacterial Priority Pathogens List (BPPL) in 2024, featuring 15 families of antibiotic-resistant bacteria grouped into critical, high, and medium categories for prioritisation [2]. The list guides the development of new and necessary treatments to stop the spread of AMR (Table 18.1).

Pathogens in the critical priority group, such as Gram-negative bacteria resistant to last-resort antibiotics and rifampicin-resistant *Mycobacterium tuberculosis*, represent significant global threats due to their high disease burden, resilience to treatment, and potential to spread resistance to other bacteria. Gram-negative bacteria are especially alarming because they can develop new resistance mechanisms and transfer genetic material, facilitating resistance in other bacteria.

High-priority pathogens, such as *Salmonella* and *Shigella,* pose a hefty burden in low- and middle-income countries (LMICs), alongside *Pseudomonas aeruginosa* and *Staphylococcus aureus*, which create significant challenges in healthcare settings.

The WHO 2024 BPPL updated list [2] removed five pathogen–antibiotic combinations from the WHO 2017 high-priority pathogens list [3], and added four new ones. Notably, *Enterobacterales* resistant to third-generation cephalosporins are now classified as a separate critical priority, emphasising their significance and the urgent need for targeted control, particularly in resource-limited settings.

Table 18.1 Bacterial priority pathogens requiring new antibiotics

Critical	High priority	Medium priority
Acinetobacter baumannii, carbapenem-resistant; *Enterobacterales*, third-generation cephalosporin-resistant; and *Enterobacterales*, carbapenem-resistant; *Mycobacterium tuberculosis*, rifampicin-resistant	*Salmonella* Typhi, fluoroquinolone-resistant *Shigella* spp., fluoroquinolone-resistant *Enterococcus faecium*, vancomycin-resistant *Pseudomonas aeruginosa*, carbapenem-resistant Non-typhoidal *Salmonella*, fluoroquinolone-resistant *Neisseria gonorrhoeae*, third-generation cephalosporin- and/or fluoroquinolone-resistant *Staphylococcus aureus*, methicillin-resistant	Group A streptococci, macrolide-resistant *Streptococcus pneumoniae*, macrolide-resistant *Haemophilus influenzae*, ampicillin-resistant Group B streptococci, penicillin-resistant

These updates highlight how AMR is constantly changing and emphasise the need for responses that are tailored to specific contexts. While the BPPL continues to serve as a crucial global standard, customising it to fit national and regional circumstances helps address variations in pathogen prevalence and resistance patterns. For example, although not yet included, antibiotic-resistant *Mycoplasma genitalium* is increasingly becoming a concern in some areas.

18.3 Development of New Antibiotics

In 2022, a WHO report [4] revealed that the global clinical pipeline included 80 new antimicrobial drugs, comprising 46 traditional and 34 non-traditional agents. Of these, 34 were in phase 1 trials, 29 in phase 2, 14 in phase 3, and three were under regulatory review. Among the traditional antibiotics, 28 (61%) targeted WHO priority pathogens (Table 18.2). The WHO highlighted that, despite the increase from 80 agents in 2021 to 97 in 2023, there remains an urgent requirement for innovative, new agents to combat serious infections and replace those losing effectiveness due to widespread use [2].

Box 18.2 Summary of WHO Review of Antibiotics Development [3]

The current pipeline contains 97 antibacterial agents.

Fifty-seven of these are antibiotics, and 40 are non-traditional agents.

Thirty-two of 57 antibiotics are intended against BPPL.

Twelve of these 32 are innovative products.

Four of these 12 are active against at least 1 WHO "critical" pathogen.

Fifteen of 32 products are β-lactam/BLI combinations.

Three non-traditional agents are faecal-based products with the potential to prevent recurrent *Clostridium difficile* infections following antibiotic treatment in adults.

Table 18.2 Novel antibiotics approved by the US FDA or under clinical trials

Drug (brand)	Class / mechanism	Main target pathogens	Route	Stage / approval year
Sulbactam–durlobactam [5]	β-lactamase inhibitor (durlobactam) + sulbactam	*Acinetobacter baumannii* complex (MDR/XDR)	IV	US FDA approved 2023
Cefepime–enmetazobactam	4th-gen cephalosporin + novel β-lactamase inhibitor	ESBL-producing *Enterobacterales*	IV	US FDA approved 2024
Pivmecillinam [6, 7]	Oral amidinopenicillin prodrug	Uropathogenic *E. coli*, other *Enterobacterales*	Oral	US FDA approved 2024
Ceftobiprole medocaril	Broad-spectrum cephalosporin (anti-MRSA activity)	*Staphylococcus aureus* (including MRSA), Streptococci	IV	US FDA approved 2024
Sulopenem etzadroxil/ probenecid [8]	Oral penem + probenecid booster	ESBL *Enterobacterales* causing UTI	Oral	US FDA approved 2024
Aztreonam–avibactam [9]	Monobactam + diazabicyclooctane BLI	MBL-producing *Enterobacterales,*	IV	US FDA approved 2025
Gepotidacin	First-in-class triazaacenaphthylene; dual gyrase/topo IV inhibitor	*E. coli* (UTI); developing for *N. gonorrhoeae*	Oral	US FDA approved 2025
Zoliflodacin [10]	First-in-class spiropyrimidinetrione; novel topoisomerase inhibitor	*Neisseria gonorrhoeae* (including MDR)	Oral (single dose)	Phase 3 positive; FDA Priority Review 2025
Cefepime–taniborbactam [11]	Cephalosporin + boronate BLI	CRE (KPC), ESBLs	IV	FDA CRL 2024; ongoing
Afabicin [12]	FabI inhibitor (pathogen-specific)	*Staphylococcus* spp.	Oral / IV	Phase 2 trial

MDR/XDR multidrug-resistant/extensive drug resistant, *ESBL* extended spectrum beta-lactamase, *MRSA* methicillin-resistant *Staph. aureus*, *UTI* urinary tract infection, *MBL* metallo-beta-lactamase producer, *CRE(KPC)* carbapenem resistant *enterobacteriales* (*Knebsiella pneumoniae* carbapenemase producers), *CRL* complete response letter

The innovation in antibacterial development is limited, mainly due to the extensive time, effort, and risks involved in R&D. Of the 32 antibiotics under development for BPPL infections, just 12 are considered innovative [3]. Among these, only four are effective against one or more of the WHO's "critical" pathogens, the highest threat level for BPPL, which surpasses the "high" and "medium" priority categories. The pipeline also has gaps, such as treatments for children, more user-friendly oral options for outpatients, and medications addressing the rising problem of drug resistance.

Between 2017 and 2024, 13 new antibiotics were approved; however, only two belong to a novel chemical class and are genuinely innovative, highlighting the scientific and technological hurdles in discovering new antibacterials that are both effective and safe for humans [3]. Highlights of the WHO review are summarised in Box 18.2.

18.4 Why New Antibiotics Still Matter?

WHO's routine pipeline reviews point out two key issues: (i) the scarcity of truly new mechanisms progressing through clinical stages, and (ii) a disconnect between current development efforts and the most urgent resistance challenges. The 2024 WHO pipeline review reaffirmed that both clinical and preclinical pipelines are "insufficient and fragile" relative to the growing needs, especially given changing resistance trends, bacterial infection patterns, and the emergence of new resistance mechanisms [1].

The WHO review clearly demonstrates that the overall number of candidate antibiotics has remained roughly steady compared to previous WHO assessments; however, truly novel classes/mechanisms are scarce, and many candidates are derivatives. The pipeline is relatively richer for *C. difficile* and specific community pathogens than for the highest-priority Gram-negative threats. Small-company sponsors dominate; attrition risks are high; and market failures persist.

At the same time, the US FDA has approved several novel products and is supervising the clinical trials of additional ones (Table 18.2).

18.5 Molecules in Early-Stage Development

While comprehensive lists are fluid, WHO's 2024 report [1] and recent reviews outline several product categories with genuine novelty (Box 18.3):

Box 18.3 Promising Novel Antimicrobials in Development Phases
Novel topoisomerase inhibitors
New β-lactamase inhibitors and combinations
Membrane/permeabilizer strategies and LPS pathway targets
Pathogen-specific agents
Adjunctive and non-traditional approaches
AI-enabled discovery and metagenomic mining

18.6 Process of Development of New Antibiotics

Developing a new antibiotic is a lengthy, complex, high-risk, and resource-demanding process, usually taking 10–15 years and costing over a billion dollars. Despite the urgent global need for new drugs to address antimicrobial resistance (AMR), only a few truly innovative antibiotics reach the market. Understanding the stages of antibiotic development highlights both the scientific rigour involved and the bottlenecks that slow innovation.

18.6.1 Discovery and Target Identification

The process starts with discovering potential bacterial targets—molecules or pathways crucial for bacterial survival or virulence. Ideal targets are unique to bacteria (reducing human toxicity), conserved across important strains, and resistant to easy mutation. Targets may involve:

- Cell wall synthesis (e.g., peptidoglycan enzymes).
- Protein synthesis (ribosomal subunits).
- DNA replication (DNA gyrase, topoisomerases).
- Metabolic pathways specific to bacteria.

Advances in genomics, bioinformatics, and structural biology have facilitated "target-based" drug discovery, which involves screening bacterial genomes for essential genes. Alternatively, phenotypic screening detects compounds that inhibit bacterial growth without initially identifying the specific target.

Sources of candidate molecules include:

- Natural products (soil microbes such as Streptomyces species).
- Synthetic chemical libraries.
- Semi-synthetic derivatives of existing antibiotics.
- Peptides and biologics.
- AI-assisted compound discovery platforms.

From thousands to millions of compounds screened, only a few "hits" demonstrate meaningful antibacterial activity.

18.6.2 Hit Validation and Lead Optimization

Once promising "hits" are identified, they undergo validation to confirm antimicrobial activity and eliminate false positives. Researchers determine spectrum of activity (Gram-positive, Gram-negative, anaerobes), minimum inhibitory concentration (MIC), activity against resistant strains, and cytotoxicity in mammalian cells.

Validated hits become "lead compounds." These are chemically modified through medicinal chemistry to improve their potency, stability, solubility, oral bioavailability, reduced toxicity, and resistance profile.

This stage consists of repeated cycles of synthesis and testing. Structure–activity relationship (SAR) studies are used to determine which molecular changes improve activity. Many potential leads may fail at this point due to toxicity, unfavourable pharmacokinetics, or the inability to penetrate bacterial membranes, particularly in Gram-negative bacteria.

18.6.3 Preclinical Development

If a lead compound demonstrates strong *in vitro* activity and acceptable safety profiles, it enters preclinical testing (Table 18.3) including *in vitro* and animal studies in animal models (usually mice or rats).

18.6.4 Clinical Development

Clinical development is conducted in three main phases, under strict regulatory and ethical oversight (Table 18.4)

Phase I: determines safety and dosage. Phase I trials typically involve 20–100 healthy volunteers (sometimes patients in severe infections). The primary objective is safety. If the antibiotic is well tolerated, it proceeds to Phase II.

Phase II: Efficacy and Dose Optimization. Phase II determines whether the antibiotic is effective in treating real infections under controlled conditions. If results are encouraging, the trial moves to its phase III.

Table 18.3 Overview of preclinical development of an antibiotic

In vitro studies to determine		Animal model studies assess
Mechanism of action confirmation Resistance development studies Synergy with other antibiotics Activity in biofilm models		Pharmacokinetics (PK): absorption, distribution, metabolism, elimination Pharmacodynamics (PD): relationship between drug concentration and bacterial killing Toxicology: acute and chronic toxicity Dose optimization
Outcomes		
Attainment of the therapeutic levels in blood and tissues without causing unacceptable harm		Feasibility on formulation work, such as creating oral tablets or IV solutions, and evaluating manufacturing feasibility.

Table 18.4 Phases of clinical development of antibiotics

Phase	Characteristic	Number of participants	Expected outcome
I	Safety and dosage determination	Usually up to 100 healthy volunteers	Safety profile Tolerability Maximum tolerated dose Pharmacokinetics in humans Drug interactions
II	Efficacy and dose optimization	Several hundred patients with specific ailments	Evaluating preliminary efficacy Confirming optimal dose Monitoring side effects Refining treatment duration
III	Large-scale confirmation	Multi-center studies involving hundreds to thousands of patients. These trials compare the new antibiotic against standard-of-care therapies.	Demonstrate non-inferiority or superiority Confirm safety in diverse populations Detect rare adverse events Assess outcomes across geographic regions
IV	Post-marketing surveillance	Entire consuming community of the patients	Long-term safety Real-world effectiveness Rare adverse events Emergence of resistance

Phase III: Large-Scale Confirmation. Phase III trials are large, multicentre studies involving hundreds to thousands of patients. These trials compare the new antibiotic against standard-of-care therapies.

In some countries, antibiotics aimed at resistant pathogens may require special regulatory pathways, such as limited-population approvals. If Phase III results are successful, the company then submits a New Drug Application (NDA) or an equivalent dossier for approval.

18.6.5 Regulatory Review and Approval

Regulatory authorities evaluate quality (manufacturing standards, consistency), safety data, clinical efficacy, risk–benefit profile and labelling and indications

Review processes typically Approval typically takes 1–2 years. However, antibiotics aimed at urgent unmet needs may be approved faster through fast-track, priority review, or breakthrough designations. Although approval permits marketing, their use may be restricted to prevent rapid development of resistance.

Post-Marketing Surveillance (Phase IV). Even after approval, monitoring continues. Phase IV studies assess long-term safety, real-world effectiveness, rare adverse events, and emergence of resistance

Pharmacovigilance systems track adverse drug reactions. Surveillance networks monitor resistance trends to ensure continued effectiveness.

18.6.6 Manufacturing and Stewardship Considerations

Unlike many other drugs, antibiotics face unique economic and stewardship challenges including short treatment durations that limit revenue, stewardship programmes restrict widespread use and resistance may reduce the drug's lifespan.

It is also essential that the manufacturing must meet Good Manufacturing Practice (GMP) standards, ensuring consistent quality and purity [13].

18.6.7 Challenges in Antibiotic Development

Antibiotic development faces scientific, economic, and regulatory hurdles such as the following:

- Rapid resistance development.
- Difficulty discovering new classes active against Gram-negative bacteria.
- High failure rates in clinical trials.
- Limited financial incentives compared to chronic disease drugs.
- Stringent regulatory requirements.

Since antibiotics should be used sparingly, conventional market-based approaches often fail to motivate research and development. Consequently, there are proposals for "push" strategies, such as grants and tax incentives, and "pull" strategies, like market entry rewards and subscription models.

18.6.8 Emerging Innovations

While adaptive clinical trial designs and pathogen-focused approvals are evolving, several new approaches aim to accelerate antibiotic development. These are shown in Box 18.4

Box 18.4 New Approaches Aim to Accelerate Antibiotic Development

- AI-assisted compound screening
- Phage therapy
- Antimicrobial peptides
- CRISPR-based strategies
- Microbiome-modulating therapies
- Anti-virulence drugs that disarm pathogens without killing them

18.6.9 Prominent Global Antibiotic Manufacturers

The companies that play major roles in global antibiotic supply chains, including active pharmaceutical ingredient (API) production and finished drug manufacturing:

1. *Pfizer Inc.*—One of the largest global pharmaceutical companies with a long history in antibiotic development and production, including APIs and finished formulations.
2. *GlaxoSmithKline plc (GSK)*—A major UK-based pharmaceutical firm with broad antibiotic offerings, especially in beta-lactams and other core classes.
3. *Sanofi S.A*—French pharmaceutical leader producing a range of antibiotics and contributing significantly to global supply.
4. *Novartis AG*—Swiss global pharma company with a presence in antibiotic APIs and formulations, including through its generics arm Sandoz.
5. *Johnson & Johnson Services, Inc*—US multinational with a diverse portfolio including antibiotics, especially through branded and hospital products.
6. *Bayer AG*—German multinational that produces a range of antibiotic products and contributes to broader anti-infective portfolios.
7. *Teva Pharmaceutical Industries Ltd.*—One of the world's largest generic medicine makers, including major supplies of antibiotic APIs and medicines.
8. *Aurobindo Pharma Ltd.*—India-based global supplier of antibiotic APIs and finished dosage forms, especially beta-lactams.
9. *Cipla Ltd.*—Indian multinational pharmaceutical company with a strong portfolio of antibiotic formulations and global export reach.
10. *North China Pharmaceutical Group Corp***.** Major Chinese producer of antibiotic APIs and finished products, including penicillins and cephalosporins at significant scale.

18.7 Challenges in Antibiotic Development

The number of new antibiotics entering the market has been declining, while resistance to existing antibiotics continues to rise. This is because of the following three major hurdles:

1. Creating new antibiotics is costly, and the potential return on investment is often lower than that for treatments of chronic diseases. Developing new antibiotics is also a laborious process. The success rate is low, with only a fraction of molecules making it to market. In fact, at the discovery stage, the chances of a molecule reaching the market are less than 1 in 200 [16]. As a result, few pharmaceutical companies or research institutes are willing to undertake the task of discovering new antibiotic molecules [14]. This lack of market incentives has led to a decline in investment in antibiotic research and development. Stringent regulatory requirements for antibiotic approval can slow down the process of bringing new drugs to market.
2. There is a lack of financial incentives for pharmaceutical companies to invest in antibiotic research and development, as the market favours drugs for chronic conditions.
3. Multiple scientific challenges hinder the creation of new molecules. The Gram-negative outer membrane and efflux pumps significantly limit chemical space. While "rule-of-penetration" heuristics (such as polar surface area, rigidity, and ionizable nitrogens) have improved hit quality, they still restrict novelty. Even for promising bacterial targets (such as LpxC, FabI, and FtsZ), on-target toxicity and resistance emergence have slowed the development of potential candidates. Recent reviews show that only a small fraction of agents in clinical development represent genuinely new scaffolds or mechanisms, and many are modified derivatives aimed at optimising exposure or resistance stability [15].

18.8 Possible Solutions and a Way Forward to Develop New Antibiotics

18.8.1 Develop New Antibiotics Through Public Funding and Public–Private Partnership

Investing in research and development of new antibiotics with novel mechanisms of action is essential. Aligning R&D efforts with public health priorities is crucial. Developing new antibiotics may need incentives. The Innovative Medicines Initiative has explored alternative economic strategies for antibiotic development and suggested global market entry rewards of about $1 billion per antibiotic as "pull" incentives [16]. In 2019, the UK launched a programme to test a payment model based on the medicine's value to the health system, separating payments from the volume of antibiotics sold. This was achieved through a trial that paid drug companies with a subscription-based model [17]. If successfully implemented, the UK's incentive approach for new antibiotics could serve as a model for other countries [18].

18.8.2 Improve Diagnostics

Rapid and accurate diagnostic tools are needed to identify the specific pathogen and its antibiotic susceptibility, enabling targeted treatment.

18.8.3 International Collaboration

Global collaboration is essential for surveillance of AMR, research, and development of new drugs and strategies.

18.8.4 Focus on Innovation

Innovation in antibiotic development is essential for fighting AMR. Breakthroughs, such as AI-based discovery and microbiome-preserving methods, show potential but require investment incentives and global access strategies to sustain research and development. Stewardship, diagnostics, and surveillance are critical for ensuring long-term clinical success.

Despite some recent progress with new antibiotics and alternative treatments, the antibacterial pipeline remains insufficient—particularly for carbapenem-resistant Gram-negative bacteria. Stronger collaboration among governments, researchers, and the pharmaceutical industry is urgently needed.

Creating a new antibiotic involves multiple complex stages, starting with target identification and lab discovery, followed by preclinical tests, phased clinical trials, and ending with regulatory approval and post-market surveillance. Each stage requires careful scientific validation, substantial funding, and regulatory compliance. As the global threat of AMR grows, bolstering antibiotic development pipelines is essential. However, scientific progress alone is insufficient; sustainable funding, global stewardship policies, and equitable access frameworks are vital to ensure that effective and accessible antibiotics remain available for future generations.

References

1. World Health Organisation. 2024 antibacterial agents in clinical and preclinical development: an overview. Geneva: WHO; 2024. Available at https://www.who.int/publications/i/item/9789240094000. Accessed 3 June 2025.
2. WHO. WHO updates list of drug-resistant bacteria most threatening to human health. Available at https://www.who.int/news/item/17-05-2024-who-updates-list-of-drug-resistant-bacteria-most-threatening-to-human-health#:~. Accessed 7 June 2025.

3. WHO. WHO publishes list of bacteria for which new antibiotics are urgently needed. Available at https://www.who.int/news/item/27-02-2017-who-publishes-list-of-bacteria-for-which-new-antibiotics-are-urgently-needed#:~:text. Accessed 13 June 2025.
4. WHO. WHO releases report on state of development of new antibiotics. Available at https://www.who.int/news/item/14-06-2024-who-releases-report-on-state-of-development-of-antibacterials#:~:text=. Accessed 3 May 2025.
5. McLeod SM, O'Donnell JP, Narayanan N, Mills JP, Kaye KS. Sulbactam-durlobactam: a β-lactam/β-lactamase inhibitor combination targeting *Acinetobacter baumannii*. Future Microbiol. 2024;19(7):563–76. https://doi.org/10.2217/fmb-2023-0248.
6. European Medicines Agency. New antibiotic to fight infections caused by multidrug-resistant bacteria. Available at https://www.ema.europa.eu/en/news/new-antibiotic-fight-infections-caused-multidrug-resistant-bacteria? Accessed 3 June 2025.
7. US FDA. FDA approves new treatment for uncomplicated urinary tract infections. Available at https://www.fda.gov/news-events/press-announcements/fda-approves-new-treatment-uncomplicated-urinary-tract-infections? Accessed 3 June 2025.
8. Fierce Pharma. After prior rejection, Iterum nabs long-sought FDA nod for oral UTI drug Orlynvah. Available at https://www.fiercepharma.com/pharma/after-prior-rejection-iterum-nabs-fda-nod-2nd-uncomplicated-urinary-tract-infection-drug-20. Accessed 23 June 2025.
9. Daikos GL, Cisneros JM, Carmeli Y, Wang M, Leong CL, Pontikis K, et al. Aztreonam-avibactam for the treatment of serious infections caused by metallo-β-lactamase-producing Gram-negative pathogens: a Phase 3 randomized trial (ASSEMBLE). JAC Antimicrob Resist. 2025;7(4):dlaf131. https://doi.org/10.1093/jacamr/dlaf131.
10. GARDP. Positive results announced in largest pivotal phase 3 trial of a first-in-class oral antibiotic to treat uncomplicated gonorrhoea. Available at https://gardp.org/positive-results-announced-in-largest-pivotal-phase-3-trial-of-a-first-in-class-oral-antibiotic-to-treat-uncomplicated-gonorrhoea/? Accessed 3 June 2025.
11. Medthority. FDA has issued a Complete Response Letter (CRL) regarding the New Drug Application (NDA) for cefepime-taniborbactam, a beta-lactam/beta-lactamase inhibitor (BL/BLI) combination antibiotic. Available at https://www.medthority.com/news/2024/2/fda-issues-complete-response-letter-for-cefepime-taniborbactam-application.%2D%2Dvenatorx-pharma%2D%2Dmelinta-therapeutic#:~:. Accessed 23 June 2025.
12. Nowakowska J, Cameron DR, De Martino A, Kühn J, Le Fresne-Languille S, Leuillet S, Amouzou Y, Wittke F, Carton T, Le Vacon F, Chaves RL, Nicolas-Metral V, Vuagniaux G. Evaluation of the microbiota-sparing properties of the anti-staphylococcal antibiotic afabicin. J Antimicrob Chemother. 2023;78:1900–8. https://doi.org/10.1093/jac/dkad181.
13. WHO: Guidelines Production. Available at https://www.who.int/teams/health-product-and-policy-standards/standards-and-specifications/norms-and-standards-for-pharmaceuticals/guidelines/production#:~:text. Accessed 1 Feb 2026.
14. Waring M, Arrowsmith J, Leach A, et al. An analysis of the attrition of drug candidates from four major pharmaceutical companies. Nat Rev Drug Discov. 2015;14:475–86. https://doi.org/10.1038/nrd4609.
15. Heimann D, Kohnhäuser D, Kohnhäuser AJ, Brönstrup M. Antibacterials with novel chemical scaffolds in clinical development. Drugs. 2025;85(3):293–323. https://doi.org/10.1007/s40265-024-02137-x.
16. Blaskovich MAT, Cooper MA. Antibiotics re-booted—time to kick back against drug resistance. npj Antimicrob Resist. 2025;3:47. https://doi.org/10.1038/s44259-025-00096-1.
17. Outterson K, Rex JH. Global pull incentives for better antibacterials: the UK leads the way. Appl Health Econ Health Policy. 2023;21:361–4. https://doi.org/10.1007/s40258-023-00793-w.
18. Dall C. UK to test new payment model for antibiotics. 2019. http://www.cidrap.umn.edu/news-perspective/2019/07/uk-test-new-payment-model-antibiotics. Accessed 3 June 2025.

Chapter 19
Alternatives to Antibiotics

Abstract Since their discovery in the twentieth century, antibiotics have been vital in reducing deaths from bacterial infections. However, their overuse and misuse have accelerated the crisis of antimicrobial resistance (AMR), rendering many treatments ineffective and posing a significant threat to global health. The slow pace of new antibiotic discovery—due to scientific, financial, and regulatory barriers—necessitates urgent exploration of alternatives. Research is ongoing on several options to antibiotics, including bacteriophages, antimicrobial peptides, probiotics, immunotherapies, and novel synthetic compounds. Phage therapy offers targeted action against resistant pathogens, while probiotics and microbiome modulation restore microbial balance and enhance host defences. Monoclonal antibodies and immunotherapies provide precise immune-based interventions, whereas novel synthetic agents and antibody-antibiotic conjugates aim to bypass conventional resistance mechanisms. Other approaches, including photodynamic therapy, gene-editing tools like CRISPR-Cas, and artificial intelligence-driven drug discovery, present innovative possibilities. In the veterinary sector, alternatives such as vaccines, probiotics, plant-derived products, and ethnoveterinary practices are gaining traction to reduce antibiotic use in livestock and safeguard One Health. While no single solution can entirely replace antibiotics, integrating these alternatives with stewardship, biosecurity, and improved animal husbandry can significantly reduce reliance on traditional drugs. Together, these innovations represent critical pathways to contain AMR and secure sustainable health systems.

Keywords Antimicrobial resistance · Bacteriophage therapy · Probiotics · Immunotherapy · Antimicrobial peptides · Artificial intelligence in drug discovery · Ethnoveterinary medicine

Antibiotics have been instrumental in reducing mortality and morbidity from bacterial infections since their discovery in the early twentieth century. Unfortunately, the widespread and often inappropriate use of antibiotics has led to a mounting crisis of antimicrobial resistance (AMR), rendering many antibiotics ineffective. The World Health Organisation (WHO) has identified AMR as one of the top ten global public

R. Bhatia, *Drug-Resistant Infections*,
https://doi.org/10.1007/978-981-92-4190-3_19

health threats, with the potential to undo decades of progress in treating infectious diseases [1]. The apparent response to the dearth of effective antibiotics and burgeoning AMR is to develop more antibiotics. However, that has not been the case in recent times.

19.1 Possible Alternatives to Antibiotics

The discovery of new antibiotics has slowed down significantly, with the last new class of antibiotics discovered over 30 years ago. This is due to a combination of scientific, financial, and regulatory hurdles (Table 19.1)

In essence, the combination of scientific complexities, financial disincentives, and regulatory burdens has created a challenging environment for antibiotic discovery, leading to a decline in research and development efforts and a shortage of new drugs to combat resistant bacteria.

Consequently, there is an urgent need to develop and implement alternative strategies to antibiotics for treating bacterial infections. These possible alternatives include bacteriophages, antimicrobial peptides, probiotics, immunotherapies, and novel synthetic compounds (Box 19.1).

Table 19.1 Factors hindering the development of new antibiotics

	Challenge	Key challenges
1	Scientific	Complexity of bacterial systems and their incredible adaptation/evolution of resistance mechanisms Difficulty in finding safe agent that can penetrate bacteria, reach the site of infection, and effectively kill the bacteria without harming the patient. Challenges in identifying new drug targets Decline in natural product research Limitation of traditional screening methods to identify novel compounds The decline in antibiotic research has led to a loss of specialized knowledge and personnel in the field. (see chapter on R&D)
2	Financial	High cost and long development time often taking >10 years Irrational use of new antibiotics making these resistant leading to reduced use and low return on investment Many companies have scaled back or abandoned their antibiotic research programmes due to the challenges and lack of profitability.
3	Regulatory	Stringent regulations for testing and approval add to the cost and time required for development. Clinical trials for antibiotics get delayed due to various regulatory compliances and other factors, including patient recruitment and logistical challenges.

Box 19.1 Major Promising Alternatives to Antibiotics and Novel Approaches

Bacteriophages
- Probiotics and Microbiome Modulation
- Immunotherapy and monoclonal antibodies
- Novel Synthetic Compounds and Adjuvants
- Photodynamic Therapy
- Antimicrobial peptides
- Antibody-antibiotic conjugate
- Gene therapy
- Artificial intelligence and machine learning

19.1.1 Bacteriophages

Bacteriophages, abbreviated as phages, are viruses that specifically infect bacteria. These were discovered independently by Frederick Twort in 1915 and Félix d'Hérelle in 1917 [2]. In some countries, phages were utilised historically for treating bacterial infections before the widespread adoption of antibiotics [2]. Their biological specificity and ability to kill bacteria made them an attractive therapeutic option, especially in cases of antibiotic-resistant infections. With the alarming rise of multidrug-resistant (MDR) bacteria, there has been a resurgence of interest in phage therapy as a promising adjunct or alternative to antibiotics [3].

19.1.1.1 Mechanisms of Action

Phages infect bacteria through a highly specific interaction, binding to unique surface receptors on bacterial cells. Once attached, they inject their genetic material—either DNA or RNA, depending on the phage type—into the host. The phage genome then hijacks the bacterial machinery to produce new phage particles (Fig. 19.1), culminating in bacterial cell lysis and the release of progeny phages [4].

The lytic cycle is the primary mechanism leveraged in phage therapy. These lytic phages produce enzymes, such as endolysins, that degrade bacterial cell walls, thereby facilitating bacterial destruction [5]. Unlike lysogenic phages, which integrate into the bacterial genome and can sometimes transfer undesirable genes, strictly lytic phages are preferred in therapeutic contexts to avoid unintentional gene transfer.

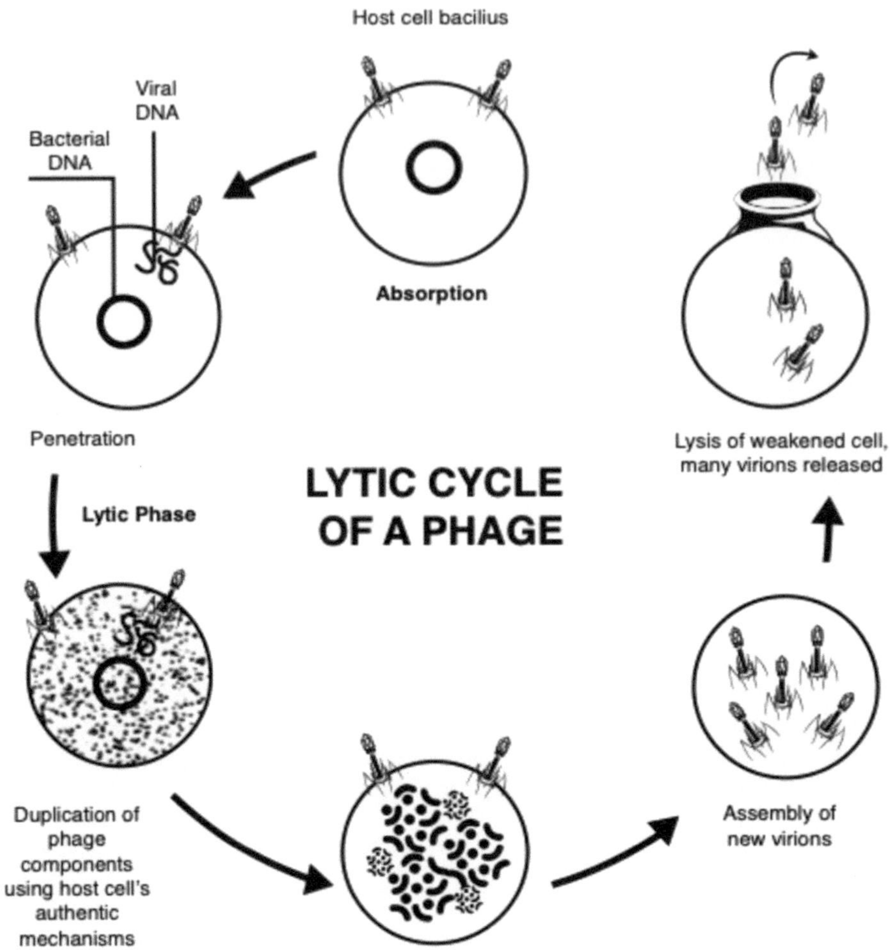

Fig. 19.1 Lytic cycle of a bacteriophage that destroys the host cell

19.1.1.2 Advantages of Phage Therapy

19.1.1.3 Specificity and Safety

One of the most notable benefits of bacteriophages is their high specificity—they target only particular bacterial strains or species, sparing beneficial microbiota [6]. This targeted approach minimises dysbiosis, a common adverse effect of broad-spectrum antibiotics, and reduces the risk of secondary infections [7], such as *Clostridioides difficile*.

19.1.1.4 Efficacy Against Biofilms

Biofilm-associated infections are more resistant to antibiotics due to the protective matrix and the reduced metabolic activity of bacteria embedded within the biofilm. Phages produce depolymerases—enzymes that degrade biofilm components—enhancing their ability to penetrate and eliminate bacteria within biofilms [8]. This attribute is beneficial in treating chronic infections associated with indwelling medical devices.

19.1.1.5 Combination Therapy

Phages can be used in combination with antibiotics to enhance treatment efficacy, particularly against bacteria that are resistant to antibiotics.

19.1.1.6 Evolution and Resistance

Bacteria can develop resistance to phages, but unlike antibiotics, phages can evolve rapidly in response to bacterial defences [9]. This evolutionary arms race means that phages can be tailored or naturally adapt to overcome bacterial resistance, making them a dynamic therapeutic tool.

19.1.1.7 Challenges and Limitations in Phage Therapy

Despite their promising features, several challenges hinder the widespread adoption of phage therapy:

Host Range Limitations: Phages typically infect a narrow spectrum of bacteria. This specificity necessitates the identification and preparation of tailored phage cocktails for each infection, which complicates clinical deployment [10]. This specificity, while beneficial for targeted treatment, complicates clinical deployment due to the need for extensive phage libraries and lengthy strain identification processes.

Bacterial Resistance to Phages: While bacteria can develop resistance to phages, combining multiple phages into cocktails can mitigate this issue. Phages that co-evolve with bacteria can adapt accordingly [11].

Regulatory and Standardisation Issues: Unlike antibiotics, which are chemically synthesised and standardised, phages are biological entities with complex production processes. Regulatory frameworks for phage therapy are not yet fully established in many countries, which complicates approval and commercialisation [12].

Immunogenicity: The human immune system can recognise and neutralise phages, reducing their therapeutic efficacy upon repeated administration. Strategies to mitigate this include encapsulation or engineering of phages [13].

Manufacturing and Storage: Producing stable, high-purity phage preparations requires sophisticated biotechnological facilities, adding to the complexity of large-scale deployment.

19.1.1.8 Clinical Evidence and Applications

Numerous case studies and clinical trials have demonstrated the potential of phages against resistant pathogens. For instance, a landmark case report involved a patient with a *Pseudomonas aeruginosa* infection resistant to all antibiotics, successfully treated with personalised phages [14]. Other applications include the treatment of multidrug-resistant (MDR) *Acinetobacter baumannii*, *Klebsiella pneumoniae*, and *Staphylococcus aureus* infections.

In recent years, several advanced clinical trials have been initiated worldwide. The PhagoBurn trial, conducted in France [15], evaluated the safety and efficacy of phage therapy in burn wound infections caused by *P. aeruginosa*, with promising results. However, technical and regulatory challenges have led to mixed outcomes, highlighting the need for further research and standardised protocols.

Phage therapy is emerging as a promising alternative to antibiotics, particularly for infections resistant to antibiotics. Phage therapy offers a targeted approach, potentially minimising disruption to the body's beneficial bacteria and reducing the risk of antibiotic-associated side effects. While not yet widely approved in many countries, phage therapy is used in some regions, particularly when antibiotics fail. It is gaining traction as a potential solution to the growing threat of AMR.

Phage therapy holds significant promise as a valuable tool in the fight against AMR, offering a targeted and potentially personalised approach to treating bacterial infections. While challenges remain, ongoing research and clinical trials are paving the way for broader adoption of phage therapy in the future.

19.1.2 Probiotics and Microbiome Modulation

The human microbiome is essential for health and helps prevent pathogen colonisation. Adjusting microbiota with probiotics, prebiotics, or faecal microbiota transplantation offers an alternative to antibiotics. Probiotics work by competing with pathogens for adhesion and nutrients, producing antimicrobial substances like bacteriocins, and boosting the immune system [16]. They restore microbiome balance, decrease the risk of secondary infections, and lessen antibiotic-associated diarrhoea [17]. However, their effects are strain-specific and outcomes can vary. Safety concerns remain, especially in immunocompromised patients [18].

Probiotics have demonstrated efficacy in preventing and treating certain gastrointestinal infections, notably *Clostridioides difficile* infections. Microbiome-targeted therapies hold promise but require further research to achieve standardisation.

19.1.3 Immunotherapy and Monoclonal Antibody Therapy

Utilising the host immune system presents an alternative method to directly target bacterial pathogens. Passive immunisation through monoclonal antibodies (mAbs), vaccines, or cytokine therapy can boost the immune response against bacteria [19]. These antibodies are specific and may help prevent infections while modulating the immune response [20]. However, their use is limited by factors such as availability, high costs, and variability in immune responses.

Human mAbs have mainly been used to treat cancer and autoimmune diseases. Palivizumab, the first human mAb proven effective against infections, was approved by the FDA in 1998 for preventing respiratory syncytial virus in at-risk infants [21]. In 2016, obiltoxaximab was approved for inhalational anthrax treatment, combined with antibiotics. These developments highlight the growing potential of human mAbs as antimicrobial therapies.

Human mAbs deliver quick and lasting antimicrobial effects through several mechanisms, such as improved opsonisation for phagocytosis, direct killing of bacteria, complement activation, antivirulence actions, and toxin neutralisation. Their high specificity helps preserve the host's natural microbiota and lowers the risk of developing cross-resistance. As of 2024, fourteen human mAb products are in development to treat infections caused by ESKAPE pathogens[1] and *Clostridioides difficile* [24].

Recent developments include mAbs targeting specific bacterial components, such as ExbB (a protein in the inner membrane of Gram-negative bacteria) or toxins, which have shown efficacy in preclinical and clinical studies.

19.1.4 Novel Synthetic Compounds and Adjuvants

Recent breakthroughs in medicinal chemistry have resulted in synthetic molecules that can suppress bacterial growth or virulence through mechanisms different from traditional antibiotics. These include antivirulence agents that block bacterial toxins or adherence factors, and quorum-sensing inhibitors that interfere with bacterial communication and biofilm development [22]. Such approaches could lessen the

---

[1] ESCAPE pathogens include six multidrug-resistant bacteria viz. *Enterococcus faecium, Staphylococcus aureus, Klebsiella pneumoniae, Acinetobacter baumannii, Pseudomonas aeruginosa,* and *Enterobacter species.*

selective pressure for resistance and may be used alone or combined with other therapies [23]. However, these options are still in early development stages and have yet to overcome regulatory hurdles.

19.1.5 Photodynamic Therapy

Photodynamic therapy involves using photosensitisers activated by light to produce reactive oxygen species, which damage bacterial cells. This is also in the development or experimental stage.

19.1.6 Antimicrobial Peptides

Antimicrobial peptides (AMPs) and antibiofilm peptides, classified as natural host defence peptides, are usually small (under 50 amino acids), positively charged, and amphiphilic molecules. Thanks to their rapid and broad-spectrum antimicrobial action—including against multidrug-resistant ESKAPE pathogens—these AMPs offer a promising avenue for developing treatments for AMR, with a low risk of inducing further resistance [24].

Specific antibiofilm AMPs exhibit remarkable broad-spectrum efficacy against biofilms, which are responsible for 65% of infections. Their advantageous characteristics result from multitargeting the integrity of membranes, biosynthesis of cell walls, cytoplasmic membranes, or a mix of these factors [25].

As of now, around 20,000 natural or synthetic AMPs have been identified [26]. FDA-approved options, such as gramicidin and polymyxins, are conventional drugs resembling AMPs. The clinical application of AMPs faces several challenges, including vulnerability to proteolysis, poor oral bioavailability, high costs, and potential toxicity. However, to date, AMPs have not demonstrated greater efficacy compared to traditional antibiotics in Phase 2 or Phase 3 clinical trials.

Over 12 peptide-based antimicrobial or antifungal agents have been approved by the FDA since the mid-twentieth century [27]. Some of these are shown in Table 19.2. Many novel AMPs (e.g. hLF1–11, C16G2, Novexatin/NP213) are currently in clinical trials but have not yet been FDA-approved.

19.1.7 Antibody-Antibiotic Conjugate

Antibody-antibiotic conjugates, inspired by antibody-drug conjugates, are advanced drugs made of mAbs chemically linked to potent antibiotics. These conjugates aim to specifically target certain antigens and deliver antibiotics directly to infection sites. In mouse models, a single dose of an antibody-antibiotic conjugate—comprising anti*S aureus* antibodies attached to

Table 19.2 FDA-approved AMPs and usage

Peptide (or Drug)	Year approved	Indications/usage
Bacitracin	1948	Topical treatment for skin, ear, and eye infections caused by gram-positive bacteria (e.g., *Staphylococcus, Streptococcus*)
Colistimethate sodium (prodrug of colistin)	1999	Intravenous/inhalation use against multidrug-resistant gram-negative bacteria, including *Pseudomonas, Acinetobacter*
Polymyxin B	Late 1950s	Topical/systemic use against gram-negative infections; historically suspended due to toxicity concerns
Vancomycin	1958	Intravenous antibiotic for serious gram-positive bacterial infections, including MRSA
Daptomycin	2003	Intravenous treatment of gram-positive infections like *Staphylococcus* and *Enterococcus* spp.
Dalbavancin	2014	IV therapy for acute bacterial skin and skin structure infections (ABSSSIs), including MRSA and *Streptococcus pyogenes*
Oritavancin	Between 2009–2014	IV treatment of serious gram-positive infections, including vancomycin-resistant strains
Telavancin	2009 and 2013	IV therapy for complicated skin/skin structure infections (cSSSI) and hospital-acquired/ventilator-associated bacterial pneumonia due to *Staph. aureus*
Teicoplanin	Not FDA-approved in U.S.	Used in Europe, Asia, South America for MRSA and other gram-positive infections; not approved by FDA

vancomycin—administered 24 h after infection, effectively eradicated intracellular methicillin-resistant *S. aureus* [28] by releasing the active antibiotics after internalisation. This approach proved significantly more effective than the standard treatment of vancomycin given twice daily.

The research highlighted the promise of antibody-antibiotic conjugates in addressing the challenges associated with unmodified antimicrobial substances, including inadequate pharmacokinetic characteristics, diminished therapeutic indices, and unwanted toxicity. Therefore, antibody-antibiotic conjugates may ultimately be used to combat tuberculosis and other challenging infections. In theory, using highly selective antibodies to target pathogens could transform broad-spectrum antibiotics into pathogen-specific or site-specific ones, mitigate the adverse effects of broad-spectrum antibiotics, and reduce the unintended elimination of beneficial microbes.

19.1.8 Gene Therapy

Bacteria use various mechanisms to defend against phages, notably the CRISPR immune system. CRISPR (acronym of clustered regularly interspaced short palindromic repeats) is a family of DNA sequences found in the genomes of prokaryotic organisms such as bacteria. Each sequence within an individual prokaryotic CRISPR is derived from a DNA fragment of a phage that had previously infected the prokaryote or one of its ancestors. These sequences are used to detect and destroy DNA from similar phages during subsequent infections. Hence, these sequences play a key role in the antiphage defence system of prokaryotes and provide a form of heritable acquired immunity.

Discovering CRISPR has paved the way for advanced genetic technologies, particularly genome editing with the CRISPR-Cas9 nuclease system [29]. Modifying Cas9 nucleases causes irreversible chromosomal damage in bacteria, leading to cell death [30]. This discovery facilitated the development of Cas9 nucleases as targeted antimicrobials, allowing for the precise removal of specific bacterial species in mixed populations. Supported by CARB-X funding, Danish microbiome firm SNIPR Biome® successfully completed a phase 1 trial of a CRISPR-based phage therapy targeting *Escherichia coli* in the gastrointestinal tract. Their product, SNIPR001, comprises four bacteriophages equipped with CRISPR/Cas DNA editing technology, containing sequences specific to *E. coli*, including antibiotic-resistant strains.

19.2 Potential Role of Artificial Intelligence and Machine Learning

Thanks to advancements in AI technologies, increased computational resources, and access to big data—including electronic health records and omics data—artificial intelligence is becoming a vital tool in combating infectious diseases and AMR. It supports activities like antibiotic susceptibility testing, AMR surveillance, antimicrobial stewardship, diagnosis, and drug discovery or development [24]. AI can analyse vast amounts of data using computers and machines, either through manual feature engineering (machine learning) or by employing representation learning methods such as deep neural networks (deep learning), including the generation of new information via generative AI.

Traditional phenotypic antibiotic susceptibility testing depends on bacterial growth measurements and usually takes 24–48 h, or longer for slow-growing bacteria like *Mycobacterium tuberculosis*, delaying the initiation of optimal antibiotic treatments. Increasingly, machine learning is used to analyse whole-genome sequencing data for quick prediction of antibiotic susceptibility and AMR surveillance. This reduces the need for extensive bioinformatics resources or expertise in sequencing analysis. Such methods hold significant potential for large-scale AMR surveillance, especially in low- and middle-income countries.

Machine learning has identified nearly 1 million antibiotic molecules within the global microbiome, covering 63,410 metagenomes and 87,920 microbial genomes. Some, such as lachnospirin-1 and enterococcin-1, have shown effectiveness in preclinical mouse models [24]. Overall, these AI-driven approaches have significantly sped up antibiotic discovery, shrinking the timeline from years to hours.

The main difficulty in applying AI to small molecules is that the compounds identified might not be synthesisable chemically. Nonetheless, recent advances in computational models are promising, as they can generate multiple outputs, enabling the modelling of toxicity, pharmacology, solubility, and activity simultaneously. For example, the generative AI model SyntheMol®, which aims to create readily synthesisable compounds from a chemical space of around 30 billion molecules, has successfully produced six new molecules with strong activity against *A. baumannii* [31].

19.3 Alternatives to Antibiotics in the Veterinary Sector

The veterinary sector is vital in combating AMR, since antibiotics are extensively used not just for treating animal infections but also for growth promotion and disease prevention in intensive farming. Overusing and misusing antimicrobials in livestock and aquaculture creates intense selective pressure, leading to resistant pathogens that can impact animal, human, and environmental health via the One Health interface (see Chaps. 5 and 7).

Key alternatives to antibiotics in veterinary use (Box 19.2) broadly resemble the products that are being advocated or researched for possible use in humans.

Box 19.2 Key Alternatives to Antibiotics in Veterinary Use

Animal species-specific vaccines

Prebiotics and Synbiotics

Prebiotics are non-digestible feed components that stimulate the growth of beneficial gut microbiota, while *synbiotics* combine probiotics and prebiotics for synergistic effects. These reduce colonisation of Salmonella and Campylobacter

Bacteriophages

Antimicrobial peptides

Plant-derived products (phytogenics) include essential oils, herbs, and plant extracts, which have antimicrobial, antiinflammatory, and antioxidant properties

Ethnoveterinary products

Immune stimulants to enhance the innate and adaptive immune responses of animals

The frequent transmission of resistant zoonotic pathogens, such as *Salmonella*, *Campylobacter*, and *Escherichia coli*, from animals to humans through food or direct contact, as well as trade and export requirements and global initiatives, particularly the WHO Global Action Plan on AMR, urge member states to reduce non-therapeutic antibiotic use in agriculture [32].

19.3.1 Ethnoveterinary Products

Ethnoveterinary products originate from the traditional knowledge of using plants and natural substances to treat animal illnesses. They provide a promising alternative or supplement to antibiotics, helping to control AMR in livestock. These practices, based on local communities' understanding of medicinal plants, can decrease dependence on antibiotics and reduce the risk of developing AMR.

Ethnoveterinary practices offer alternative treatments for common livestock ailments like mastitis, diarrhoea, and wound infections, helping to decrease reliance on antibiotics, a key factor in driving AMR.

Many ethnoveterinary products can be made at home with easily obtainable ingredients, offering an affordable and accessible solution for farmers, especially in low- and middle-income countries [33]. Ethnoveterinary medicines can be used for both preventing diseases and treating existing infections, offering a holistic approach to animal health management.

Ethnoveterinary Products commonly used include a paste made from betel leaves, black pepper, and jaggery for treating lumpy skin disease. Other oral preparations may consist of garlic, coriander seeds, cumin, cinnamon leaves, black pepper, chireta leaf powder, sweet basil, neem leaves, and turmeric.

A mixture of *Acalypha indica* leaves, garlic, neem leaves, coconut or sesame oil, turmeric powder, henna leaves, and tulsi leaves can be used as a fomentation for swollen areas and wounds. Aloe vera, turmeric powder, and lime paste can be applied to areas affected by mastitis.

Research is ongoing to understand the active components of these plant-based remedies and their mechanisms of action, further validating their effectiveness and safety. In India, the National Dairy Development Board has been actively promoting the use of ethnoveterinary medicine in the Indian dairy sector through its Mastitis Control Popularisation Programme [34].

These products require policy backing and ongoing research and development to be incorporated into national programmes. Promoting ethnoveterinary medicine allows the livestock sector to adopt more sustainable and responsible approaches, supporting the global fight against AMR. Alternatives work best when paired with enhanced biosecurity, hygiene, nutrition, and animal welfare measures.

Alternatives to antibiotics in veterinary medicine are crucial for protecting animal health, supporting sustainable food supplies, and mitigating public health risks from AMR. Although no single alternative can completely substitute antibiotics, using a mix of vaccines, probiotics, bacteriophages, phytogenics, immune boosters, and better husbandry practices can greatly lower reliance on antimicrobials. Advancing research, streamlining regulations, and encouraging stakeholder collaboration are key to integrating these options as standard tools in contemporary animal care.

19.4 Regulatory Requirements for the Use of an Antibiotic Alternative

Introducing alternatives to antibiotics for human or animal health involves a complex regulatory process that differs based on whether the product is a vaccine, probiotic, bacteriophage therapy, antimicrobial peptide, immunomodulator, phytochemical, or diagnostic-linked therapy. Nonetheless, the fundamental principles remain consistent: demonstrating safety, efficacy, quality, and dependable manufacturing to achieve market approval.

19.4.1 Product Classification and Regulatory Pathway

The initial step is to determine the product's classification under national regulations. Accurate classification is essential because it impacts data requirements, trial design, manufacturing standards, and approval timelines.

In human health, alternatives might be classified as:

- Biological products (e.g. vaccines, monoclonal antibodies, bacteriophages).
- Small-molecule drugs.
- Medical devices (e.g. antimicrobial coatings).
- Probiotics or microbiome-based therapeutics.
- Combination products.

In animal health, the categories include veterinary medicinal products, feed additives, biologics, or immunological veterinary products, with specific pathways defined by regulatory agencies.

19.4.2 Preclinical Development

Before starting human or animal trials, sponsors need to conduct laboratory and animal studies to show the product's mechanism of action, in vitro effectiveness against targeted pathogens, toxicity profile, pharmacokinetics (absorption, distribution, metabolism, elimination), and environmental impact—particularly for veterinary and agricultural products.

For veterinary alternatives, additional assessments, such as residue studies in food animals, are needed to ensure safety for human consumption. A regulatory submission (like an Investigational New Drug application (see Chap. 18)) is then filed to request approval for clinical trials.

19.4.3 Clinical or Field Trials

For human health, trials typically proceed in phases as have been described in Chap. 18. These include the following:

- Phase I: Safety and tolerability in healthy volunteers
- Phase II: Preliminary effectiveness and dose optimisation in patients
- Phase III: Large-scale comparisons with standard therapy or placebo

Adaptive trial designs may be used for non-traditional options like bacteriophages, particularly when targeting resistant infections.

In animal health, products require target animal safety studies, dose confirmation, farm-condition efficacy trials, residue depletion analyses (for food animals), and environmental risk assessments. Regulators assess if the product reduces disease, decreases antibiotic usage, and maintains animal productivity.

19.4.4 Quality and Manufacturing Standards

Manufacturers must follow Good Manufacturing Practices (GMP), including:

- Process validation
- Batch consistency
- Stability testing
- Sterility assurance (if relevant)

Biologics and probiotics require additional strain or component characterisation to ensure reproducibility.

19.4.5 Regulatory Review and Permission

The national regulatory authorities evaluate alternative product's safety and efficacy data, quality and manufacturing documents, risk–benefit analysis and labelling and usage instructions.

Withdrawal periods for food animals must be specified for veterinary products. Some regions offer accelerated pathways specifically for products targeting antimicrobial resistance or addressing unmet needs.

19.4.6 Post-approval Monitoring

Post-market, the manufacturer must monitor adverse effects, long-term effectiveness, the development of resistance, and environmental impacts. Veterinary products also require monitoring for residues in food.

Approval doesn't guarantee adoption; guidelines, stewardship policies, and reimbursement plans influence usage. For alternatives that aim to cut antibiotic use, integration into national AMR strategies is key.

Introducing an antibiotic alternative fundamentally involves precise classification, thorough preclinical and clinical data, strict manufacturing standards, and extensive regulatory assessment. As addressing antimicrobial resistance becomes increasingly vital globally, regulatory systems are evolving to balance safety and efficacy with innovation.

Alternatives to antibiotics for humans and animals are increasingly crucial in combating AMR. They help decrease dependence on traditional drugs, whose effectiveness is quickly declining. Approaches such as vaccines, bacteriophages, probiotics, immune-modulating agents, and antimicrobial peptides can prevent infections, target specific pathogens without harming the microbiome, and reduce the selective pressure that fosters resistance. By expanding our options for preventing and treating infections in humans, animals, and agriculture, these alternatives not only protect public health but also preserve the long-term effectiveness of existing antibiotics. This makes them essential for sustainable AMR management.

References

1. World Health Organization. Antimicrobial resistance; 2020. Available at https://www.who.int/news-room/fact-sheets/detail/antimicrobial-resistance. Accessed 5 July 2025.
2. Aswani VH, Shukla SK. An early history of phage therapy in the United States: is it time to reconsider? Clin Med Res. 2021;19(2):82–9. https://doi.org/10.3121/cmr.2021.1605.
3. Liu C, Hong Q, Chang RYK, Kwok PCL, Chan HK. Phage-antibiotic therapy as a promising strategy to combat multidrug-resistant infections and to enhance antimicrobial efficiency. Antibiotics (Basel). 2022;11(5):570. https://doi.org/10.3390/antibiotics11050570.
4. Batinovic S, Wassef F, Knowler SA, Rice DTF, Stanton CR, Rose J, Tucci J, Nittami T, Vinh A, Drummond GR, Sobey CG, Chan HT, Seviour RJ, Petrovski S, Franks AE. Bacteriophages in natural and artificial environments. Pathogens. 2019;8(3):100. https://doi.org/10.3390/pathogens8030100.
5. Alisigwe CV, Ikpa CS, Otuonye UJ. examining alternative approaches to antibiotic utilisation: a critical evaluation of phage therapy and antimicrobial peptides combination as potential alternatives. The Microbe. 2025;6:100254. https://doi.org/10.1016/j.microb.2025.100254.

6. Palma M, Qi B. Advancing phage therapy: a comprehensive review of the safety, efficacy, and future prospects for the targeted treatment of bacterial infections. Infect Dis Rep. 2024;16(6):1127–81. https://doi.org/10.3390/idr16060092.
7. Cusumano G, Flores GA, Venanzoni R, Angelini P. The impact of antibiotic therapy on intestinal microbiota: dysbiosis, antibiotic resistance, and restoration strategies. Antibiotics (Basel). 2025;14(4):371. https://doi.org/10.3390/antibiotics14040371.
8. Mayorga-Ramos A, Carrera-Pacheco SE, Barba-Ostria C, Guamán LP. Bacteriophage-mediated approaches for biofilm control. Front Cell Infect Microbiol. 2024;14:1428637. https://doi.org/10.3389/fcimb.2024.1428637.
9. Oromí-Bosch A, Antani JD, Turner PE. Developing phage therapy that overcomes the evolution of bacterial resistance. Ann Rev Virol. 2023;10:503–24. https://doi.org/10.1146/annurev-virology-012423-110530.
10. Kim MK, Chen Q, Echterhof A, et al. A blueprint for broadly effective bacteriophage-antibiotic cocktails against bacterial infections. Nat Commun. 2024;15:9987. https://doi.org/10.1038/s41467-024-53994-9.
11. Jdeed G, Kravchuk B, Tikunova NV. Factors affecting phage–bacteria coevolution dynamics. Viruses. 2025;17(2):235. https://doi.org/10.3390/v17020235.
12. Yang Q, Le S, Zhu T, Wu N. Regulations of phage therapy across the world. Front Microbiol. 2023;14. Available at https://www.frontiersin.org/journals/microbiology/articles/10.3389/fmicb.2023.1250848/full https://doi.org/10.3389/fmicb.2023.1250848.
13. Loh B, Gondil VS, Manohar P, Khan FM, Yang H, Leptihn S. Encapsulation and delivery of therapeutic phages. Appl Environ Microbiol. 2021;87(5):e01979–20. https://doi.org/10.1128/AEM.01979-20.
14. Onallah H, Hazan R, Nir-Paz R, Michael J, Brownstein JR, Fackler B'AH, et al. refractory Pseudomonas aeruginosa infections treated with phage PASA16: a compassionate use case series. Med. 2023;4:600–11. https://doi.org/10.1016/j.medj.2023.07.002.
15. ClinicalTrials.gov. Evaluation of phage therapy for the treatment of Escherichia coli and pseudomonas aeruginosa wound infections in burned patients (PHAGOBURN). Available at https://clinicaltrials.gov/study/NCT02116010. Accessed 5 July 2025.
16. Latif A, Shehzad A, Niazi S, Zahid A, Ashraf W, Iqbal MW, et al. Probiotics: mechanism of action, health benefits and their application in food industries. Front Microbiol. 2023;14:1216674. https://doi.org/10.3389/fmicb.2023.12.16674.
17. Kopacz K, Phadtare S. Probiotics for the prevention of antibiotic-associated Diarrhea. Healthcare (Basel). 2022;10(8):1450. https://doi.org/10.3390/healthcare10081450.
18. Boyle RJ, Robins-Browne RM, Tang MLK. Probiotic use in clinical practice: what are the risks?. 2. Am J Clin Nutr. 2006;83:1256–64. https://doi.org/10.1093/ajcn/83.6.1256.
19. Marcotte H, Hammarström L. Passive immunization: toward magic bullets. Mucosal Immunol. 2015:1403–34. https://doi.org/10.1016/B978-0-12-415847-4.00071-9.
20. Both L, Banyard AC, van Dolleweerd C, Wright E, Ma JK, Fooks AR. Monoclonal antibodies for prophylactic and therapeutic use against viral infections. Vaccine. 2013;31(12):1553–9. https://doi.org/10.1016/.vaccine.2013.01.025.
21. Garegnani L, Styrmisdóttir L, Roson Rodriguez P, Escobar Liquitay CM, Esteban I, Franco JV. Palivizumab for preventing severe respiratory syncytial virus (RSV) infection in children. Cochrane Database Syst Rev. 2021;11:CD013757. https://doi.org/10.1002/14651858.CD013757.pub2.
22. Fleitas Martínez O, Cardoso MH, Ribeiro SM, Franco OL. Recent advances in anti-virulence therapeutic strategies with a focus on dismantling bacterial membrane microdomains, toxin neutralization, quorum-sensing interference and biofilm inhibition. Front Cell Infect Microbiol. 2019;9:74. https://doi.org/10.3389/fcimb.2019.00074.
23. Garg P, Malhotra J, Kulkarni P, Horne D, Salgia R, Singhal SS. Emerging therapeutic strategies to overcome drug resistance in cancer cells. Cancers (Basel). 2024;16(13):2478. https://doi.org/10.3390/cancers16132478.

24. Ho CS, Wong CTH, Aung TT, Lakshminarayanan R, Mehta JS, Rauz S, et al. Antimicrobial resistance: a concise update. Lancet Microbe. 2025;6(1):100947. https://doi.org/10.1016/j.lanmic.2024.07.010.
25. Ting DSJ, Li J, Verma CS, et al. Evaluation of host defense peptide(CaD23)-antibiotic interaction and mechanism of action: insights from experimental and molecular dynamics simulations studies. Front Pharmacol. 2021;12:73149. https://doi.org/10.3389/fphar.2021.731499.
26. Kang, X • Dong, F • Shi, C • et al. DRAMP 20, an updated data repository of antimicrobial peptides Sci Data 2019; 6:148. doi:https://doi.org/10.1038/s41597-019-0154-y.
27. Al Musaimi O. FDA-approved antibacterials and echinocandins. Antibiotics (Basel). 2025 Feb 7;14(2):166. https://doi.org/10.3390/antibiotics14020166.
28. Lehar SM, Pillow T, Xu M, et al. Novel antibody-antibiotic conjugate eliminates intracellular *S. Aureus*. Nature. 2015;527:323–8. https://doi.org/10.1038/nature16057.
29. Wong F, de la Fuente-Nunez C, Collins JJ. Leveraging artificial intelligence in the fight against infectious diseases. Science. 2023;381:164–70. https://doi.org/10.1126/science.adh1114.
30. Citorik RJ, Mimee M, Lu TK. Sequence-specific antimicrobials using efficiently delivered RNA-guided nucleases. Nat Biotechnol. 2014;32:1141–5. https://doi.org/10.1038/nbt3011.
31. Swanson K, Liu G, Catacutan DB, Arnold A, Zou J, Stokes JM. Generative AI for designing and validating easily synthesizable and structurally novel antibiotics. Nat Mach Intell. 2024;6:338–53. https://doi.org/10.1038/s42256-024-00809-7.
32. O'Neill J. Tackling drug-resistant infections globally: Final report and recommendations. Review on AMR; 2016. Available at https://amr-review.org/sites/default/files/160518_Final%20paper_with%20cover.pdf. Accessed 5 July 2025.
33. Akinbobola JS, Kumuyi OA, Olusoji JA, Omeje JN, Dare TA, Jolayemi KO. Antibiotics use and ethnoveterinary practices in pig farming: an insight from federal capital territory, Nigeria. BMC Vet Res. 2025;21(1):418. https://doi.org/10.1186/s12917-025-04865-y.
34. National Dairy Development Board, India. Ethoveterinary products for mastitis. Available at https://nddb.coop/node/1593. Accessed 3 Sept 2025.

Part V
Advocacy, Communication, and Future Directions

Chapter 20
Communication Strategy to Combat AMR

Abstract Antimicrobial resistance (AMR) poses a significant global health threat, requiring effective communication strategies to drive awareness and behavioural change among diverse stakeholders. Communities, being the most affected and simultaneously the most complex to engage, are central to risk communication and community engagement (RCCE). A strategic framework for AMR communication is mandatory to emphasise principles of rights-based, evidence-based, people-centred, and culturally sensitive approaches. The 3Ts—technical accuracy, transparency, and trust—are highlighted as foundational pillars for effective communication. Objectives of RCCE include raising awareness, promoting responsible antibiotic use, enabling behaviour change, fostering collaboration, and strengthening health systems. Implementation demands context-specific, participatory methods to counter misinformation and overcome cultural, linguistic, and structural barriers. Tailored messages for communities, professionals, and policymakers are vital to inspire action and sustain change. Various tools—ranging from educational campaigns and social media to stakeholder engagement—are available, though they have challenges and pathways to impactful outreach. Ultimately, RCCE aims to simplify AMR complexities and catalyse sustained behavioural transformation for rational antimicrobial use across human, animal, and environmental health.

Keywords Antimicrobial resistance · Risk communication · Community engagement · Behavioural change · Trust and transparency · Health communication tools · Multisectoral collaboration

Antimicrobial resistance (AMR) is a complex issue with numerous stakeholders. Human health, animal health and the environment sector—apart from many other diverse settings contribute to this global problem. Most importantly, the role of human beings needs to be better understood. They are not only bearers of the impact of resistant pathogens, but they also significantly compound the problem through indiscriminate self-medication and non-compliance with the recommended dose and duration of antimicrobial therapy. It is essential to have an effective communication strategy, plan, and programmatic approach to create awareness and drive

R. Bhatia, *Drug-Resistant Infections*,
https://doi.org/10.1007/978-981-92-4190-3_20

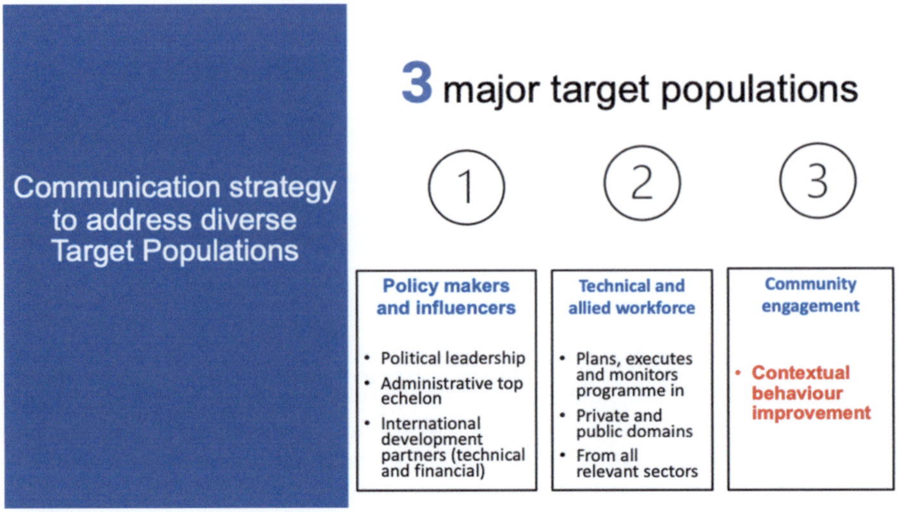
Communication strategy to address diverse Target Populations
3 major target populations
1
2
3
Policy makers and influencers
• Political leadership
• Administrative top echelon
• International development partners (technical and financial)
Technical and allied workforce
• Plans, executes and monitors programme in
• Private and public domains
• From all relevant sectors
Community engagement
• Contextual behaviour improvement

Fig. 20.1 Target population for communication on AMR containment

action among various stakeholders, including health administrators, technical professionals across different sectors, and communities (Fig. 20.1).

The effectiveness of health communication increases when the communication strategy addresses different levels.

Of various target populations, the most difficult with diverse knowledge and behavioural practices are the communities, some of whom may not be adequately educated to understand the nuances of AMR. Any AMR communication strategy, therefore, must place greater emphasis on engaging these communities appropriately.

20.1 Strategic Approach for Risk Communication and Community Engagement

Communities are at the heart of every public health response. Effective risk communication and community engagement (RCCE) supports communities and individuals in understanding the risks they face and making informed decisions about how to protect themselves and the people around them. Accurate information, provided to communities in ways they understand and respect, builds trust, and supports the success of prevention, response, and recovery efforts for health issues.

Social sciences—including sociology, psychology, and anthropology, among other disciplines—are an essential part of developing effective RCCE interventions that are sensitive to the cultural, historical, and behavioural perspectives of communities [1]. The fundamentals of social sciences must be applied to build trust and ensure that communities are equal partners in developing solutions before, during and after burgeoning health emergencies, including AMR.

Risk communication is the real-time exchange of information, advice, and opinions between experts or officials and people who face a hazard or threat to their survival, health, or economic or social well-being. The purpose of risk communication is to enable people at risk to make informed decisions to mitigate the effects of a threat (hazard)—such as a disease outbreak and AMR—and take protective and preventive measures.

Community engagement is the process of developing relationships and structures that engage communities as equal partners in creating appropriate responses and solutions that are acceptable and workable for those they impact. The goal of community engagement is to empower communities to confidently share the leadership, planning, and implementation of initiatives throughout the persistence of risk.

RCCE plays a vital role in controlling AMR by fostering awareness, promoting behaviour change, and enabling the development of context-specific solutions. By actively involving communities in the process, communities can enhance the effectiveness and sustainability of AMR control efforts.

RCCE focuses on engaging the affected communities in taking informed decisions based on facts and evidence to reduce adverse health effects and better protect themselves from risky behaviours.

According to UNICEF [2], any RCCE strategy should embrace the following key principles:

- Rights-based.
- Evidence-based.
- Systems strengthening.
- People-centred.
- Accountable to affected populations.
- Do-no-harm.

20.2 Fundamentals of a Successful AMR Communication Strategy: 3Ts

Any successful AMR communication strategy shall require the following three fundamental ingredients, which must be built into the implementation process.

- *Technical accuracy*
  Communication messages must carry technical accuracy
- *Transparency*
  Information conveyed should be transparent
- *Trust*
  The strategy activities should create and sustain trust in all target population.

20.3 Objectives and Major Activities of RCCE for AMR

Community engagement should have well-defined objectives (Table 20.1), which can be achieved through several major activities on a programmatic and sustainable basis within the specific community context [3]. Priority needs to be accorded to the

Table 20.1 Objectives and major activities for an effective community engagement on AMR

	Objective	Major activities
1	Raising Awareness and Understanding	Increase awareness and understanding of AMR within communities, including how it develops and spreads
		Provide clear and accessible information, communities can better grasp the importance of appropriate antibiotic use and the consequences of AMR
		Launch educational campaigns, workshops, and community dialogues
2	Promoting Behaviour Change	Facilitate behaviour change related to antibiotic use, infection prevention, and hygiene practices
		Ensure that solutions are tailored to local contexts and cultural norms, increasing the likelihood of adoption
		Promote community-based interventions for appropriate use of antibiotics for humans and animals, and encourage better hygiene practices to prevent infections
3	Developing Context-Specific Solutions	Allow for the co-creation of solutions with communities, recognising that AMR is a complex issue with diverse drivers
		Involve community members in identifying problems, developing interventions, and evaluating their effectiveness, and formulating solutions that are relevant, acceptable, and sustainable
		Tailor interventions to address specific challenges faced by different communities, such as antibiotic use in agriculture or healthcare settings
4	Strengthening Health Systems	Strengthen local health systems by integrating community perspectives and needs into health programmes and policies
		Engage communities in the design and implementation of health interventions to improve access to healthcare, enhance the quality of services, and promote community ownership of health initiatives
		Support effective and sustainable health systems that are better equipped to address AMR
5	Fostering Collaboration and Partnerships	Promote collaboration and partnerships between various stakeholders, including communities, healthcare providers, researchers, policymakers, and other relevant actors
		Bring together diverse perspectives and expertise to foster a shared understanding of AMR and facilitate the development of comprehensive and coordinated responses
		Establish platforms for dialogue, joint planning, and collaborative action to address AMR

vulnerable populations in the community. A system for measuring the progress and assessing the impact should be instituted.

20.3.1 Implementation Approach

A systematic and locally relevant approach through RCCE is crucial. When developing RCCE for communities, especially in developing countries with diverse cultures, social norms, educational levels, languages, faiths, beliefs, and demographics, it is vital to identify and properly address the common practical concerns of the communities in responding to AMR containment. The WHO guidelines [4] on ethical considerations in developing a public health response to an influenza pandemic can be adopted to create strategies in the local AMR context that align with relevant cultural values.

The RCCE should systematically address the multisectoral, multidimensional risks and impacts of AMR, and devise communication tools to promote prevention and response to the silent pandemic of AMR [3]. Multiple drivers collectively tend to increase risk vulnerability and reduce societal resilience; all these factors need to be factored into the implementation plan. Trust and transparency are essential for achieving widespread public engagement. There is no "one-size-fits-all" approach. Communication strategies and actions must address the multitude of factors that influence the dissemination of actionable messages to the public. At the same time, these messages must bust the myths and misinformation, ensuring that stigma and discrimination are strongly rejected.

Effective AMR RCCE implementation, which is crucial for successful behavioural change in the targeted population, involves building trust through strategic communication and co-developing solutions with affected communities. RCCE is not just about disseminating information, but also about fostering two-way communication and understanding community needs and perceptions.

Following the template of a step-by-step approach (Fig. 20.2) can be considered while designing RCCE:

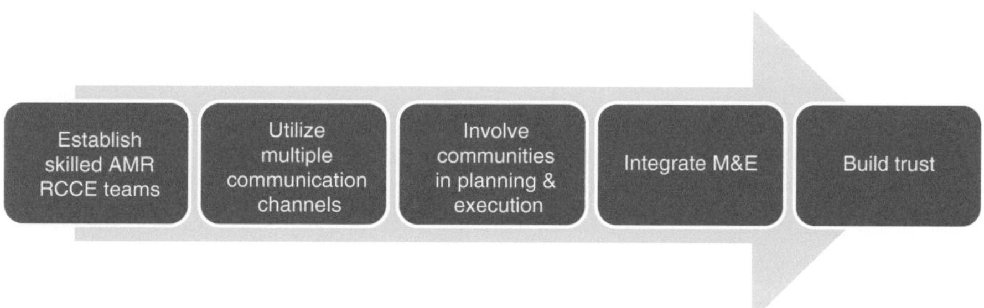

Fig. 20.2 Template of a step-by-step approach for AMR RCCE

The most important component of any communication strategy is earning the trust of the individual or the group with whom communication has been initiated.

20.3.2 Messages for AMR Behavioural Change

Being a complex and multisectoral issue, AMR requires a broader approach in terms of building a consensus on the messages and the potential target audience. Large campaigns are sometimes effective in creating awareness among the general public and professional groups, but the efforts involved may be disproportional to the impact of the strategy [5].

Effective communication plays a crucial role in enhancing community awareness about significant healthcare issues. But increasing awareness alone does not result in significant behaviour change unless the issues are addressed holistically [6].

Effective communication about AMR requires clear, tailored messages for diverse audiences. Key aspects include explaining what AMR is, how it impacts human, animal, and environmental health, and the importance of responsible antimicrobial use. Messages should also highlight the consequences of inaction and inspire behaviour change.

The messages should explain the problem, define AMR in the simplest possible language and highlight its impact on human, animal, and environmental health. The messages should emphasise the growing threat of AMR and the potential consequences of inaction, such as the loss of effective treatments. The communication through brief, unambiguous messages must promote appropriate use of antibiotics in humans, animals, and agriculture. Awareness alone is not adequate. Sharing examples of successful interventions and behavioural changes, aided by a visual presentation, may carry a greater impact in inspiring others. Messages should empower and motivate individuals to take steps to combat AMR.

The language used in messages should be simple, relatable, and focus on the personal impact of AMR, such as the risk of infections becoming harder to treat. While communicating with policymakers, it is prudent to highlight the economic and social costs of AMR and the need for effective policies and regulations.

Messages should be coordinated, consistent, and tailored to align with the specific cultural context and values of the target audience. They are essential for effective communication, allowing multiple stakeholders to speak with a unified voice and engage the public and communities across all channels. Simply providing technical information, even in simple, understandable language, is unlikely to lead to significant behaviour change. Beyond delivering critical, actionable health information, messages and their delivery interventions must be thoughtfully designed to reflect community values, convey care and concern, and consider local context, culture, and potential stigma related to the AMR. They should be part of a responsive, two-way communication process with those at risk.

The WHO has, in comprehensive guidelines [7], articulated the characteristics of possible achievements through various messages for the general public and for health professionals (Table 20.2).

The communities consist of individuals, and usually, messages need to be created that target individuals. These basically respond to the question a person asks about what they can do to contain AMR. Figure 20.3 shows a possible and representative message with doable and straightforward actions by an individual.

Table 20.2 Expected outcomes of messages delivered through communication tools

General public	Health professionals
Understand the importance of acquiring antimicrobials by prescription only, from a qualified professional who is authorised to prescribe them Understand that antimicrobials are not for treating headaches or viral infections (such as colds or common flus), which account for a large percentage of community infections Understand the importance of the proper use and acquisition of antimicrobials Refrain from sharing antimicrobials with others Understand that they should not pressure healthcare professionals to prescribe antimicrobials when told they do not need them Refrain from self-medicating to treat symptoms they recognise from previous experience. A healthcare provider should always be consulted before purchasing antimicrobials Know that antimicrobials can be harmful when not used properly Understand that self-medication is dangerous to health	Support and provide the means for patients to always acquire properly prescribed medicines from known and reliable sources Be prepared to educate their patients when asked to prescribe antimicrobials they do not consider necessary Educate their patients on how to use antimicrobials Have access to materials they can learn from and use to teach others, such as brochures, a list of FAQs, and posters with simple, clear images and messages Receive continuing education on prescribing antimicrobials When diagnosing patients, be certain about either prescribing antimicrobials or deciding not to prescribe them Have access to evidence-based guidelines for prescribing and dispensing antimicrobials Know that some antimicrobials should be restricted to very specific instances Comply with and support the implementation of regulations on the dispensation of prescription antimicrobials

Working individually WE can
contribute immensely to combat AMR

Follow hand hygiene, teach it to friends and families.		Take the antibiotics as prescribed.
Cover your mouth while coughing or sneezing.		Do not skip prescribed doses of antibiotics.
Improve sanitation and prevent spread of infection.		Do not save antibiotics for possible future use.
Get vaccinated and nutritious food.		Do not take antibiotics prescribed for someone else.
Reduce unnecessary use of antibiotics in agriculture and their dissemination into the environment		

Fig. 20.3 Representative message for actions by an individual to contain AMR

20.4 Tools for Communication

AMR communication tools refer to the various methods and resources used to raise awareness, educate, and promote behaviour change related to the responsible use of antibiotics and the prevention of AMR. These tools can range from public awareness campaigns and educational materials to social media engagement and media outreach [8]. Some of these are described in Table 20.3.

By utilising a combination of these communication tools, organisations can effectively raise awareness, promote responsible antibiotic use, and combat the growing threat of AMR.

In the modern era, apart from conventional tools, several others, mainly electronic, have gained immense importance. Developing countries are now at par with the developed world in the use of these tools, which must be tapped for spreading messages of AMR containment [9].

20.5 Challenges in RCCE Implementation

Communication strategies for bringing about changes in the behaviour of implementers, users and affected populations are rarely high on the agenda of the responsible authorities [10]. Technological tools drive AMR control programmes and are hardly ever people-centred. WHO has recently developed a people-centred approach for AMR in health settings [11]. Plans created based on such documents should have communication as a cross-cutting intervention in AMR action plans. In addition, the programme should expect the following challenges while implementing its plans.

- *Misinformation and rumours*
  Rapidly spreading misinformation can undermine trust and hinder response efforts.

Table 20.3 Different categories of AMR communication tools

	Category	Material
1	Educational materials	Leaflets and posters that provide basic information about AMR, its causes, and how to prevent it
		Campaign videos used to grab attention and effectively convey key messages about AMR to a wider audience
		Social media content including Facebook, twitter, Instagram, and WhatsApp can be used to share information, engage with the public, and disseminate campaign materials
		Website banners and graphics to create a central hub for information about AMR, including downloadable resources and campaign updates
		Information, education, and communication (IEC) materials that can be specifically designed for veterinary hospitals, animal producers, and other relevant groups
2	Media engagement	Media engagement toolkit that has developed by organisations like the quadripartite (FAO, WHO, WOAH, and UNEP), provides resources and guidance for media professionals to improve their coverage of AMR
		Media outreach programmes through engagement with journalists to enhance their understanding of AMR and equip them to report accurately on the topic Evidence-based reports can be used to advocate for policy changes and resource allocation related to AMR
3	Stakeholder engagement	Community and religious leaders can help disseminate information and promote positive behavioural changes within communities
		Primary and high school teachers can educate future generations about the importance of responsible antibiotic use by including AMR in the curriculum
		University students and lecturers particularly those in health-related fields, can foster a deeper understanding of AMR among future healthcare professionals
		Veterinary professionals and manufacturers to encourage the responsible use of antibiotics in animals and promote alternative methods for animal health
		Policymakers who can be communicated with evidence-based reports can be used to influence policy changes and resource allocation related to AMR
4	Other tools	Online collaboration tools which can facilitate communication and collaboration among different stakeholders involved in AMR prevention and control

- *Lack of resources and capacity*
  Insufficient funding, staffing, and training can limit the effectiveness of RCCE activities.
- *Cultural and linguistic barriers*
  Reaching diverse populations with culturally appropriate and linguistically accessible information can be challenging.
- *Coordination and collaboration*
  Effective RCCE requires coordination among various stakeholders, including government agencies, health organisations, and community groups.

Table 20.4 Overview of using communication for moving forward to impact AMR

From		To
Conceptual and implementation approach on one health	➡	Impact oriented field action
Total government programme	➡	Whole-of-society engagement including private sector and communities
Passive messaging to public	➡	Affirmative and active community partnership leading to behaviour modification
	⬇	
Improved human and animal health, along with safer environment		

Notwithstanding these challenges, all efforts should be made to attain the objectives of RCCE. Table 20.4 summarises the essence of moving forward.

20.6 Expected Outcome of RCCE

The single expected outcome of efficiently implemented RCCE is a change in behaviour of the individual and the community on rational use of antibiotics for themselves, families, community, animals, and animal husbandry practices.

Communities typically start unaware of an issue or health behaviour. Through communication efforts, individuals become aware, reflect on the intervention or behaviour change, adopt it, repeat it, and advocate for it, encouraging this behaviour within themselves and their community.

20.7 Recommendations for NAP Programme Manager for RCCE

Risk communication and community engagement (RCCE) plays a vital role in the successful implementation of a national action plan (NAP) on Antimicrobial Resistance (AMR), especially in developing countries where antibiotic misuse often results from behavioural, systemic, and socio-economic factors. For a NAP manager, RCCE is not just a communication campaign; it is a structured, ongoing, multisectoral effort that raises awareness, fosters trust, encourages behaviour change, and ensures accountability across human health, animal health, agriculture, and environmental sectors.

20.7.1 Strategic Vision for RCCE in AMR

A strong approach starts with understanding that AMR is a "silent pandemic." Unlike sudden outbreaks, AMR develops slowly, making it hard to generate public urgency. Hence, the NAP manager should frame RCCE around:

- Protecting families from infections that cannot be treated.
- Preserving essential medicines for future generations.
- Protecting livelihoods dependent on livestock and poultry.
- Ensuring food safety and maintaining export credibility.

RCCE should align with the One Health framework, which highlights the interconnectedness of human, animal, and environmental health.

20.7.2 Situational Assessment and Audience Segmentation

Before starting activities, the NAP manager should conduct a quick knowledge, attitudes, and practices (KAP) assessment. This will identify:

- Patterns of antibiotic use and misuse.
- Sources of antibiotics (pharmacies, informal vendors, veterinary outlets).
- Cultural beliefs influencing self-medication.
- Farmer practices regarding prophylactic antibiotic use.
- Gaps in awareness among healthcare providers.

Audience segmentation is key. Messages tailored for urban pharmacists will differ from those for rural poultry farmers. RCCE must be customised for:

- Clinicians and veterinarians.
- Pharmacists and drug sellers.
- Livestock and poultry farmers.
- Community leaders.
- Policymakers.
- Media professionals.
- School children and youth.

20.7.3 Clear, Contextualised Messaging Is Critical

Effective RCCE messaging should be straightforward and action-oriented (e.g. "Use antibiotics only with a prescription"), relevant to local contexts (translated into regional languages), culturally sensitive, evidence-based, and not overly technical. Messaging should avoid blame. Instead, it should empower stakeholders with practical alternatives.

Core themes may include:

- Antibiotics do not treat viral infections.
- Completing prescribed courses.
- Avoiding sharing medicines.
- The importance of vaccination and hygiene.
- Responsible antibiotic use in livestock.

20.7.4 Multichannel Communication Strategy

In developing countries, depending on a single communication channel is ineffective. A combined strategy should include:

- Mass media campaigns (radio, TV, community FM stations).
- Social media engagement (focusing on urban youth).
- Outreach through community health workers.
- Farmer field schools and veterinary extension services.
- Posters and job aids in clinics and pharmacies.
- Integration into school curricula.
- Religious and community gatherings.

Traditional channels, like local leaders or village meetings, are often more influential than national media in rural areas.

20.7.5 Active Community Engagement

RCCE needs to go beyond just sharing information. Community involvement requires dialogue, feedback mechanisms, and participation. This can be achieved through community advisory groups, village health and sanitation committees, farmer cooperatives, feedback hotlines or digital platforms, and participatory workshops. Engaging communities in identifying problems and designing solutions increases ownership and promotes sustainable behavioural change.

20.7.6 Integration with Health and Veterinary Systems

RCCE should be part of existing service delivery platforms rather than a separate activity. In human health, it can be linked to antimicrobial stewardship programmes in hospitals and involve primary healthcare providers in patient counselling.

In veterinary and agriculture sectors, RCCE can be incorporated into livestock vaccination campaigns and promoted alongside biosecurity practices through extension workers. Pharmacists and drug retailers should also be trained to support responsible dispensing.

20.7.7 Capacity Building

The NAP manager should focus on training spokespersons and frontline workers, including public health officers, veterinary officers, community health workers, pharmacists, and media professionals. Training should cover the basics of AMR, communication skills, rumour management, and risk messaging during outbreaks involving resistant pathogens.

20.7.8 Monitoring and Evaluation

RCCE effectiveness must be measurable. Indicators may include:

- Changes in antibiotic prescription rates.
- Reduction in over-the-counter antibiotic sales.
- Increased vaccination uptake.
- Improved public awareness levels.
- Farmer adoption of biosecurity measures.

Periodic KAP surveys and prescription audits can provide evidence of behavioural shifts.

20.7.9 Crisis Communication Preparedness

AMR-related outbreaks (e.g. drug-resistant infections in hospitals or food chains) require rapid and transparent communication. Pre-developed communication templates, designated spokespersons, and media protocols are essential to maintain public trust and avoid panic.

20.7.10 Sustainability and Institutionalisation

RCCE should not be limited to annual awareness weeks. Sustainable approaches include incorporating AMR education into school curricula, establishing annual national AMR awareness campaigns, partnering with civil society organisations and securing budget lines within the NAP.

Public–private partnerships can amplify outreach, especially through pharmaceutical associations and livestock industry groups.

20.7.11 Active Stakeholders in RCCE for AMR

A successful RCCE strategy requires coordinated action from multiple stakeholders. These have been summarised in Table 20.5.

20.7.12 Actions to Be Avoided for Community Engagement

For national action plan (NAP) managers working on antimicrobial resistance (AMR), community engagement can either build trust and ownership—or unintentionally create resistance, confusion, and fatigue. Avoiding common pitfalls is just as important as implementing good strategies. Below are key practices that NAP managers should avoid in community engagement.

Table 20.5 Active stakeholders in RCCE for AMR

No	Broad category	Active stakeholders
1	Government ministries	Ministry of Health Ministry of Agriculture/livestock Ministry of Environment Ministry of Education Drug regulatory authority
2	Health sector	Hospitals and primary healthcare centres Professional medical and nursing associations Pharmacist associations
3	Veterinary and agriculture sectors	Veterinary councils Livestock and poultry associations Farmer cooperatives Feed industry representatives
4	Academia and research institutions	Public health institutes Universities conducting AMR research
5	Civil society and community Organisations	NGOs working in health and agriculture Women's self-help groups Youth organisations Religious leaders
6	Media and communication partners	Journalists Radio broadcasters Social media influencers
7	Private sector	Pharmaceutical companies Veterinary drug suppliers Food industry stakeholders
8	International development partners	WHO, FAO, WOAH country offices Development partners supporting AMR programmes
9	Celebrities	Sportspersons Film/TV stars Political leaders

Avoid One-Way Communication RCCE is not a lecture. Top-down messaging without listening to community concerns reduces credibility and limits behaviour change. Communities must have space to ask questions, express doubts, and share local realities (e.g. lack of access to qualified doctors or veterinary services). Engagement should be dialogic, not prescriptive.

Avoid Technical and Fear-Based Messaging Overly technical language about "multidrug-resistant pathogens" or "genomic surveillance" alienates the public. Similarly, fear-based messaging ("antibiotics will stop working tomorrow") can create panic or fatalism. Communication should be simple, practical, and solution-oriented.

Avoid Blaming Communities or Providers Blaming farmers, pharmacists, or patients for antibiotic misuse undermines collaboration. In many developing settings, inappropriate use stems from structural issues—limited access to diagnostics, weak regulation, or financial pressures. Messaging should acknowledge systemic constraints and promote shared responsibility.

Avoid Ignoring Cultural and Socioeconomic Context Generic national campaigns that do not account for local language, literacy levels, gender roles, or livelihood patterns are ineffective. For example, advising farmers to "stop preventive antibiotic use" without offering alternatives like vaccination or biosecurity support will not work. Contextualization is essential.

Avoid Short-Term or One-off Campaigns Community engagement should not be limited to annual AMR awareness weeks. One-time campaigns generate temporary awareness but rarely change behaviour. Sustainable engagement requires integration into ongoing health services, agricultural extension programmes, and school curricula.

Avoid Excluding Key Stakeholders Failure to involve pharmacists, informal drug sellers, private practitioners, livestock traders, or community leaders weakens impact. These actors often influence antibiotic access and decision-making. Inclusive stakeholder mapping is crucial.

Avoid Misinformation and Mixed Messages Conflicting guidance—such as promoting antibiotic stewardship while allowing unregulated sales—erodes credibility. Messaging must align with regulatory policies and enforcement. NAP managers should coordinate across ministries to ensure consistency.

Avoid Over-Promising Outcomes Claiming that "antibiotic resistance will be solved" through awareness alone creates unrealistic expectations. RCCE should clearly state that AMR control is a long-term effort requiring multiple interventions, including surveillance, stewardship, vaccination, and regulation.

Avoid Neglecting Feedback Mechanisms Community engagement without mechanisms for feedback (hotlines, community meetings, surveys) becomes tokenistic. NAP managers should actively collect and respond to community concerns to maintain trust.

Avoid Lack of Monitoring and Evaluation Engagement activities must be measured. Without indicators such as changes in antibiotic sales, prescribing patterns, or vaccination uptake, it is impossible to determine whether communication efforts are effective.

Avoid Politicisation of AMR Messaging AMR should be framed as a public health and livelihood issue, not a political agenda. Associating messages with partisan interests may reduce public trust and stakeholder cooperation.

Avoid Ignoring Equity Considerations Marginalised groups—rural populations, smallholder farmers, women, and informal workers—may have limited access to information or services. Excluding them widens inequities and undermines national efforts.

For a NAP manager in a developing country, RCCE is both a technical and social endeavour. The most effective approach combines evidence-based messaging, community dialogue, multisectoral coordination, and continuous monitoring. Active stakeholder engagement ensures shared responsibility across human health, animal health, agriculture, and environmental sectors. When RCCE is institutionalised and adequately resourced, it transforms AMR from an abstract scientific concern into a collective national priority, enabling sustainable behaviour change and stronger implementation of the national action plan.

For NAP managers, effective community engagement requires humility, inclusiveness, cultural sensitivity, and long-term commitment. Avoiding one-way communication, blame, technical jargon, short-term campaigns, and exclusion of key actors is critical. When engagement is participatory, transparent, and aligned with practical solutions, communities become active partners in combating antimicrobial resistance rather than passive recipients of information.

To sum up, the communication strategy or the AMR RCCE should simplify AMR complexity, ultimately leading to behavioural change among all stakeholders, especially the communities, for rational use of antibiotics and reduce the impact of AMR.

References

1. Godinho N, Bezbaruah S, Nayyar S, Gautam J, Sachdeva S, Behara I, Vong S. Antimicrobial resistance communication activities in South East Asia. BMJ. 2017;358:j2742. https://doi.org/10.1136/bmj.j2742.
2. UNICEF. Risk communication and community engagement. Available at https://www.core-commitments.unicef.org/rcce. Accessed 7 July 2025.

3. Mitchell J, Hawkings H, Latham S, Fieroze F, Arjyal A, Barrington DJ, et al. Addressing antimicrobial resistance through community engagement: a framework for developing contextually relevant and impactful behaviour change interventions. JAC Antimicrob Resist. 2023;5(6):dlad124. https://doi.org/10.1093/jacamr/dlad124.
4. World Health Organization. Ethical considerations in developing a public health response to pandemic influenza. WHO; 2007. Available from: https://iris.who.int/bitstreams/46f6a29c-b584-495a-9860-7dc0543aadee/download. Accessed 17 July 2025.
5. Seymour J. The impact of public health awareness campaigns on the awareness and quality of palliative care. J Palliat Med. 2018;21:S30–6. https://doi.org/10.1089/jpm.2017.0391.
6. Mathew P, Sivaraman S, Chandy S. Communication strategies for improving public awareness on appropriate antibiotic use: bridging a vital gap for action on antibiotic resistance. J Family Med Prim Care. 2019;8(6):1867–71. https://doi.org/10.4103/jfmpc.jfmpc_263_1.
7. WHO. Handbook for communication on the rational use of antimicrobials for the containment of resistance. Washington, D.C.: Pan American Health Organization; 2021. License: CC BY-NC-SA 3.0 IGO. https://doi.org/10.37774/9789275123683.
8. FAO. Launch of a Quadripartite toolkit: Enhancing the role of media for effective Antimicrobial Resistance (AMR) communication. Available at https://www.fao.org/brussels/events/events-detail/launch-of-a-quadripartite-toolkit%2D%2Denhancing-the-role-of-media-for-effective-antimicrobial-resistance-(amr)-communication/en#: Accessed 27 July 2025.
9. Bhatia R. Public engagement is key for containing COVID-19 pandemic. Indian J Med Res. 2020;151(2 & 3):118–20. https://doi.org/10.4103/ijmr.IJMR_780_20.
10. Almutairi KS, Okmi EA, Alnofaiei SS, Alshamari WK, Almutairi SH, Alsuwailem SI, Alkhaldi EH. The effects of health education on the awareness of antimicrobial resistance among high school students in Riyadh, Saudi Arabia during 2023: a quasi-experimental study. Cureus. 2023;15(7):e41639. https://doi.org/10.7759/cureus.41639.
11. WHO. WHO people-centred approach to addressing AMR in the human health, 2023. Available at https://www.who.int/publications/i/item/9789240082496 Accessed 7 July 2025.

Chapter 21

A to Z of Combating Antimicrobial Resistance

Summarised Actions for Control of AMR

Abstract Ensure continuous Advocacy with all stakeholders especially national policy makers

A	Ensure continuous **A**dvocacy with all stakeholders especially national policy makers
B	Collate **B**est practices from all over the world and disseminate for adaptation and wider use in local settings
C	**C**ommunicate frequently and effectively with all collaborators to guide and coordinate actions targeted for minimizing AMR
D	Develop, design, and utilize national and comprehensive **D**ata management system to analyse the dynamics of AMR
E	**E**stimate and fulfil the financial and technical needs of the national programme
F	Articulate, emphasize, and encourage active role of **F**orgotten stakeholders: Environment, industry, private sector, researchers
G	Phase out use of antimicrobial agents as **G**rowth promoters in animal sector
H	Ensure stringent infection control practices in all **H**ealthcare facilities and animal farms and emphasize **H**and washing
I	**I**nnovate and improvise to achieve the core objective of combating AMR
J	Undertake **J**oint planning, programme development, implementation and monitoring with other stakeholders including animal health, environment, private sector, research institutes, industry, and civil society
K	Improve **k**nowledge and behaviour of the professionals and paraprofessionals in all sectors on AMR and rational use of antimicrobials
L	Strengthen **L**aboratory-based surveillance to generate reliable data on magnitude of AMR, monitor trends, strengthen knowledge and evidence
M	Integrate and utilize outcomes of **M**&E in improving programme efficiency
N	Use **N**ational Action Plan as the guiding document for steering country ahead in reducing AMR
O	Make **O**ne health approach central to national and local activities
P	Foster interaction between various **P**artners including international development agencies and utilize their support for enhancement of national activities
Q	Ensure strong regulatory system across the country to make available **Q**uality antimicrobials and diagnostics
R	Reduce gaps in knowledge and promote development of new interventions through **R**esearch & Development
S	Make antibiotic **S**tewardship applicable in all health facilities
T	Implement comprehensive multisectoral training plan and impart **T**rainings on AMR for all key stakeholders as an essential component of the phased NAP implementation

R. Bhatia, *Drug-Resistant Infections*,
https://doi.org/10.1007/978-981-92-4190-3_21

U	Optimize **U**se of antimicrobials in humans and animals
V	**V**accinate human and animal populations with available antigens to reduce burden of infectious diseases
W	Develop national framework for surveillance of antibiotic residues and contaminants in **w**aste from farms, factories, industry, veterinary, and human healthcare settings and to detect antimicrobial residues/contaminants in food and environment
X	Develop e**X**pertise and institutionalise national surveillance system for antimicrobial use (AMU) in humans, animals, agriculture, and food sectors
Y	Engage **Y**outh and school children in disseminating interventions that reduce disease burden and prevent spread of AMR including hygiene and sanitation
Z	Ensure **Z**ero irrational use of antimicrobials in all sectors and make rational use as the cornerstone of entire programme

Glossary of Important Terms

Antimicrobial Resistance (AMR) The ability of microorganisms to resist medicines that once treated them effectively.

Antimicrobial Stewardship (AMS) Coordinated strategies to optimize use of antimicrobials.

Antimicrobial Susceptibility Testing (AST) Lab test to determine sensitivity of microbes to drugs.

Antimicrobial Use (AMU) Usage of antimicrobial drugs in humans, animals, and agriculture.

AWaRe Classification The WHO system categorizing antibiotics into Access, Watch, and Reserve groups.

Biosecurity Measures to prevent the introduction and spread of harmful organisms.

Broad-Spectrum Antibiotic Drugs are effective against a wide range of bacteria.

Extended-Spectrum Beta-Lactamase (ESBL) Enzymes that confer resistance to multiple beta-lactam antibiotics.

Healthcare-Associated Infections (HAI) Infections acquired during medical care.

Infection Prevention and Control (IPC) Measures to stop spread of infections.

Low- and Middle-Income Countries (LMICs) Nations classified by the World Bank with constrained healthcare resources.

Methicillin-Resistant Staphylococcus aureus (MRSA) A dangerous multiple antibiotic-resistant bacterium.

Multidrug-Resistant (MDR) Resistant to multiple antimicrobial classes.

National Action Plan (NAP) National-level framework to address AMR.

Nosocomial Infections Hospital-acquired infections.

One Health An integrated approach to human, animal, and environmental health.

Pharmacovigilance Monitoring of medicine use and side effects.

Plasmid A genetic element in bacteria that can carry resistance genes.

Public Health Emergency of International Concern (PHEIC) WHO declaration of an extraordinary health event.

R. Bhatia, *Drug-Resistant Infections*,
https://doi.org/10.1007/978-981-92-4190-3

Standard Treatment Guidelines (STGs) Evidence-based clinical practices for prescribing.
Surveillance Continuous monitoring of antimicrobial use and resistance trends.
Vaccination Preventive measures against infectious diseases.
Vector-Borne Diseases Infections transmitted by vectors such as mosquitoes.
Zoonotic Infections Diseases transmitted between animals and humans.

MIX
Papier aus verantwortungsvollen Quellen
Paper from responsible sources
FSC® C105338

If you have any concerns about our products,
you can contact us on
ProductSafety@springernature.com

In case Publisher is established outside the EU,
the EU authorized representative is:
Springer Nature Customer Service Center GmbH
Europaplatz 3, 69115 Heidelberg, Germany

Printed by Libri Plureos GmbH
in Hamburg, Germany